Lifestyle Counselling and Coaching
for the Whole Person:

Or how to integrate nutritional insights, physical exercise and sleep coaching into talk therapy

By Jim Byrne DCoun FISPC

With Renata Taylor-Byrne BSc (Hons) Psychol

Hebden Bridge: The Institute for E-CENT Publications, in collaboration with the CreateSpace Platform (Amazon)

Copyright © Jim Byrne and Renata Taylor-Byrne, 2018

Published by: The Institute for Emotive-Cognitive Embodied-Narrative Therapy, 27 Wood End, Keighley Road, Hebden Bridge, West Yorkshire, HX7 8HJ, UK

Telephone: 01422 843 629

~~~

All rights reserved.

The right of Jim Byrne and Renata Taylor-Byrne to be the exclusive creators of this book, and its exclusive owners, have been asserted. This book is the intellectual property of Dr Jim Byrne and Renata Taylor-Byrne (at ABC Coaching and Counselling Services, and the Institute for E-CENT). No element of this work may be used in any way, without explicit written permission of the authors. The sole exception is the presentation of brief quotations (not for profit), which must be acknowledged as excerpts from:

Byrne, J.W. (2018) *Lifestyle Counselling and Coaching of the Whole Person: Or how to integrate nutritional insights, physical exercise and sleep coaching into talk therapy.* Hebden Bridge: The Institute for E-CENT Publications.

Website: https://ecent-institute.org/

~~~

Cover design: Charles Saul. Website: http://www.charles-saul.co.uk/

~~~

ISBN-13: 978-1986462174

Copyright © Dr Jim Byrne and Renata Taylor-Byrne, March 2018

~~~

About the authors

Lead author: Jim Byrne has a doctoral degree in counselling and a master's degree in education; plus a diploma in counselling psychology and psychotherapy, and a number of counselling certificates and accreditations. He has been involved in counselling psychology and psychotherapy (private practice) for almost twenty years; and he's studied optimum nutrition and balanced exercise approaches to improve his own physical and mental health for decades. He is the creator of Emotive-Cognitive Embodied Narrative Therapy (E-CENT), which emphasizes the interactionism of body-brain-mind-environment as a whole system, which is what underlies the phenomenon which some see as 'the life of the individual', and which he has characterized as *the embodied and embedded social-self*.

~~~

Contributing author: Renata Taylor-Byrne did most of the research and writing on the diet, exercise and sleep elements of this work. She has an honours degree in psychology, plus diplomas in nutrition, stress management, CBT and other systems of coaching and counselling. She taught health and nutrition courses, as well as counselling, stress management, self-assertion, and other personal development courses, in further education, with adult students, during a thirty-five year teaching career. As a Lifestyle Coach, she has a very strong interest in the link between diet, exercise, sleep, health, and emotional wellbeing.

~~~

Disclaimer

This book is intended for educational purposes only, and does not claim to be a medical text, nor to promote any medical prescriptions or processes. We discuss the relationship between physical health and emotional wellbeing, especially in relation to diet, exercise, sleep, nutritional supplements, meditation and relaxation. While every care is taken in preparing this material, the publishers cannot accept any responsibility for any damage or harm caused by any treatment, advice or information contained in this book. You should consult a qualified health, fitness or nutritional practitioner before undertaking any treatment.

~~~

Lifestyle Counselling and Coaching for the Whole Person:

Or how to integrate nutritional insights, exercise and sleep coaching into talk therapy

Contents

PREFACE..XIII
PROLOGUE...XVII
CHAPTER 1: INTRODUCTION..1
1.1 Counsellors and their clients..1
1.2 What is E-CENT counselling?..3
1.3 Our unique perspective..5
1.4 The status of E-CENT theory...6
1.5 An accidental evolution of theory...7
1.6 Views of science..7
1.7 The case against using case studies..8
1.8 Subjectivity of case studies..10
    Figure 1.1: The subjectivity of observation...11
1.9 Narratives and stories..12
1.10 The E-CENT approach...14
    A client's case summarized..15
    Analysis...16
    Self-reflection..17
1.11 Defining Attachment Theory more clearly...18
1.12 The role of the individual's social environment.......................................19
1.13 The centrality of relationship..20
1.14 The need for emotional availability, and sensitive caring......................20
1.15 Attachment in psychotherapy...21
1.16 Attachment in E-CENT..23
    Figure 1.3 – Modelling the *good* and *bad wolf* states....................................24
1.17 Brief summary of the E-CENT models..25
    Figure 1.4: The elements of the SOR model...27
    Figure 1.5: The full Six Windows Model..28

Figure 1.6: The Jigsaw-story model 29

Postscript: On the body-brain-mind-environment complexity 31

CHAPTER 2: KEY ELEMENTS OF THE EMOTIVE-COGNITIVE COUNSELLING APPROACH 35

2.1: Overview 35

2.2: Basic description and origins 37

2.3: Basic theory of E-CENT 38

2.4: The importance of emotion 40

Figure 2.1: Interpenetrating minds of the mother-baby dyad 43

Figure 2.2: The most basic model of CENT: 44

Figure 2.3: How the ten elements of the PAC model - (4 P's, 4 C's, 2 A's) - emerge within the dialectical ego space between the mother and child 45

2.6: The client's problems and tasks of counselling 46

CHAPTER 3: CORE BELIEFS OF THE EMOTIVE-COGNITIVE PHILOSOPHY OF COUNSELLING 49

The 20 core principles of human development 49

CHAPTER 4: OVERVIEW OF DIET AND EXERCISE IMPACTS UPON MENTAL HEALTH 59

4.1: Introduction 59

4.2: The psychobiological model of E-CENT and the impact of diet and exercise 59

4.3: The importance of food for the body-brain-mind 61

4.4: Balanced diet and toxic foods... 63

What is a balanced diet? 63

Personalized diet 64

Beware toxic foods 65

4.5: The importance of nutritional supplements for mental health 68

4.6: The link between food and anger, anxiety and depression 69

4.7: The conclusion regarding diet and mental health 72
4.8: Physical exercise and emotional wellbeing 73
4.9: Anxiety and physical activity 74
4.10: Exercise and anger 75
4.11: Depression and physical exercise 75
4.12: Exercise for stress reduction 77
4.13: Yoga and Chi Kung for emotional self-management 78
4.14: Summary of research on diet and exercise for mental health 78
4.15: Dr Jim's Stress and Anxiety Diet 79
4.16: The science of nutritional deficiency and mental health 81

CHAPTER 5: THE IMPACT OF SLEEP ON MENTAL HEALTH AND EMOTIONAL WELLBEING 83

5.1 Introduction 83
5.2: The primary importance of sleep 84
5.3: Common sense views of sleep 85
5.4: Distractions from sleep 86
5.5: Problems of sleep insufficiency 87
    Why we need sleep 87
    How much we need, and the effects of not getting it 88
    Seven major negative results of sleep insufficiency 89
5.6: Famous cases of sleep-deprived individuals and the negative consequences 92
5.7: The benefits of sleep 94
5.8: Insomnia: the curse of sleeplessness, and how to treat it 96

CHAPTER 6: REFRAMING EXPERIENCES WITH THE SIX WINDOWS MODEL 101

6.1: Introduction 101
    6.1(a) Context: 102
    6.1(b) Elaboration of the theory: 103

6.1(c) Re-framing: 103

    Figure 6.1(b): The Six Windows Model of E-CENT 104

6.1(d) Frame theory 106

6.2: Defining, describing and justifying this approach 107

6.3: The Mind Hut Model...108

    Window No.1...109

    Window No.2...111

    Window No.3...114

    Window No.4...115

    Window No.5...116

    Table 6.1: The controllable and the uncontrollable......................117

    Window No.6...118

6.4: Case illustration 119

CHAPTER 7: UNDERSTANDING AND MANAGING HUMAN EMOTIONS - INCLUDING THE INTEGRATION OF TALK THERAPY AND DIETARY AND EXERCISE GUIDELINES 121

7.1: Introduction 121

7.2: Buddhism and Stoicism on emotion 123

    7.2(a). Regarding Buddhist theory: 123

    7.2(b). Regarding Stoic theory:..125

7.3: Another point of departure – Evolutionary psychology................127

7.4 The origin of human emotions 129

7.5 The proximal cause of emotional disturbance 130

7.6 The evolutionary view..131

7.7 Understanding emotive-cognitive interactionism 133

7.8 Language and mentation..138

7.9 The social individual 140

7.10 Managing human emotions 146

7.11 Managing anger, anxiety and depression 148

7.11(a). Anger: 148
    Managing anger with diet and nutrition 151
    How anger can be reduced by exercise: 152
7.11(b). Anxiety: 153
    Practical strategies for managing anxiety 154
    Anxiety management: The impact of diet and nutrition 155
    Anxiety management: How anxiety can be reduced by exercise: 157
7.11(c). Depression: 158
    Depression: How diet and nutrition can reduce and eliminate it 160
    Depression: How it can be reduced by exercise 161

CHAPTER 8: COUNSELLING INDIVIDUALS USING THE E-CENT APPROACH 163

8.1: Quick introduction 163
8.2: Validity of our models and processes 165
8.3: Imaginary 'typical' session structure 166
    8.3(a): Confession 166
    The RCFP model: 167
    Questioning strategies: 168
    8.3(b): Elucidation 170
    Using the Holistic SOR model 173
    Figure 8.2: The E-CENT holistic SOR model 173
    The exploration process 174
    Other instruments 175
    Questioning strategies 175
    Dangers of questioning! 176
    Figure 8.3 Gerard Nierenberg's question grid 178
    8.3(c): Education 180
    General teaching points, including diet and exercise 180
    Applying the Six Windows Model 182

Using the EFR model 183
Narrative inquiry 184
Teaching the client about human disturbance 184
The APET model: 185
Fragments of disconnected story 186
Figure 8.4: The Jigsaw-story model 186
The Parent-Adult-Child model 187
Figure 8.5: The PAC Model of TA 187
The OK Corral (from TA): 188
Figure 8.6: The OK Corral 188
8.3(d): Transformation 189
Six main therapy-deepening processes 190
Use of the Gestalt Chair-work model: 190
Gradual desensitization: 190
Cutting the Ties that Bind: 191
Meditation: 191
Attachment system work: 191
Exploring personality: 192
1. The Keirsey Temperament Sorter: 192
2. Personality Adaptations 192
Additional processes: 192
8.4 Summing up 192

CHAPTER 9: HOW TO INCORPORATE LIFESTYLE AND HEALTH COACHING INTO TALK THERAPY ... 195

9.1 Introduction 195
9.2 Guidance for those who feel they need it 196
1. Who to teach 196
(i) Teaching strategies: 197
(ii) Learning styles and learning readiness: 198

Or how to integrate nutritional insights, exercise and sleep coaching into talk therapy

    2. What to teach 199
       (a) Coaching for sleep improvement 199
       (b) Coaching for nutritional and dietary improvement 200
       (c) Coaching for physical fitness 202
    3. When to teach it 203
    4. How to teach it 204

CHAPTER 10: CONCLUSION 207
10.1 Overview 207
10.2 The core theory of E-CENT 207
10.3 Key Learning Points and Applications 208
    (a) For therapists and counsellors: 208
    (b) For individuals interested in self-help and personal development: 210
    (c) For counselling and psychotherapy students: 212

REFERENCES 215
INDEX 233
ENDNOTES 241

Lifestyle Counselling and Coaching for the Whole Person:

Or how to integrate nutritional insights, exercise and sleep coaching into talk therapy

Preface

The contents

In this book, you will find a very clear, brief, easy to read introduction to a novel approach to *'counselling the whole person'*. This emotive-cognitive approach does not restrict itself to mental processes. We go beyond what the client is 'telling themselves', or 'signalling themselves'; or what went wrong in their family of origin. We also include how well they manage their body-brain-mind in terms of diet, exercise, sleep, and emotional self-management (including self-talk, or inner dialogue). And we propose that it is better for counsellors and therapists to operate in *a primarily right-brain modality*, and to use the left-brain, cognitive processes, secondarily.

The most important, and novel, chapters in this book are as follows:

> Chapter 4, which summarizes our research on the impact of diet/nutrition and physical exercise on mental health and emotional wellbeing.
>
> Chapter 5, which reviews the science of sleep hygiene, plus common sense insights, and presents a range of *lifestyle changes* to promote healthy sleep, and thus to improve mental and emotional wellbeing.
>
> Chapter 9, which explains how to incorporate the learning from chapters 4 and 5 into any system of talk therapy or counselling.

There is also a chapter (8) on counselling individuals using our Emotive-Cognitive approach, in which there is a section (8.3(b)) on using the Holistic SOR model to explore many aspects of the lifestyle of the client.

To be more precise: The holistic SOR model states that a client (a person) feels and reacts, at point 'R' (Response), to a (negative or positive) stimulus at point 'S' (Stimulus), on the basis of the current state of their social-body-mind (or their whole Organism). Important variables include the following:

> How well rested are they? How high or low is their blood-sugar level (which is related to diet and nutrition)?
>
> How well connected are they to significant others (which is a measure of social support)?
>
> How much conflict do they have at home or at work? What other pressures are bearing down upon them (for examples: from their socio-economic circumstances; physical health; home/ housing; work/ income; security/ insecurity; etc.)
>
> And how emotionally intelligent are they? (Emotional intelligence is, of course, learned, and can be re-learned!)

Within the Holistic-SOR model (as shown in Figure 8.2 below), in the middle column, what we are aiming to do is to construct a balance sheet (in our heads) of the pressures bearing down on the client (person), and the coping resources that they have for dealing with those pressures.

In addition, there is Chapter 6, which teaches how to help the client to re-frame any negative experience, using six perspectives, or frames, or lenses. These Six Windows mostly conform to some of the best insights among the philosophical propositions shared by moderate Stoicism and moderate Buddhism. But we discard the harsh and unworkable elements of extreme Stoicism and extreme Buddhism. This 'Six Windows' Model, which was created by Jim Byrne, with a contribution from Renata Taylor-Byrne, is easy to understand and easy to use.

Chapter 7 deals with how to understand and manage human emotions. This chapter reviews a wide range of perspectives, including: Darwin and the evolutionary psychology perspective; the Buddhist and Stoic views; and many modern perspectives, including: neuroscience; cognitive science; interpersonal neurobiology; attachment theory; and affect regulation theory. And that chapter includes a good deal of guidance on how to manage anger, anxiety and depression using a multifactorial approach which straddles diet, exercise, sleep, stress management, emotional self-management, mind-management, and so on.

And the book includes a quick review of a whole range of models and tools which we use in Emotive-Cognitive counselling, and which can be incorporated into the practices of integrative and holistic counsellors, psychologists and psycho-therapists.

The origin of this book

Much of the material in this book was originally published in Byrne (2016) – *Holistic Counselling in Practice*. However, that book turned out to be too expensive, partly because of its number of pages; but even more because we included a lot of full-colour illustrations. And we put a lot of supportive material in a set of appendices at the back of the book.

Because that book was so over-full, we decided, in 2016, to omit any material on sleep deprivation and its effects upon mental health; apart from some passing references. However, we now believe that was a mistake, as it seems likely that seriously disturbed individuals may often have to fix their sleep pattern *before* they can fully concentrate upon making dietary changes or committing to regular physical exercise.

The title of the original work also was a bit opaque. It did not clearly indicate the treasures contained within its pages, or how useful they could be to counsellors across the whole spectrum of counselling schools.

Because of the problems outlined above, we have now decided to republish some of the original material under a new, more descriptive title, and omitting the material which had been in the appendices, plus most of the illustrations. We also deleted a chapter (which was number 9) on holistic self-management strategies for self-help enthusiasts. That material will be incorporated into a subsequent book on how to manage our emotions.

We have now, in this new edition,

- added a brief chapter (5) on fixing sleep hygiene problems,

- plus a briefer summary of our recommendations regarding diet and exercise than was contained in the original edition.

- And we have added a brief chapter on how to integrate lifestyle coaching into any system of talk therapy.

Goals for this book

Furthermore, we have come to terms with the fact that most readers want a *manageable amount of material* which does not overload them in terms of the amount or changing and learning and growing involved. They do not want a *comprehensive* book, which covers *everything* about the holistic approach to counselling the whole person, all in one volume. They want to get that learning in digestible chunks, spread out over time.

Therefore, in this volume, we have tried to emphasize our presentation of the following issues:

(1) How to *understand some core ideas about the impact of poor quality sleep, inadequate nutrition and lack of physical exercise upon the body-brain-mind of the counselling client.*

(2) How holistic or integrative counsellors can *integrate elements of sleep, diet and exercise coaching into their talk therapy about broader emotional problems with life difficulties.* And:

(3) How to teach the broader picture of the causes and cures of emotional distress, including reframing strategies.

We hope you enjoy working with the material in this book, whether you are a counsellor/ psychotherapist/ psychologist; a student of those disciplines; or a self-help enthusiast who wants to improve your own body-brain-mind functioning for a better life. And regardless of which school of counselling, or psychotherapy tradition, to which you belong.

Jim Byrne, Doctor of Counselling

Hebden Bridge, March 2018

~~~

Lifestyle Counselling and Coaching for the Whole Person:

Prologue

In these pages you will find a detailed introduction to the theory and practice of one of the most recent, and most comprehensive, forms of holistic counselling and psychotherapy.

This new system (for helping people to optimize their positive experiences of life, and to process their negative experiences), necessarily deals with emotions, thinking, stories and narratives, *plus* bodily states; and thus is called Emotive-Cognitive Embodied Narrative Therapy (E-CENT). But we do not wish to proselytize for this system. We would be happy to have individual counsellors and therapists, from all the schools of counselling and therapy, experimenting with adding some small elements of our innovations into their own, idiosyncratic systems for helping their own clients.

This book has been designed to be helpful for three audiences:

(1) Counsellors, psychotherapists, coaches, psychologists, psychiatrists, social workers, educators and others;

(2) Students of counselling, psychotherapy, psychology, psychiatry, social work and related disciplines; and:

(3) Self-help and personal development enthusiasts.

The content of this book has been a long time incubating, at the very least since 2001 when I first tried to defend the ABC model of Rational Emotive Behaviour Therapy (REBT) by relating it to the three core components of Freud's model of the mind (or psyche):

(1) the Id (or **It** [or baby-at-birth]);

(2) the **Ego** (or sense of self, or personality); and

(3) the **Superego** (or 'internalized other', including social and moral rules).

The more I tried to defend REBT, the more its core models fell apart in my hands! See Byrne (2017) in the References near the back of this book.

At the same time, I was studying thirteen different systems of counselling and therapy, from Freud and Jung, via Rogers and Perls, and the behaviourists, to the cognitivists and existentialists.

Later, I considered Plato's model of the mind, alongside the Buddhist and Stoic philosophies of mind.

Into this mix, at some point, Attachment theory arrived, and that helped to make more sense of the emerging model of mind: (Gerhardt, 2010). Attachment theory, and Object relations theory – (Gomez, 1997) - eventually formed the core of my model of the mother-baby dyad, and the way in which the mind of the baby was born out of the interpenetration (or overlapping interactions) of the *physical baby* and the *cultural mother*.

And this gave rise to a greater awareness of the individual counselling client as a 'social individual', who is 'wired up' (neurologically) by social stories (about social experiences) to be a creature of habit, living out of historic scripts; and viewing the world through non-conscious frames (or lenses) which dictate how things 'show up' in their automatic (cumulative-interpretive) apprehension of the external world.

As these developments were reaching fruition, I also discovered the insights of interpersonal neurobiology (IPNB – Siegel, 2015) and Affect Regulation Theory (Hill, 2015).

~~~

But even beyond those developments, I also became increasingly aware that, because *we are body-minds*, our experience of sleep, diet, exercise, alcohol, water consumption, and socio-economic circumstances – (in addition to current and historic relationships) - have as much to do with our emotional disturbances (very often) as do our psychological habits of mind. And, in any event, our psychological habits of mind cannot be totally separated from the states of our body-brain-mind.

And in Chapter 4 below, Renata Taylor-Byrne and I present brief but compelling evidence, from reliable sources, that (1) dietary changes and physical exercise can produce dramatic reductions in levels of anger, anxiety and depression; (2) anti-depressants are not nearly as effective as has been claimed (and that physical exercise alone is as effective at curing depression as are antidepressant drugs); (3) that drug companies hide negative trial results; (4) that the real pills often fail to outperform placebo (sugar) pills; (5) that the real pills are often totally ineffective; (6) that they seem to be addictive, and difficult to get off in some cases; and (7) they have serious side effects (in some cases involving suicidal ideation).

And in addition, we agree with those theorists who have argued that *physical exercise* is *at least as effective as anti-depressants;* and also that some forms of *dietary change* can and do reduce and/or eliminate depression, and also reduce anxiety and anger. (See Chapter 4, below).

Counselling and therapy systems have normally ignored the convincing evidence that exercise and diet can change our emotional states. For example, in Woolfe, Dryden and Strawbridge's (2003) book on counselling psychology, there are *no references* in the index to diet or physical exercise[1]. As in the case of McLeod (2003)[2], there is a *'virtual* postscript' (in Chapter 29 [of 32] of Woolfe, Dryden and Strawbridge) on *counselling psychology and the body* – which is essentially about using bodily experience in counselling and therapy – as in *breath work*, and *body awareness* – though the chapter author (Bill Wahl) also includes a consideration of *body-work as such*. However, in our emotive-cognitive (E-CENT) counselling approach, we consider that *direct physical touch* is too problematical (ethically) to include in our system of counselling. What we do include, because it is now clearly *an essential ingredient of the health and well-being of the whole-client* (body-brain-mind), is awareness of *the role of diet and exercise* and *sleep patterns* in determining or influencing the level of emotional disturbance of the client; and an awareness of the need to teach the client that their diet, sleep and exercise practices have a significant impact upon their emotional and behavioural performances in the world. (See Chapter 4).

~~~

This then is a story of counselling and therapy revolution: the radical reformulation of most of our major theories of therapy; and their integration into a completely new view of *the social individual* as *a body-brain-mind-environment whole*.

Talk therapy has a lot to offer the social individual, but talk therapy *alone* cannot cure most of the ills of the modern world, many of which are related to *the lifestyle* of the client. (Interestingly, *lifestyle coaching* and *lifestyle medicine* are beginning to emerge in various quarters, including among some psychiatrists, [who are experimenting with diet – 'Holistic psychiatry']; some neurologists ['Holistic neurology']; and some medical doctors ['Integrative medicine', and 'Nutritional therapy']. But none of these approaches is nearly as complete or holistic as E-CENT theory and practice).

The world of counselling and therapy is being transformed (once again!). And in this book, in Chapter 3, we have summarized the core insights arising out of those various revolutions which have already occurred, which have relevance for counselling today. We have also explored the very latest thinking about how to understand and manage human emotions – especially anger, anxiety and depression, in Chapter 7.

Chapter 4 presents an overview of our research on diet and exercise, and how those two lifestyle factors impact on mental health and emotional wellbeing.

Chapter 5 is a brief review of the impact of sleep on mental health.

Chapter 6 deals with our approach to helping clients to *reframe* their unavoidable problems – using our Six Windows Model – which draws on the insights of moderate Buddhism and moderate Stoicism.

Chapter 8 explores some of the most important and helpful models we use in E-CENT, to guide our counselling sessions, and to *help the client to perfink* (perceive, feel and think) more self-supportingly.

The core beliefs of Emotive-Cognitive Embodied Narrative Therapy (E-CENT) are summarized in twenty principles, in Chapter 3.

Counselling and therapy have been in a constant state of evolution and revolution since the creation of psychoanalysis by Sigmund Freud, in the late nineteenth century. This book represents one of the most recent, and most comprehensive, reformulations; influenced as it is by attachment theory, affect regulation theory, personality adaptation theory, and interpersonal neurobiology.

I hope you enjoy this volume, and that you find some useful theories, techniques, tools and models within: for use in your own way, in your own life, and/or with the people you aim to help.

Dr Jim Byrne
Doctor of Counselling, Hebden Bridge
March 2018

~~~

Chapter 1: Introduction

1.1 Counsellors and their clients

Good counsellors and psychotherapists devote their lives to caring for the minds of their clients – the *lives* of their clients. They wrestle with difficult situations, challenging goals, and with dysregulated emotions (like grief and loss; anger and panic; relationship conflict, and mental confusion).

Innovative counsellors are constantly looking for new ways to help their clients. They mostly begin their careers with a single model of counselling, and many of them add in techniques and models and ideas from any source that seems likely to help their client. (There are of course a few 'purists' who will not deviate from their original training). However, after a few years of practice, in most cases, counsellors end up practicing a hybrid of many different approaches. Although they normally begin with a very simple model of counselling, and the nature of the counselling client, those perceptions change and evolves over the years.

For example: almost twenty years ago, I would sit in my consulting room, waiting for a counselling client. I had little to think about, because I *already knew* what their problem would be – the client's 'irrational beliefs' – and my only challenge would be how to get the client to change to more 'rational' beliefs.

Today, more than nineteen years later, when I sit in my counselling room waiting for a new client, I sometimes run through a checklist in my head. It goes something like this:

1. I do not know who this client will turn out to be; or how complex their case might be; or how I should begin to think about them. I have to wipe my mind as clear as possible of preconceptions, which, of course, is *an impossibility* for a human being. (Our *preconceptions* reside at the non-conscious level, and we most often do not know what they are! And without our preconceptions we would be gaga! We would literally not know what anything *was*).

2. This client will be a body-brain-mind, linked to a familial social environment (in the past) and a set of relationships (in the present).

3. They will be subject to a range of stressors in their daily life, and those stressors will be managed by a set of coping strategies (good and bad – resulting from the degree to which their emotions are habitually regulated or dysregulated).

4. This client will have been on a long journey through space-time, sometimes learning something new, and often repeating the habitual patterns of their past

experience/conditioning. They will be aware of some of their emotional pain, and unaware of much of it.

5. This client will have some kind of problem, or problems, for which I have been identified as an aid to the solution.

6. This client will come in and tell me a story; and another story; and another; and will want me to make sense of those stories; so they can escape from some pain or other. And that is part of my job. But a more immediate, and important part may be to be a 'secure base' for them[3] – to re-parent them.

7. This client may or may not be aware that their body and mind are one: a body-mind. They may not realize that, to have a calm and happy mind, they need to eat a healthy, balanced diet; exercise regularly; manage their sleep cycle; drink enough water; process their daily experiences consciously (and especially the difficult bits [preferably in writing, in a journal]); have a good balance of work, rest and play; be assertive in their communications with their significant others; have good quality social connections; and so on.

8. This client may have heard of 'the talking cure', and believe that all we have to do is *exchange some statements*, and then I will say 'Take up thy bed and walk!' And they will be healed.

They may not know that the solution to their problems is most likely going to involve them taking **more** *responsibility* for the state of their life; being **more** *self-disciplined*; learning to *manage* the 'shadow side' of their mind (or 'bad wolf' state); learning to *manage* their own emotions; *manage* their own relationships better; *manage* their physical health, in terms of diet, exercise, sleep, relaxation, stress, and so on; and to *manage* their minds also.

~~~

About the only things I do know for sure, in advance, are as follows:

1. This client will be a largely non-conscious creature of habit, wired up in early childhood to be secure or insecure in their relationships;

2. It will take some time to reach some kind of agreement about the nature of their main problems; and:

3. Our communications will be relatively difficult, because all human communication is very difficult. This is so because they will have to *interpret* what I say and do in the light of **their** previous experiences, and I will have to *interpret* what they say and do in the light of **my** previous experiences. So the grounds for misunderstanding are vast!

4. A lot of what will be communicated between us will go directly from my right brain to their right brain, non-verbally.

5. They will know *how I feel about them* long before they know any of my ideas.

6. I will have to have my wits about me, like Hercule Poirot, sailing through a dark night, on a choppy river, watching for shadows in the bushes on either bank! But I love the challenge. And now that I have developed E-CENT counselling, I have a broad range of models and theories and strategies in my toolbox to help me on my journey through the therapeutic relationship with any client who consults me in the future.

~~~

If I reflect upon some of my clients from recent years, and how I worked with them, I might conclude that:

1. Their problems ranged from couple conflict, anger management and anxiety/panic, and *an anxious-clinging attachment style* - on the one hand - to grief and depression, guilt and shame, lack of self-confidence, and an *avoidant attachment style* on the other. In other words, some of them were troubled by hyper-aroused emotions, and others were troubled by low or hypo-arousal. (I have more to say on this subject in section 2.6 below, where I present a more extensive list).

2. Although they were (and are) *primarily emotional beings* – (as am I) - nevertheless we had to communicate with each other through our *socialized, largely language-based communication interface habits*. (This, of course, includes a good deal of paralinguistic signals [or body language], and emotional leakages [or 'tells'], which are beyond our control!)

3. My main *modus operandum* consisted of: (a) Providing the client with a secure base; (b) Exploring their current life situation, including their lifestyle habits; and (c) Attempting to teach them those models and theories and techniques which I have used in the past (and those I use today) to keep my emotional arousal *in the middle ground* between too high and too low. (For more on the tasks undertaken in E-CENT counselling, please see section 2.6 below).

4. In the process of working with me, over time, they mainly seemed to become *more adult* – without losing sight of the value of their **Nurturing Parent** and **Playful Child** parts (or 'ego states' – or states of their ego, or personality variations). They learned to perceive-feel-think in a less extreme mode, and to keep their affects (or emotions/feelings/actions) on an even keel.

1.2 What is E-CENT counselling?

E-CENT counselling is one of the newest, most comprehensive systems of holistic counselling. But this is something of a paradox, because, as John McLeod writes: "There are no new therapies." (From page ix of McLeod 1997/2006). Of course, what he means here is that most new systems of counselling are a result of experiencing and knowing about older systems of counselling, which coalesce and mingle and transform and evolve over time.

For example, E-CENT theory has some of its roots in the moderate teachings of the Buddha, and the moderate teaching of the Stoic philosophers; though I also have criticisms of both of these schools of thought.

I have reviewed models of mind from Plato and Freud, and John Bowlby and the post-Freudian, 'object relations' tradition[4].

And I have incorporated many ideas from the very latest thinking in affective neuroscience and interpersonal neurobiology. I stand on the shoulders of giants!

Furthermore, as argued by Hill (2015), in describing other innovations, I am participating in the development of "major advances in psychotherapy", via the "integration of disciplines". (Page 98).

It should be stated quite clearly, however, that I am critical of as many aspects of those disciplines as those I favour!

I am wary of taking anything on board too readily, without adequate testing and critical analysis. And I encourage you to do the same with the content of this book!

~~~

E-CENT counselling theory is about *the whole individual client* – the body-brain-mind-environment - and not just the *mind* of the client. It involves integrating the body-mind of the social-individual with their social environment.

It arose out the integration of various pre-existing theories and models of counselling and therapy - including the rational-emotive; cognitive-behavioural; emotive/psychodynamic; and person-centred approaches. Plus attachment theory; and moral philosophy; narrative analysis; and some moderate Buddhist and Stoic principles.

Our ultimate aim was to integrate - as potentially equal contributors to personal happiness and mental tranquillity – the following elements:

    (a) The body, (diet and exercise [plus sleep, relaxation and meditation]);

    (b) The brain, (brain food, blood sugar, and brain/mind development);

    (c) The environment, (relationships, right livelihood, living conditions);

    (d) Family of origin and childhood experiences, including traumatic experiences;

    (e) Personal narratives, (or stories, scripts, frames, beliefs, attitudes, values, which were learned from family and society); and:

    (f) A sense of "something bigger than the self", (a spiritual or moral practice, or a social/political/community involvement).

1.3 Our unique perspective

E-CENT counselling has a full title which benefits from being broken down into its constituent elements, for ease of presentation!

The 'E' stands for **Emotive**. We believe that humans are *primarily feeling beings*, with an innate set of emotional control systems, which are subject to development over time, in the context of social modelling and social shaping. (Panksepp 1998; and Siegel 2015).

The 'E-C' (or Emotive-Cognitive) juxtaposition was necessitated because of 'the cognitive turn', which began back in the 1950's, when psychology researchers began to lose faith in the models of behaviourism. When it became obvious, for example, that experimental animals had their own 'goals and agendas', separate and apart from the behavioural shaping conducted by the observing researchers, then those disillusioned neo-behaviourists concluded: "Ah, there must be something going on inside of those animals: like *thinking*!" And thus the *cognitive turn* occurred. Now we were all thought to be 'cognitive beings', where cognition was thought to be dominated by *thinking*. Some of the major researchers (from the 1930's and '40's) who laid the foundations for this field - like Jean Piaget and Lev Vygotsky - *overlooked human emotion*. They also did not notice that our so-called cognitive processes, of attention, perception, memory, etc., are (apparently) strongly *guided by emotional control systems*. (Panksepp 1998; Siegel 2015; and Hill 2015[5]).

I have come up with the E-C (Emotive-Cognitive) formulation to emphasize that we are *primarily emotional, feeling beings*, who also have a (limited) capacity to engage in *relatively cool* reasoning processes. In addition, those reasoning processes seem to **depend upon** our ability *to form emotional evaluations of our choices and options* (Damasio, 1994)[6]. Indeed, I dislike speaking or writing about 'thinking'; preferring to use the term 'perfinking', to indicate that *we perceive, feel and think (or perfink) all in one grasp of the mind*.[7] Those apparently separate processes (like 'thinking') cannot ever be clearly and wholly separated out from each other (though we can perhaps *distinguish* between them for certain theoretical purposes).

~~~

So much for the 'E-C' element of our acronym. Now for the 'E-N' element:

The *E-N element* stands for **Embodied-Narrative**. Again, this is an attempt to get away from some unhelpful ideas from the past: this time some ideas that have become prevalent in Rational and Cognitive therapies (REBT/CBT), to the effect that we have **automatic thoughts, or beliefs**, which are *completely disconnected from the state of our bodies*. **This is not true**. The REBT/CBT approaches lead therapists and counsellors to relate to their clients as 'floating heads', which they are not.

For examples: An *inebriated body* will produce different thoughts and beliefs and narratives than a *sober* body.

A *hungry* body (with exceptionally low blood sugar levels) will produce different (and more negative) thoughts and beliefs and narratives than a *well fed* body (given a balanced diet at regular intervals throughout the day).

A *well exercised* body will produce different (more positive, constructive) thoughts and beliefs than *a 'couch potato' body*, all other things being equal.

An excessively *stressed* body will produce different thoughts and beliefs than a suitably *relaxed* body. And so on.

Hence the importance of the concept of **_Embodied-Narratives_**.

So, our system of Emotive-Cognitive Embodied-Narrative Therapy (E-CENT) exists because of some of the most obvious errors in the therapies which preceded us.

1.4 The status of E-CENT theory

Most of the models and processes which went into forming the theoretical foundations of E-CENT counselling come from one or more of the ten systems of therapy which were evaluated by Smith and Glass (1977), and found to be not only *effective*, but fairly **equally effective**![8] So I do not feel any need to waste resources funding a Randomized Control Trial to 'prove' the efficacy of E-CENT. (West and Byrne, 2009[9]).

The main types of therapy validated by Smith and Glass (1977, 1982)[10], and also by later studies[11], and used in E-CENT counselling, are: Transactional analysis; Rational emotive therapy; Psychodynamic approaches; Gestalt therapy; Client-centred; and Systematic desensitization.

The *main exceptions* to this rule – that E-CENT has been constructed from *validated* systems of counselling and therapy (validated by the Common Factors School of research – Smith and Glass [1980]; Wampold and Messer [2001]; and others) – include the use of:

> 1. Elements of **Attachment theory** (which is perhaps the most researched and validated approach to developmental psychology in use today) – See: Wallin (2007); and Bowlby (1988)[12].
>
> 2. Aspects of **the most popular approaches** to Moral philosophy (including The Golden Rule; Rule utilitarianism; Duty ethics; and Virtue ethics.)[13]
>
> 3. Aspects of *moderate* Buddhist philosophy, including elements of the Zen perspective on language; and some of the insights of the Dhammapada.[14]
>
> 4. The **Narrative approach** to counselling and therapy, which has become increasingly popular, mainly as a result of the work of White and Epston; and Kenneth Gergen; plus Theodore Sarbin.[15]

5. And some *moderate* elements of Stoicism, especially those parts that overlap *moderate* Buddhism.

1.5 An accidental evolution of theory

I did not go seeking to *invalidate* any particular theory, but rather to *validate* REBT (and I had *no reservations* about Zen Buddhism or Stoicism – which I do now!) In practice, however, as I worked at trying to validate the ABC model of REBT[16], (between 2001 and 2007/8), our reflective learning increasingly drew attention to flaws and weaknesses in Rational Emotive Behaviour Therapy theory and models.

In one of my papers on REBT - (Byrne 2009a) - I was trying to validate the ABC model by comparing and contrasting it with:

(1) Elements of Freud's theory of the tripartite psyche (or mind): (Comprising the **It** [or organism]; the **Ego** [or socialized personality] and the **Super-ego** [or internalized mother-father-other]);

(2) Aspects of Transactional Analysis (TA) theory – including how the so-called *Parent, Adult* and *Child* 'ego states' (or 'ways of being') could be accommodated within the ABC model;

(3) The *Object Relations* emphasis on the relationship of mother and baby; and:

(4) Some cognitive science (including Hofstadter 2007, Le Doux 1996, and Damasio 1994 and 2000); some Zen koans; and some general theory of emotions from mainstream psychology.

In practice, REBT fell apart in our hands, and E-CENT emerged from the debris.

In 2009, six years before Daniel Siegel produced his book on Interpersonal Neurobiology (IPN), I had constructed a model of the 'social individual' who grows out of the interaction of mother-and-baby in the context of socialization and education (or induction into a culture – Byrne 2009b).

In this development, I had been influenced by the neuroscientific insights of Douglas Hofstadter's (2007) view of the human brain-mind[17], and the other elements mentioned in sub-paragraphs (1)-(4) above.

1.6 Views of science

I am not claiming that "E-CENT is right, and everybody else is wrong!" This would contradict the *Common Factors* theory that all systems of counselling and therapy that are designed to be therapeutic produce broadly equivalent outcomes for clients (on average).

I take the view that all science is *tentative and propositional*. (Of course, a few sciences [when closely related to technology, or to other physical referents that are easy to explore] prove to be *more verifiable*. But psychological science tends to be harder to verify; and verifications are often overturned with time. Indeed, the very idea of 'verification' in the human sciences is problematical. The positivistic approach is to apply the model of the hard (technological and physical) sciences to the world of psychology and therapy. But a more sustainable approach is to see the theories of psychology and psychotherapy as *social constructions*, in *a world of social constructions about a 'concrete reality'* – the human brain-mind - which is *difficult to explore.*

E-CENT theory is such a social construction, which should be continually tested in practice, and modified in the light of experience. Like **all** human science products, E-CENT theory was produced by "blokes and birds (or guys and gals) trying to make sense of stuff".

I have used the best theories, models and evidences available to us in the most relevant literature. I have tried to avoid turning our theories into 'facts' – which is very hard for humans to do. We humans believe so strongly in our ideas that we tend to project them out into the world and 'find them' there. For example, Panksepp (1998) has said that what cognitive scientists think of as the **cognitive** functions of *attention, perception*, etc., *are thought to be controlled by our emotional control systems.*

However, in practice, I may sometimes seem to be firming that up into *an incontrovertible fact*. But in terms of my intentions, I intend to say: It **seems** to me (based on my literature reviews, and my own 'clinical' experiences) that we humans are *primarily* emotional beings, for the whole of our lives. It **seems**, from work conducted by Antonio Damasio, Jaak Panksepp, Allan Schore, Daniel Siegel, and others, *that our thinking **depends upon** our feelings*. And it **seems** to us that this should reverse the *cognitive revolution*, and usher in *an era of emotional revolution* in counselling and psychotherapy.

1.7 The case against using case studies

You will not find *a pivotal case study* at the foundations of E-CENT.

It is impossible to write a case study, or case studies, which would illustrate the essence of Emotive-Cognitive Embodied-Narrative Therapy (E-CENT) – at least in the sense of revealing *what is going on inside the counsellor and the client*. How could a case study reveal the *non-conscious* workings of the mind of the client, and the equally *concealed mental processes* of the counsellor?

If Sigmund Freud's case studies reveal anything, they show the *conscious formulations of cause and effect* that Freud **deduced**, *in the form of subjective **interpretations*** from his conversations with, and thoughts about, his individual clients. They tell us *nothing* of what went on at the most important level of body-mind in either the analyst or the client.

If you read the case study at the beginning of Albert Ellis's original version of his book, *Reason and Emotion in Psychotherapy* (1962)[18] – pages 22-33 (with context provided in pages 18-22) - what you will mainly learn (from the creator of Rational Therapy) is *Albert Ellis's* **theory** *of the human condition*, and **not** anything *real* about the client. I now have good reasons to conclude that Dr Ellis had decided (as a child, probably mainly non-consciously), as an after-effect of the fact that he had been largely abandoned and emotionally neglected by his parents, that *humans should be cool and detached*.[19] (This was evidenced by his lifelong avoidant attachment style, and his tendency to emphasize thoughts over feelings; and the fact than some of his closest colleagues considered him to be "somewhat Aspergerish", or slightly autistic).

He also believed that there were *no really good* **objective reasons** *for anybody to be disturbed* (which was what he had learned from reading the *extreme views* of the major Stoics, Marcus Aurelius and Epictetus).

And in his case study (from 1962), mentioned above, concerning a disturbed female client, Ellis states quite clearly that "…every human being who gets disturbed really is *telling himself a chain of false sentences*…" (Page 28). This is very far from the truth, as you will find if you take one hundred ordinary citizens at random, and expose them to a rattle snake or a mad dog in a confided space in which they are captive. Most of them will become *highly disturbed,* no matter what they 'try to tell themselves' – because the reasoning centres of the mind can only damp down emotional disturbance at low levels of intensity. And the fearful things which we could imply they are 'telling themselves' (or emotively signally themselves) about these threats are, in any case, *far from being false!* Snakes really *are* dangerous, and a threat to our survival, in some contexts.

People *are* affected by their environments, and especially their social environments (which contradicts the extremist view expressed by Epictetus in his most famous dictum: where he states, in the *Enchiridion*, that "people are **not** disturbed by what happens to them, but rather by **the attitude** they adopt towards what happens to them"). Most often, our emotional reactions are *automatic,* very *fast,* and *non-conscious* (Goleman)[20]. The emotional arousal occurs in a fraction of a second, which is far too fast for any thinking to take place. And very often, the strong emotional reaction is 'self-preserving' or *self-protective,* or *survival oriented,* and not at all 'irrational'.

The way Albert Ellis constructed his case study, above, allowed him to *mislead* his readers into becoming less sensitive and less empathic towards their clients and other people. The clients' feelings are treated as *an irrelevant epiphenomenon* contingent upon *what the clients are telling themselves* – which is now seen by us – or now *seems to us* – to be a **false** theory of human mental functioning. More often than not, *the feeling comes* **before** *the thought*, and the thought is coloured by the feeling! (See the APET model from the Human Givens tradition, in chapter 8 below).

Here's another example where a case study is used to justify an approach to counselling. Take a look at the case study at the beginning of Aaron Beck's (1976) book on cognitive therapy[21]. In a section titled 'The discovery of automatic thoughts' (in pages 29-35), Beck presents 'an autobiographical note' which claims to be a description of a conversation with a client, during which Beck *discovered* - by getting the client to *introspect* about (or look into) his own thought processes - that the client had 'two streams of thought'. Beck admits that he had *earlier formulated the theory* that 'clients in general withheld certain kinds of ideas' that passed through their minds. Beck (1976) was **hunting** for just such ideas when this particular client "volunteered the information" (page 30) that he had been having *a second stream of automatic thoughts* while expressing the first stream verbally. Since we know that *introspection into our thought processes is unable to reveal most of our moment to moment processing of our environment* – as demonstrated by: Gladwell (2006); Gray (2003); Bargh and Chartrand (1999); Maier (1931) – and we also know that introspection was *dumped* by the world of psychology at the end of the nineteenth century as being *unreliable* - we can infer that this client was (*unintentionally* and *non-consciously*) 'making up plausible stories' (Maier 1931; and Hill 2015) to satisfy Beck's questions. He was giving Beck *what he asked for!*

So case studies seem to be a poor source of ***objective*** data, telling us more about the *author's ideas* than anything real about the subjects of the study.

1.8 Subjectivity of case studies

Back in 2005, I had a research associate (let's call him Charles) who wanted us to collaborate on the question of ***what he did*** in his counselling sessions that benefitted his clients, and ***how*** he did it.

He wanted me to review a few of his counselling sessions, recorded on video tape, and to write down a case study of: "....what I (Charles) did, and what my clients gained from particular interventions".

I said I'd think about it. And I did. In fact, I created *a thought experiment*, which went like this:

Imagine this: (a) Charles is in a small counselling room with an individual client; (b) there are four one-way mirrors – one on each wall of that room; and (c) behind each one-way mirror there is an observer.

Now let us suppose that each of those four observers come from *a different school* of counselling and therapy theory. When each of them submits their written report of 'what happened' in the room, how good will the correspondence be between the four reports? ***Not very good***, I am sure you will agree. (Because people do not see with their eyes, but rather with their interpreted, and interpretive, *life experiences* stored in their body-minds!)

My thought experiment is a bit like asking a rugby league (RL) player, a rugby union (RU) player[22], a soccer player and a Gaelic Athletic Association (Irish Football) player to evaluate a game of ladies netball, and to identify *the three key events* in the game which seemed to have determined the outcome.

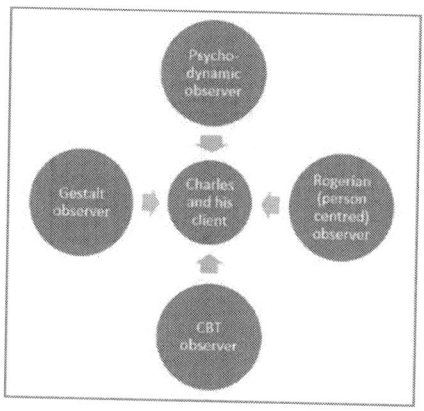

Figure 1.1: The subjectivity of observation

Clearly there would be very little agreement between the reports – because we do not see with our eyes, but rather with our *mental maps of the world*. And each distinct school of counselling and psychotherapy teaches a distinct map of the psychological world.

So, if we want to know about Charles's approach to doing counselling and therapy work, might it not be better to find out what his **theory** is? What **models** he uses? What **processes** he promotes? His **concept** *of the mind* of the client, and so on? And we could also try to get some testimonials from his clients regarding their experience of his counselling skill.

If we knew those things, we could then decide whether or not they **seemed** *credible to us*. We could experiment with his approach to see how it works in practice (for us!) And we could incorporate into our lives those elements that worked for us, and discard the rest.

That is what I intend to do in this book – to describe the key principles, models and theories upon which E-CENT counselling is based; and to describe how E-CENT is applied in individual counselling; and in self-management.

I will **not** try to develop case studies of clients and what they got from E-CENT, for the reasons outlined above, although I might quote **illustrative** examples, occasionally; or cite a client **testimonial** regarding what they got from E-CENT counselling.

E-CENT counselling sees our clients as *primarily emotional*, with some cognitive (thinking) abilities, which are underpinned by automatic, non-conscious emotional control systems (Panksepp, 1998; and Siegel, 2015).

Their narratives, or stories of their experiences, are encoded in their body-brain-minds. They are not just 'floating heads'.

~~~

1.9 Narratives and stories

> *"Clients ... come in and, one way or another, tell their story and discover or construct new stories to tell. Therapists do not usually disclose stories of their own personal troubles, but instead offer their clients more general, almost mythic stories of how people change or what life can be like. Implicit in the therapist's story is an image of the 'good life'."* (McLeod, 1997/2006).

E-CENT counselling is interested in the stories of our clients, and we have helpful stories to share with them; and also ways of helping them to explore and re-write their stories. Some of this is described in Chapter 8, where I introduce **the Jigsaw story model**, which is a guide to focusing on the client's stories, and to remember to relate the various bits of their stories to each other, and to look for patterns and inconsistencies.

But first, let us review the 'narrative' approach of E-CENT, by comparing and contrasting it to some of the more traditional approaches.

(i) <u>Similarities</u>: E-CENT accepts that human beings are immersed in social narratives, and that they apprehend their environments in terms of narrative elements of characters, plots, dramas, stories, cause and effect imputations, etc. (See: Perry, 2012, pages 71-88. And McLeod, 1997/2006). I believe humans function largely non-consciously, and view the world – non-consciously – through *frames* of reference derived (interpretively and automatically) from their past (social) experiences. And *these narratives are **emotive** or feeling stories*, which provide meaning and structure to the life of the social-individual.

(ii) <u>Differences</u>: E-CENT does not subscribe to the White and Epston (1990) strategy for dealing with narrative disturbances[23]. Instead I have created my own processes of narrative therapy. I also avoid using McLeod's commitment to *postmodern* perspectives. The E-CENT perspective on narrative is grounded in our conception of the human being as *a socialized body-mind-environment-whole*. So there is a real, physical 'me', and a real physical environment in which I am embedded. We do not advocate the view which says "all there is is story!" And the stories I tell myself are dependent upon not only my physical existence in a physical/social world, but also upon how well I slept last night; how well I have eaten today; how much physical exercise I have done recently; how hydrated my body-brain-mind is today; how well connected I am to people in significant relationships; how much pressure I am under (actually and experientially) – and what my coping resources are (or seem to me to be); and so on.

So E-CENT theory only deals with grounded narratives: or embodied-narratives.

~~~

It is now widely accepted in psychology and social science that narratives and stories are central to how humans make sense of the world, and communicate with each other about their lives. Professor Theodore Sarbin was one of the main and earliest of the American theorists who raised objections to positivist psychology, and argued that 'emotions are narrative emplotments'. (Sarbin, 1989, 2001)[24]. Kenneth Gergen (1985, 2004)[25] is another theorist of this 'narrative turn' in the field of psychology. White and Epston (1990) are probably the best known theorists of Narrative Therapy today. However, there are three pre-existing approaches to narrative therapy - as described by John McLeod (2003), pages 227-238[26]; plus McLeod (1997/2006), chapters 3 to 5. These are: (1) the psychodynamic approach; (2) the cognitive/constructivist approach; and (3) the social constructionist approach.

(1) The psychodynamic approach to the use of narratives in counselling and therapy focuses on the ways that the client's stories can reveal habitual ways of relating; and the counsellor can thus use those stories to help the client to 're-author' their lives: (Strupp and Binder, 1984[27]; Luborsky and Crits-Christoph, 1990)[28]. The main emphasis in the psychodynamic approach to the use of narrative in counselling and therapy is in helping to identify the *Core Conflictual Relationship Theme* (CCRT). This CCRT then provides the basic agenda for their work of counselling.

(2) The cognitive/constructivist approach to the use of narratives in counselling and therapy focuses on two strategies:

(a) Identifying stories that conflict with each other, which provides the possibility of using 'cognitive dissonance' to help with the challenge of rewriting and integrating conflicted schemas (or frames, scripts, stories) in the client's long-term memory[29]; and:

(b) The use of metaphor. For example: If your read my Story of Origins[30], you will find I use the metaphor of being a 'little mouse' to describe a period of my life when I was passive and withdrawn, and then 'a big moral cat', when I discovered a form of political expression that allowed me to safely express my anger towards my father. Metaphors can be depowering and empowering, and the therapist can help the client to develop more empowering metaphors for the problem roles, themes, or characters in their most difficult stories[31].

(3) The social constructionist approach to narrative therapy is based on the idea that we are social beings born into a story-telling culture; that we are surrounded by stories, myths, legends; that these stories preceded our existence; and we take on some of the story roles and themes into which we are *thrown* at birth. According to Alasdair MacIntyre, we are primarily story-telling animals[32].

The best known contributors to the development of this tradition were White and Epston, a couple of Australasian family therapists: (White and Epston, 1990)[33]. Since people are seen as occupying a family- or community-generated narrative or story, the solution is to 'externalize' this story, and get the client to see it as *not part of them*, so they can step away from the roles specified in the story; or to re-author their story in various ways.

Like E-CENT therapy, this form of therapy uses both spoken dialogue and written narratives to help the client to unearth their dominant narratives and to change them.

1.10 The E-CENT approach

E-CENT theory does not fit comfortably within any of the three narrative traditions outlined above. Neither was E-CENT directly inspired by the creators of any of those three traditions. Nevertheless, E-CENT involves, or echoes – *primarily* - an integration of elements of traditions (1) and (3) – the psychodynamic and the social constructionist.

But E-CENT is much more than that; and is a completely unique approach to narrative, in that I have integrated many different systems to develop and explicate our understanding of human development and individual functioning.

And even more than that, I have developed a form of counselling and therapy for dealing with *embodied-narratives about something (tangible and meaningful!)* And that embodied narrative approach is informed by affective neuroscience and interpersonal neurobiology. (Panksepp, 1998; Schore, 2015; Siegel, 2015).

The core foundation stones of E-CENT are these:

Element 1: A physical baby (or body-mind) in its mother's arms, internalizing her language and culture; her behaviour and speech; her values and attitudes; and her relational approach to the baby.

Element 2: A developmental history of the mother-baby dyad, resulting in:

(a) A *grown-up form* of that 'baby', which is a physical organism (dependent upon diet, exercise, relaxation, relationship connection and support, and so on); with…

(b) all of its cumulative-interpretive experiences; including:

(i) internalized representations of significant others (e.g. mother and father, etc.; called 'objects' for short); and:

(ii) all of its good and bad adaptations towards - and reactions and rebellions against - those internalized 'objects';

(c) which gave rise to its 'internal working models'[34] of relationship - (secure and/or insecure);

(d) all of which (in paragraphs 'b-c' above) is stored in long-term memory, in the form of electro-chemical equivalents of schemas, scripts, stories, frames and other narrativized *and non-narrativized* elements;

(e) below the level of conscious awareness; and:

(f) permanently beyond **direct** conscious inspection. (Byrne 2009b; and Bowlby 1988).

So *narrative* is only *part* of what is going on in the world of E-CENT theory. The larger picture is of a **real**, **physical** body, travelling through **real** space-time, in a **real** socioeconomic culture – all of which can be interpreted to some degree; but there are limitations to the degree of interpretations. (This is *Element 1* plus *Element 2* above). It would be very difficult, for example, for very many working class individuals, living and working in London or New York today, to interpret their circumstances as *living in Paradise!* Reality exerts *some constraints* upon the potential shape of our stories!

Different schools of thought have their own *theories of human story-telling*. For examples;

(a) In constructivism, the individual **makes up** their own story, as they explore their environment (Piaget).

(b) In social-constructionism, the individual **is socialized** into a belief system which is not their own (Vygotsky).

(c) In the Freudian world, the individual is a sexy organism which **makes up phantasies** about its love objects.

But in E-CENT, there is more going on than is described in (a) to (c) above.

And now, to try to firm up that E-CENT perspective, I feel compelled to do something that I have argued against: to give a case example. This is intended to *illustrate* E-CENT, rather than to *'prove'* anything about it.

A client's case summarized

Sharon is a woman who phoned me recently to say she needed help with a problem. Her husband had been in hospital to have major surgery on his intestines, during which he almost died. Now her husband (Frank) had made a shaky recovery, but with permanent impairment resulting from the surgery, which had drastically changed their relationship. And her husband (stupidly in her view) planned to return to his stressful job, which could quickly kill him off. Understandably, Sharon felt traumatized; was experiencing undigested grief; was anxious about Frank's return to work; and depressed about some of the ways in which she had lost out in life.

I assumed I might end up doing some grief work with her: helping her to get in touch with the tears and letting them out. I discussed that possibility with her.

I also thought it was possible that, instead, she might want to do some desensitization around the trauma of her husband's surgery and near death experience.

And we had also discussed on the phone the possibility that Sharon was reliving a trauma from her fifth year of life, stimulated by recent experiences.

In the event, we had one counselling session, during which fragments of stories fitted together badly, and, while some grieving came up, desensitization seemed to recede into the background.

Analysis

In trying to put Sharon's story together (the **Jigsaw-story** approach of E-CENT: See Chapter 8) I came up with these fragments:

1(a). While Sharon thought her husband's intestinal problems probably 'fell from the skies' - ('just bad luck') – I suggested that their love of a highly spicy and sugary diet might have precipitated Candida Albicans, which can in turn precipitate the form of intestinal disease Frank suffered from. (These insights come from reading alternative heath books and articles; and taking responsibility for 'becoming our own physicians'. See, in particular, Taylor-Byrne and Byrne, 2017; and Dr Mercola's website[35]. (See also Chapter 4 below).

1(b). I made sure Sharon understood that I was **not** dispensing medical advice, but rather modelling the importance of understanding our own physical and mental health; and the links between our bodies and minds; and the connections between what we eat, how we maintain our guts, and our physical health and emotional wellbeing.

2(a). Sharon had never thought about diet before; but she now realized that she also has intestinal discomfort, though it does not stop her eating hot and sweet chilli meals (yet!). (I recommended that she see a good nutritionist, or an alternative health practitioner, or a holistic medical doctor; and that she subscribe to a helpful journal which educates the general public regarding cutting edge medical science that is not normally disseminated by general medical practitioners (GPs)[36].)

2(b). Some aspects of Sharon's diet may be undermining her psychological condition. For example: Eight cups of strong, fresh-ground coffee each day; skipping breakfast; sugary foods. (I shared this insight with her. She was very surprised, as she subscribed to the common social delusion that 'eating is a form of recreation', with no health implications. In E-CENT we say: "Eating is for health and nutrition. Recreational eating can kill you!") 'How to have fun with (bad) food' is a common (irresponsible) social narrative. (See Chapter 4 for information about foods to eat and foods to avoid; and Chapter 9 on how to teach this subject).

2(c). It became apparent to me that Sharon was not getting enough sleep, because she stayed up late, watching TV, as a way of alleviating her anxiety about Frank's health. So I taught her some key insights into the science of sleep (as in Chapter 5 below).

3. She was aware of the Stoic and Buddhist injunction to **give up trying to control the uncontrollable**, but she was really upset because she could not figure out **how to stop Frank** going back to work; or **how to stop herself** trying to stop Frank going back to work. So I introduced her to my Six Windows Model, as a strategy for re-framing challenging problems. (See Chapter 6 below).

4. I told her a story of a recent dream I'd had, which had helped me to complete some longstanding grief of my own, possibly from around the same time as her age-five trauma. (Some of this proved to be 'feeling talk' – which probably was mainly right-brain to right-

brain communication, running alongside the left-brain to left-brain story-talk). She was amazed by the terrain of my dream, because it paralleled a recent dream she had had. Her dream involved walking through a particular landscape (which she described in detail), and having particularly traumatic things happen (which again were detailed by her).

I suggested that we work on that dream, using a fusion of Gestalt therapy and psychodrama.

I got her to **identify with** each element of the dream; and then, because she found it so hard to dis-identify (or dissociate) from **herself as the traumatized subject** (or viewer) of the dream, I got her to act out the process of 'stepping out of herself', and then watching herself from a safe distance – from the side-lines.

In the process, she discovered a deeply unhelpful aspect of her character and temperament, which might have been driving some of her attitudes towards her husband's illness and his plan to return to work. (As a result of that discovery, she apparently 'changed her [feeling] story' - [or rewrote or revised it] - about who she was, and how she has to act!)

By the end of the session, Sharon was "re-moralized"; more confident; less shaky. She went away saying she would think about what I'd said about the connection between diet and health. I don't think she'll be back, because I believe she has enough Stoical capacity to handle whatever is up ahead. (If she does come back, we should talk about the role of exercise in damping down anxiety and panic. See Chapter 4, section 4.9; and Chapter 9, section 9.2(2)).

Her weakness comes mainly from the coffee (which, in large amounts, usually causes stress and anxiety) and her use of sugary foods (which can cause an overgrowth of Candida Albicans, which is depression-inducing)![37] And I have asked her to look at changing those, and some other aspects of her diet, with the support of a professional nutritionist.

The rest she can handle through the normal processes of **grieving**, which I have helped her to accept as okay.

"It's okay to cry, Sharon!" I told her near the beginning of the session, when she was resisting crying openly.

"If I told you a joke, you would laugh out loud", I said.

"So when you feel sad, I **want** to see your **sad** face, **and** your tears!" I think she got it!

E-CENT has one root in narrative; one root in the body-mind (where narrative is stored); one root in the environment (where the nutrients and love and stories come from – and where the physical exercising is done [or not!]).

~~~

Self-reflection

Of course, I can redeem 'the purity' of my stance on the *limitations* of case studies, like this:

I am the only person who saw Sharon when she came to Hebden Bridge that day.

I cannot offer you any corroboration of the veracity of my story about Sharon's visit. I believe the story recounts some key elements of the counselling session we shared.

But I do not know the extent to which I might have inadvertently steered the conversation, based on my subconscious commitment to various ways of understanding Sharon (and other humans in her situation).

So my story is a 'just-so' story. It *might* be helpful to you to explore some of its inferences and implications. But it is still *just my story about Sharon*.

1.11 Defining Attachment Theory more clearly

Because Attachment theory is a significant component of E-CENT theory and practice, it is important to provide some background.

What is attachment theory? How does it relate to post-Freudian or neo-Freudian approaches to psychotherapy? And how are these ideas used in E-CENT?

Firstly, attachment theory was originated by Dr John Bowlby, a British psychoanalyst, based on his observations of the negative impact of protracted separation of young children from their parents, especially their mothers[38]. This is how it was described by Gullestad (2001)[39]:

> In a documentary film made by Dr John Bowlby for the World Health Organization, he reports on "...the mental health of homeless children in post-war Europe. The major conclusion was that to grow up mentally healthy, 'the infant and young child should experience a warm, intimate, and continuous relationship with his mother (or permanent mother substitute) in which *both* find satisfaction and enjoyment...'."

Secondly, attachment theory seems to be part of the post-WW2 movement away from classical Freudianism: (Gomez, 1997). The British Object Relations School of psychoanalysis – involving Melanie Klein, Ronald Fairbairn, Donald Winnicott, Michael Balint and Harry Guntrip – seems to have been a big part of the cultural milieu in which John Bowlby arose and developed. However, there were significant differences between all of these post-Freudian psychoanalysts, some of whom were never tolerated by Anna Freud and the heirs to Sigmund Freud, and some of whom, like Winnicott, straddled both camps.

Thirdly, some of the Object Relations theorists emphasized the role of the *inner working* of the individual's psyche in causing their emotional problems – which was the classical Freudian approach – and some emphasized the role of *the environment* – which was not. Bowlby, like Karen Horney in the USA, was adamant that people were strongly shaped by their environment, and especially by their formative relationships with their mothers (and fathers) – or their main carers[40].

Fourth, Bowlby's ideas on attachment were subjected to empirical enquiry and further elaboration by Mary Ainsworth (1967, 1969), who developed the 'strange situation' research model, in which mothers withdraw from a room in which their toddler is playing, a stranger enters, then mother returns after three minutes, and the toddler's reaction to mother is assessed. This work gave rise to the categories of:

- *secure* attachment', where the child has a basic trust in the enduring love and availability of the mother;

- *avoidant* attachment', where the child does not trust the mother to be available consistently; and:

- *resistant* (or *anxious-ambivalent*) attachment' in which the child clings to the mother, but often in punitive or angry ways.[41]

When clients come to see us in E-CENT counselling, we try to identify their attachment style, and to relate to them on the basis of re-parenting those who are avoidant or anxious-ambivalent.

1.12 The role of the individual's social environment

Paradoxically, Albert Ellis – the creator of Rational Emotive Behaviour Therapy - had his training analysis in the Karen Horney school of Object Relations in New York City, which emphasized *the role of the environment* in harming and/or helping the individual. When Ellis split from psychoanalysis, he represented himself as *splitting from Sigmund Freud* (and did not mention differences with Horney).

In fact, in developing his ABC model, he argues that it's not what happens to the client - (the Activating **Adversity** [or the 'A']) - which is upsetting, but rather their **Beliefs** about it - (which he labels as the 'B'). And it is assumed to be the **interaction** of the A and the B which causes the **Consequent emotion** (which he labels as the 'C'). (However, in practice, he normally dumps the role of the 'A' quite quickly, and focuses on the role of the 'B'. "People are always and only upset by the 'B'", is his core message! And this is a *false* conclusion! See Byrne, 2017).

In creating this A>B>C model, Ellis was leaving Horney's A>C model behind, and re-joining Freud's "ABC model", in which Freud assumes that it is the child's (or patient's [or client's]) **mentation** (or **phantasies**) which cause their upsets, and **not** the noxious behaviours of their mother/father (or other elements of their social environment)!

Both Ellis and Freud attach primary significance to the **inner workings** *of the individual* (their B, or beliefs; or drives and phantasies), and *relatively little or no importance to their* **actual** *environments*. Horney and Bowlby, on the other hand, thought the environment was **primary**. For Horney and Bowlby, young children have little or nothing to do with how they are shaped by their 'good' or 'bad' parents: (or should I say "good enough" or "not good enough" parents).

E-CENT theory takes a middle position between Freud/Ellis on the one side, and Horney/Bowlby on the other. I believe that the relationship between the mother and child is dialectical; that the child internalizes working models of how mother relates to him; how father relates to him; and he then relates to them and the world on the basis of those models. The character/personality of the child is driven by his/her cumulative, interpretive experience of encountering 'good enough' or 'not good enough' carers, and significant others (like siblings, relatives, neighbours, teachers, etc.) But the *mother/father/others* have more power and control, and more shaping impact, in this interactive encounter, than the baby ever could.

1.13 The centrality of relationship

Whereas Sigmund (and later Anna) Freud emphasized the sexual tensions between parents and children, during the child's biologized stages of development, as the seat of neurosis, some post-Freudians, such as Melanie Klein, Ronald Fairbairn, Donald Winnicott, and others, went back to **the relationship between mother and child in the early months of life** to look for the seat of emotional mal-adaptations[42]. This was the beginning of the Object Relations School of psychoanalysis.

The 'object' in Object Relations theory can be *the actual mother* (or father, or carer) of the perceiving child; or *an internalized image* or *memory* of the mother (or father, or carer) in the child's mind; or *a part* of a significant other (such as mother's breast).

One of the central ideas of Objects Relations is that children split their world up into 'good' and 'bad' *objects*, based on their experiences of pleasure and pain in relationship, and then project those splits into their social environments. And the more painful experiences they have as children, the more disturbed their later lives will prove to be, all other things being equal[43].

In the USA, Margaret Mahler and her associates conducted observational research on young children and their mothers, to develop a theory of ego development[44]. This research demonstrated a clear connection between the quality of the relationship between mother and child, on the one hand, and the degree of emotional disturbance of the child, on the other.

John Bowlby, in the UK, created his theory of Attachment on the basis of his wartime experiences of dealing with children separated from their parents by war, or hospitalization, or other forms of institutionalization. He argued that children who are separated from their parents at a young age are likely to be disturbed in ways that will affect their later adult functioning. This thesis has been extensively researched and validated.

1.14 The need for emotional availability, and sensitive caring

However, it is not **just** separation that can damage the relationship between mother and child, but also any form of *absence, neglect*, or *abuse* (including physical, sexual or emotional abuse), or lack of *sensitive attunement*. (Wallin, 2007).

A child's emotional wellbeing can be protected by 'good enough' mothering, and 'good enough' fathering, and the provision of a 'secure base'. In this connection, 'good enough' means: sensitive, caring, attuned and supportive; and a *secure base* means a person to return to when problems are encountered, to 'refuel' or calm down emotionally, and to gain reassurance and restore self-belief. According to Bowlby (1988)[45], children develop an 'internal working model' of their relationship with mother, then father, and so on. These then become templates for their later relationships. Thus, if there are significant disturbances or distortions in their earliest relationships, the child will take them into later relationships, including adult relationships, because those are the only 'maps of the territory' (or 'schemas' for relationship) that they possess. And this is why Bowlby (1988) argues that one of the tasks of a psychotherapist is to provide their client with *a secure base from which to explore (their issues), and 'good enough' substitute-parenting*. This calls for 'emotional communication' between client and therapist, and not just logical and rational, 'cognitive' or thinking-based communications. (See Hill, 2015).

1.15 Attachment in psychotherapy

This development of Attachment theory has had a profound effect on the shape of E-CENT counselling practices. In particular, I place more emphasis on my *emotional attachment* to the client, than I do on the quality of my *thinking*[46] and *philosophical teachings*, and this change makes my work quite different from REBT/CBT counselling approaches. I assume that my relationship with my client is being largely conducted on the basis of implicit, automatic, non-conscious communication from my right brain to my client's right brain. (Hill, 2015).

A 'good enough' E-CENT counsellor will seek to provide a 'secure base' for his/her clients; to treat them with concern, care and sensitivity; and to model mindfulness, body awareness, and emotional intelligence for the client to copy, or internalize. In short, a 'good enough' E-CENT counsellor should be prepared to extend 'maternal love' (or something like it) to their clients, as a matter of course. (But they also need to have an equivalent of 'paternal love' in the background, to *set **boundaries*** and be the 'reality principle' for the client). In time, the client can outgrow this re-parenting process, and move into a more equal peer-to-peer relationship with their therapist.

The subject of how to integrate Attachment theory and psychoanalysis has been taken up by David Wallin (2007)[47]. David's work, and the E-CENT perspective, will change how the self is seen in counselling and psychotherapy. The conventional view of a self is that it is a 'separate', 'individual', 'discrete entity'. However, in my E-CENT models, the individual is seen to be *a social being*, 'connected (healthily or dysfunctionally) to others' - especially the mother, and then the father, and later significant others. (This lines up with the Interpersonal Neurobiology [IPNB] model of Siegel [2015], who describes the mind [or personal identity, personality, etc.] emerging out of the interaction of the baby's brain and external relationships [especially, initially, with mother].)

I have some reservations about some aspects of Wallin's presentation. However, there is little doubt that David's model has some significant validity. For example, his emphasis on the 'somatic self' (or embodied identity) as the foundation of the person, seems intuitively right, and fits into the E-CENT model. The 'emotional self' is an extension and refinement of the somatic self - a self that is felt in the viscera (or heart, lungs and guts) and based in the limbic system (or emotional centres) of the brain. And, of course, we also have our 'narrative self', or our story of who we are; and where we came from; and where we are trying to get to!

Wallin cites Fonagy et al (2002)[48], Schore (2003)[49] and others as proposing "...that regulation of emotions is fundamental to the development of the self and that attachment relationships are the primary context within which we learn to regulate our affects (or emotional attitudes) - that is, to access, modulate, and use our emotions. The relational patterns that characterize our first attachments are, fundamentally, patterns of affect regulation that subsequently determine a great deal about the nature of our own unique responsiveness to experience - that is, about the nature of the self."

Wallin (2007) continued: "Correspondingly, in the new attachment relationship that the therapist is attempting to generate, the (client's) emotions are central and their effective regulation - which allows them to be felt, modulated, communicated, and understood - is usually at the very heart of the process that enables the (client) to heal and to grow". (Page 64).

This is a most important area for consideration by all counsellors and psychotherapists, psychologists and psychoanalysts. And this time, what I notice to be missing from David's presentation is how 'good and evil' get into human behaviour. (See Appendix H of Byrne [2016] for the E-CENT position on good and evil tendencies in humans. Also, see Figure 1.3 below, in section 1.16).

The third element of David's model of the self is the 'representational self', about which he says: "Bowlby argued that it was an evolutionary necessity to have a representational world that mapped the real one". That is to say, that we have a map in our heads of the spaces in which we live, and the experiences we have had in those spaces. "To function effectively, we needed (and still need) knowledge of the world and of ourselves, and this knowledge must be portable. We derive such knowledge from memories of past experience, and we use this knowledge to make predictions about present and future experience. Hence, the internal working model. But the map, as they say, is not the territory". (Page 64).

That is a very important point. All of our stored representations are cumulative and interpretive, as shown in the E-CENT models – which are described in Byrne (2009b). And in Chapter 8, and, more briefly, in the next section below.

Our internal working models are not images or templates for individuals we have known, but rather what Douglas Hofstadter (2007)[50] called 'strange loops' - and which I have clarified in my E-CENT writings as 'strange loops of experience of encountering others' in which our sense of the other and our sense of self get braided together into one.

This suggests that at our very foundations are *strange loops of experience* of being changed by others and changing them, in which it is impossible to separate out an 'individual-I'.

(And those 'strange loops' are not abstract thoughts or beliefs. They are based in strongly potentiated neuronal connections [Panksepp, 1998]. They can, presumably, be articulated into narratives [as 'the narrative self'], but they are not 'mere linguistic constructions'. They are physical entities which drive our existence in the world. We do not 'have' a narrative self, which drives us; we 'are had' by a 'narrative self', which is *an articulation* or our *physical-experiential-historical self*).

1.16 Attachment in E-CENT

The E-CENT model seems to somewhat overlap the position being developed by Fonagy and Wallin, but it is also significantly different. One difference seems to be that in E-CENT, I see the new baby arriving with both good and bad tendencies, in potential. Thus the baby's innate urge to attach is not its only urge. Bowlby's biggest area of weakness was his neglect of the inner world of the child, and how to understand "...how the child builds up his own internal world..." (Holmes, 1995[51], cited in Gullestad, 2001).

Attachment theory seems to be closely related to object relations theory, both of which seem to agree that "the child's need for human contact is a human one". (Gullestad, page 6).

Gullestad also draws attention to a controversial question, as to whether the drive towards relationship in the object relations and attachment theory approaches replaces or merely supplements the original theory of drives presented by Freud.

In E-CENT theory, I take the view that drive theory is one side of the coin, and attachment the other.

In practice, what that means is that there are two major components that go into creating the personality of a human being:

(1) Their physical existence, with innate urges and developmental capacities.

(2) Their social environment, of which mother, or the main carer, is the most important element.

This is illustrated in Figure 1.2 below, where I show the overlapping minds of the mother and child, where the child is seen to have innate drives, and the mother has a social-shaping role. And it is the interaction of those two forces that give rise to the baby's 'personality adaptation'; or 'ego'; or 'self'; or personality and character.

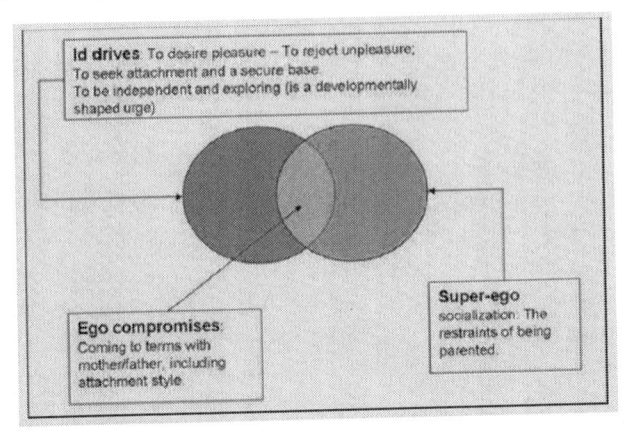

Id drives: To desire pleasure – To reject unpleasure; To seek attachment and a secure base. To be independent and exploring (is a developmentally shaped urge)

Super-ego socialization: The restraints of being parented.

Ego compromises: Coming to terms with mother/father, including attachment style

Figure 1.2: Attachment style complements the innate urges theory

Out of the interaction of the two major overlapping and interacting components, shown in Figure 1.2, a third component is 'grown' – the mind/self of the baby. (This is in line with the interpersonal neurobiology theory. See Daniel Siegel, 2015).

This is how I modelled that conceptualization, back in 2009:

4. Baby's Good Wolf side. (Potential)

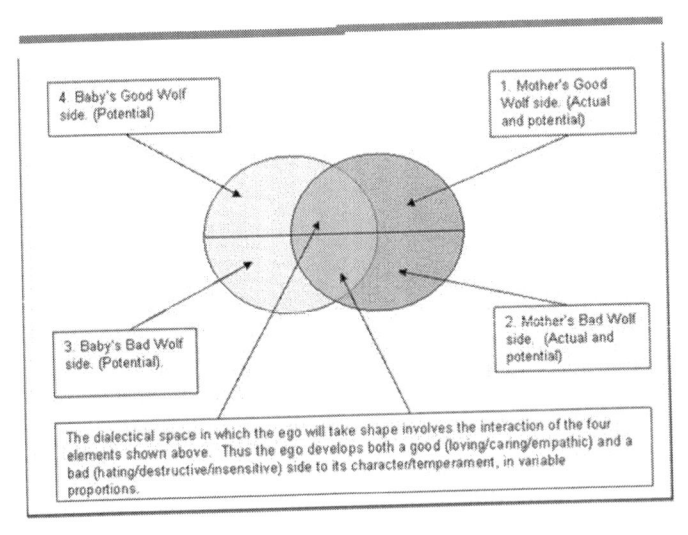

1. Mother's Good Wolf side. (Actual and potential)

3. Baby's Bad Wolf side. (Potential).

2. Mother's Bad Wolf side. (Actual and potential)

The dialectical space in which the ego will take shape involves the interaction of the four elements shown above. Thus the ego develops both a good (loving/caring/empathic) and a bad (hating/destructive/insensitive) side to its character/temperament, in variable proportions.

Figure 1.3 – Modelling the good and bad wolf states

For us in E-CENT, attachment is not just about security and comfort, but also about *desire* and *a will to power*. And as shown in Byrne (2010)[52], both the mother and the child have a good and bad side to their nature. See Figure 1.3 above. This view, of the baby as having an innate moral sense, is supported by empirical research showing that five month old babies have a preference for prosocial behaviour and an aversion to antisocial behaviour. (Bloom 2013)[53].

In E-CENT theory, we argue that each human has, innately, a good and bad side to their nature (or to their 'heart').

These "*good* and *bad wolf* states" – to borrow a concept from the Native American Cherokee people - are inherent in human nature, and in human culture, and the proportions are variable in each individual over time, and from situation to situation. The way they shape up depends a lot on the skill of the parents, and the nature of the wider social environment – and good and bad luck, in terms of peer group encounters, and so on.

When we encounter clients who have not had a good training in moral behaviour, and this is impacting their capacity to live a happy life, we teach our clients the importance of living from the Golden Rule – of never treating anybody any less well than we would desire them to treat us, if our roles were reversed.

~~~

According to Bowlby's (1988) book of lectures, republished in 2005[54], "...attachment theory (is) widely regarded as probably the best supported theory of socio-emotional development yet available (Rajecki, Lamb, and Obmascher, 1978; Rutter, 1980; Parkes and Stevenson-Hind, 1982; Sroufe, 1986)". (Page 31).

Therefore, in E-CENT, I think it is hugely important that counsellors and psycho-therapists should learn to apply Attachment theory insights to their therapeutic work, as one (fundamental) dimension of their understanding of the client's emotional wiring.

For this purpose, counsellors need to attend to any problems that exist with their own attachment style; and also learn how to be a 'secure base' for the client. (See Wallin, 2007).

1.17 Brief summary of the E-CENT models

In chapter 8, I have tried to illustrate the nature of an individual counselling session, using E-CENT theory, models and processes - in so far as that is possible.

In order to facilitate that outline, I used the standard four-part, Jungian session structure, of: Confession; Elucidation; Education and Transformation.

In practice, however, no two E-CENT counselling sessions are ever likely to be the same – since the agenda is set by where the client is 'at' on that occasion, in terms of their perfinking (perceiving, feeling and thinking); their personal history and life circumstances; and how this affects their agenda for the session.

And each session is affected and shaped by the way in which the counsellor manages to respond, non-consciously, spontaneously; and taking into account the unique shape of the client; and the unique flavour of their communication, 'in the present moment'.

In the process I clarified the status and role of some of the most important models used in E-CENT counselling, including:

The Holistic SOR Model, which is shown on the next page.

1. **The holistic SOR model.** This model helps us to focus upon the fact that the client is a socialized-body-mind in an environment (which is physical and social), and that there are *many factors* that go into shaping the client's emotional and behavioural experiences, apart from their beliefs and thoughts. (Our exploration of those many factors is supported by effective, systematic questioning strategies – quite unlike the so-called 'Socratic Questioning' which is used in REBT/CBT – as well as the teaching of mind-body health promotion strategies). See Figure 1.4 on the next page.

2. **The Six Windows Model**, which allows us to educate the client regarding various *alternative ways* of viewing their current problems – which allows them to reframe their experience and to generate reduced levels of emotional arousal, and better forms of behavioural response.

The Six Windows Model is derived from a fusion of some of the most important principles of moderate Buddhism and moderate Stoicism. For examples, the first two windows are as follows:

1. Life is difficult for all human being, at least some of the time, and often much of the time; so why must it not be difficult for me right now?

2. Life often proves to be significantly less difficult is we stick to picking and choosing modestly, moderately, realistically. (Many upsets are caused by 'choosing' to have the option which is **not** available!)

And, in this windows mode, there are four further windows – or frames – or lenses – or ways of looking at problems - which can be explored in Chapter 6, below.

The key process involved in the use of the Six Windows is about helping the client to *re-frame their problematical situations and experiences*, so that those problems 'show up' in a better light, and become more manageable and tolerable over time. But it is not just about re-framing. It also involves what Daniel Siegel (2015) calls "naming it to tame it".

Feelings arising on the right side of the brain can be named and understood by the left side of the brain. Or as Dr James Pennebaker writes: "When we translate an experience into language we essentially make the experience graspable." And in so doing, we can free ourselves mentally from being tangled in old "undigested traumas"[55].

The Holistic Stimulus-Organism-Response Model (H-SOR)		
Column 1	Column 2	Column 3
S = Stimulus	O = Organism	R = Response
When something significant happens, which is apprehended by the organism's (or person's) nervous system, the organism is activated or aroused (positively or negatively)	The organism responds, well or badly. The incoming stimulus may activate or interact with: (1) Innate needs and tendencies; (2) Family history and attachment style; (3) Recent personal history; (4) Emotive-cognitive schemas (as guides to action); (5) Narratives, stories, frames and other storied elements (which may be hyper-activating, hypo-activating, or affect regulating); (6) Character and temperament; (7) Need satisfaction; goals and values; (8) Diet and supplementation, medication, exercise regime, sleep and relaxation histories; (9) Ongoing environmental stressors, state of current relationship(s), and satisfaction with life stages, etc., etc.	The organism outputs a response, in the form of visible behaviour and inferable emotional reactions, like anger, anxiety, depression, embarrassment, etc.

Figure 1.4: The elements of the SOR model

This process – of naming and taming - is what Bucci (1993)[56] calls 'referential activity' in which the person (or counselling client) "…is involved in making links and connections between the non-verbal/affective and the verbal/symbolic domains of experience". (McLeod, 1997/2006. Page 65).

The Six Windows Model is supported by various other models, which will be explored more fully in Chapter 8. See figure 1.5 below for a quick overview.

These other models include:

(1) *The E-CENT-created EFR model* (which looks at the sequence of:

    E = an **Event**; and how it is

    F = **Framed**, or viewed through an interpreting lens; and how that framing shapes the

    R = emotional **Response**).

~~~

But here, first of all, is the promised overview of the six windows model:

Window No.1: Life is difficult and frustrating, and involves some suffering	Window No.2: Life is much less difficult if you avoid picking and choosing unrealistically.
for all human beings much of the time (regardless of wealth, fame, gender, race, age, etc).	(Choosing what does not exist causes most difficulties in life!)
Window No.3: Life is BOTH difficult and non-difficult (so remember to include	Window No.4: Life could always be more difficult than it is (so stop exaggerating it!)
the non-difficult bits in your picture of your life!)	Don't make the mistake of thinking it's 100% bad when it's actually 10% bad!
Window No.5: There are certain things about life that we can control,	Window No.6: If life was a school, what positive lesson could you learn
and certain things we cannot control. (Accept the things you cannot change, and change the rest).	from your present negative experiences of frustration, difficulties and suffering?

Fig 1.5: The full Six Windows Model

In applying the Six Windows model with a counselling client, the E-CENT counsellor helps the client to form a clear image of their problem, which is visual. The client is then asked, "On a scale of 1-10, where 10 is as bad as could be; just how bad is this problem in your estimation?"

Once that Subjective Unit of Disturbance (SUDs rating) is known, the client is then asked to look at the same image through Window No.1, and asked to assume that the slogan around Window No.1 is a true statement.

Then the client is asked: "Looking at the image of your current problem, through Window No.1, does that re-framing help you to reduce the SUDs rating?"

(Normally *it comes down a little* for each window through which the client looks! And those little reductions in disturbance add up over the six windows!)

~~~

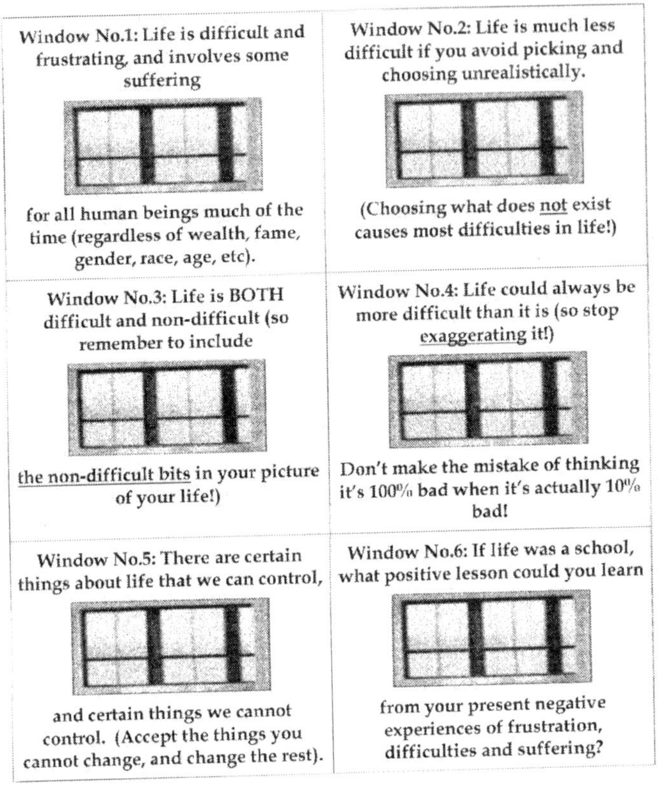

Some other models that we use include:

(2) **The APET model** from the Human Givens school (which deals with an

> 'A' (Activating event, or stimulus); which is subject to a habit-based
>
> 'P' (Pattern-matching process in the mind of the perceiver); which leads to an
>
> 'E' (Emotional response); and then to
>
> 'T' (Thoughts, about the feelings or the situation).

Plus

(3) **The Parent-Adult-Child** (or PAC) model and other models (such as *the OK Corral model*) from Transactional Analysis [TA].

In addition, we use about another dozen or more explicit models to guide our work with clients.

In this brief foretaste of the E-CENT models, let us introduce one more:

(4) **The Jigsaw-story model**, which helps us to keep track of the stories told to us by our clients, so we can spot patterns, gaps, tensions, contradictions, and so on; which we can use to help the client to revise and update their stories, and to integrate them; and to get a better life from living within a more accurate set of narratives of their life.

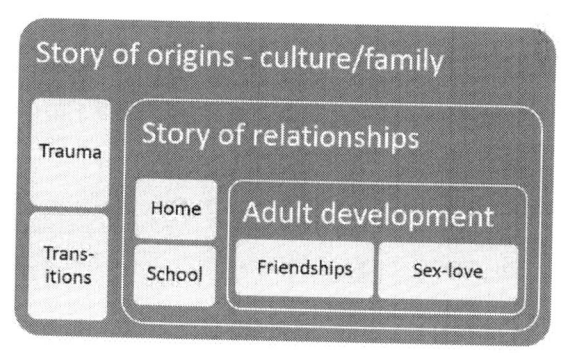

Figure 1.6: The Jigsaw-story model

The Jigsaw-story model is really a set of place-holders for potential stories to emerge in therapy.

It is based on the therapist's litany of possible stories. For examples: the story of origins; the story of childhood; the story of relationships; the story of early trauma; the story of transitions (school, puberty, college, work, marriage, having children, and so on); and/or the story of personal failure, or stuckness, or lost-ness; and so on.

The emergence of this model was necessitated by two factors:

(a) The insight from Bandler and Grinder (1975)[57] that counselling clients have their life experiences, and then – non-consciously and unwittingly - engage in *deletions*, *distortions* and *generalizations*, resulting in a 'just-so' story which they tell to their counsellor. The counsellor has to try to help the client to correct those stories. (In other words, the counsellor looks for contradictions between stories, and points those tensions out to the client, who is invited to rethink their story. The counsellor might feel that a particular story sounds highly selective, brief and patchy. 'What are the missing pieces here?' might be the obvious question.

'Did anything good happen?' is a powerful question in the context of an overgeneralized, bleak and despairing narrative.)

And:

(b) While Piaget believed that our various stories (or schemas [or schemes]) - which are in conflict with each other – will tend *to 'equilibrate' over time* (which means that he expected that the stories, or packets of information, that we have stored in long-term memory, would tend to *correct each other*, and come into line with each other) - this idea has been rejected by Lunzer (1989)[58]; and I agree with Lunzer. For example: I have noticed that a client will tell me one story about their key relationship in the first half of a counselling session, and another story in the second half, and not notice that those two stories are in contradiction, or at least in serious tension with each other. This discovery links back, I believe, to the concept of 'sub-personalities', and ego states, whereby a person may believe one thing whilst in one ego state or sub-personality, and something altogether different when in another of their ego states or sub-personalities. (Drawing the client's attention to their ego state shifts can be very helpful, in facilitating '*conscious* equilibration of schemas').

The Jigsaw-story model is a reminder and a challenge to the counsellor or therapist to watch out for the flaws and faults in the client's stories, and to help the client to come up with a new, more integrated story. As McLeod (1997/2006) writes, describing the theory of Omer and Strenger (1992)[59]:

"… the theory of therapy espoused by a therapist acts as a kind of general or overarching story through which the client learns to frame his or her life narrative. Every reflection or interpretation made by a therapist acts as a vehicle for the therapist to communicate, bit by bit, a story of what life is about". (Page 22).

I sincerely believed that I had invented the idea of creating a jigsaw of stories, using our Jigsaw-story model. Much later, I was surprised to find a very similar idea in McLeod (1997/2006) where he writes about how firefighters, at the end of a call out to a fire, have to talk among themselves in order to come up with a composite story of what happened during their call-out. This is necessary because each individual may have noticed different aspects of the event, sometimes because they were in different parts of the building; but also because of their different mental maps based on past experience; and so on. McLeod quotes Docherty (1989)[60] to the effect that this process is called, by the firefighters, 'jigsawing'.

I do this kind of jigsawing with my clients to make sense of their various stories; or to integrate fragments of a single story; or to clarify my own understanding of the client's life, which I then feed back to them.

~~~

A broad range of other models is available in E-CENT counselling, which can be used to support the work done with the Six Windows model, and those other models mentioned in sections 1-4 above. (See Chapter 8 for more).

~~~

Postscript: On the body-brain-mind-environment complexity

But please bear in mind that the client is a complex body-brain-mind-environment-whole: and therefore the following factors are as important as the client's story: Diet, exercise, and sleep patterns; home living conditions, relationships in the present, and relationships in the past; the original relationship with mother/father; current age, and stage of development; life stressors, including those related to socioeconomic circumstances; coping mechanisms and capacities; and so on.

~~~

It might seem that the models briefly introduced above mainly deal with what Hill (2015) calls "the secondary system of affect regulation" – which is, *the use of left brain to left brain, language-based communication from counsellor to client*. But in fact, we cannot ever stop communicating right brain to right brain, which involves the use of implicit, non-conscious, nonverbal communication. This goes on outside of our conscious awareness and control, no matter who we are, and no matter how long we practice counselling and psychotherapy. The reason a good counsellor is more effective than other individuals in the life of the client – at helping the client to change at deep, emotional levels – is that the good counsellor has worked on their own therapy, and their own attachment style, so that they are able to be available as 'good enough substitute parents' for the client, and help the client to achieve 'earned security' – which they can then transfer into their daily lives outside of therapy.

We do not need to develop special systems of right brain to right brain communication. Humans cannot help but communicate right brain to right brain (through nonverbal communication [including body language and facial expressions]). And the healthy counsellor cannot help but change the way the client experiences the world, given enough time, thus rewiring (or helping to rewire) that part of the client's orbitofrontal cortex (OFC) which is, and was, the source of *over-arousal* or *under-arousal* of their automatic emotional affects; and which, after effective therapy, *will* **automatically** *keep their emotional responses well-regulated at appropriate levels of arousal*.

However, the less enamoured we are of 'cognitive approaches', the more we are able to just 'be' in our encounter with our clients; to just be *human beings* in a caring encounter!

But, of course, it is important to be able to think critically – or to *perfink* (perceive, feel and think) with **Adult ego state** in the *Executive position* of our personality; supported by **Nurturing Parent ego state**. And a bit of **Playful Child** can lighten the mood of the most difficult counselling session.

There are times for dealing with the 'thinking' component of the client's 'perfinking' – or perceiving, feeling and thinking – and times to deal with the 'feeling' component of their *perfinking*. We learn how to make those judgements, of which modality to use, through practice and experience. But the main guideline may be this: The mother's relationship with her child begins in a mainly non-verbal modality. It's all smiles, and coos, and handling and helping and comforting. In a later stage of development, the mother uses more languaging, guidance, and advice. But even so, when necessary, she can always swap back to mainly being in a caring, accepting, understanding modality. A *similar strategy* may be the best a counsellor ever gets to 'knowing' how to respond to any particular client.

But finally, we should note that, in E-CENT counselling, we are not just interested in the so-called 'thinking' side of the client; or the so-called 'feeling' side of the client. We are also interested in these questions:

> *How well do you sleep? How many hours per night do you sleep?*
>
> *Do you get up in time to have a slow and gentle start to the day, or do you begin late, with time deadlines, which push up your stress level?*
>
> *What do you have for breakfast, and is it the healthiest option possible/ (It is never a good idea to skip breakfast!)*
>
> *How well do you manage your time and your stress, in your daily working life?*
>
> *How good are your relationships with your significant others? At home and in work?*
>
> *How much physical exercise do you do, and how many days per week do you do it?*
>
> *How much water do you drink during the day?*
>
> *What do you eat for lunch?*
>
> *What snacks do you have mid-morning and mid-afternoon?*
>
> *How much alcohol do you drink?*
>
> *Do you consume any of these toxic foods: sugar; alcohol; caffeine; gluten; trans-fats (or hydrogenated fat, in junk foods); and highly-processed foods (with added sugar, salt, trans-fats, colours, flavours, and other denatured components)?*

> *Tell me about your childhood? Was it broadly happy? Or not? Are you secure or insecure in your relationships?*
>
> *What is the problem that brought you here today? And how does it relate to the questions I have asked above?*

~~~

In Chapter 8, I will try to illustrate a typical E-CENT counselling session, which will not be easy, because each session is unique. But there are some ways in which I can suggest some of the kinds of things that might come up in an 'averaged' session.

~~~

Or how to integrate nutritional insights, exercise and sleep coaching into talk therapy

Chapter 2: Key elements of the emotive-cognitive counselling approach

2.1: Overview

Chapter 1 set the scene for this brief chapter, which begins with a summation of a few key features of the Emotive-Cognitive Embodied Narrative Therapy (E-CENT) approach.

This is then followed by:

(1) A basic description of E-CENT counselling and its origins;

(2) The importance of emotions;

(3) E-CENT models of the social individual; and his/her emergence from the interactions of a physical baby and a cultural mother; plus:

(4) Typical client problems and counselling tasks.

E-CENT theory sees humans as essentially ***physical-emotional story tellers*** - to ourselves and others - and storytellers who live in a concrete world of narratives and scripts; which include reasonable and unreasonable elements; logical and illogical elements; and defensible and indefensible elements.

These stories are not primarily made up by us, ***individual humans***, though we do embellish them, and produce our own variants of them. But, in essence, these are ***social stories*** – stories from our parents, our families, our school and our communities and nations (e.g. via mass media channels).

These are the stories that constitute our *social identity*, and locate us in a historical web of relationships linked to the past. And these are the stories we inevitably use to *interpret* our actual, social experiences of our ***very real*** lives in the present moment!

One of the basic functions of the central nervous system and perceptual apparatus of a human being (or any mammal) is to help us to ***classify*** and ***evaluate*** our environmental stimuli (or experiences) into those that we experience as 'good' (pleasurable) and those we experience as 'bad' (or un-pleasurable).

Humans most often tend to push away (or repress out of conscious awareness) their unpleasant experiences; to refuse or fail to process them; and to then become the (non-conscious) victims of those repressed, denied and undigested experiences. We do this - 'pushing away' (or rejecting), and repressing (out of conscious awareness) of our unpleasant experiences - because we are wired up by nature to seek pleasure and to avoid pain (or un-pleasure.) But the solution to most of our problems, paradoxically, resides in our courageous willingness to face the pain of unpleasant experiences (which we ***cannot*** avoid); to reframe them; to feel them; and to fully digest them. Only then can they disappear. You cannot, as Albert Ellis foolishly believed, "forget the god-awful past". You cannot forget it because it is *hardwired* into your neurology, and your physiology/ musculature. And it manifests in your *daily habits* today. To get rid of it, you have to digest it; complete it, and then file it away.

And there are no therapists who can "extract" your pain! And no medications that can permanently dissolve your pain (as opposed to *hiding it* for a while!) *Unavoidable Pain* has to be faced and processed. Those individuals who attempt to run away from unavoidable pain by taking recreational or prescription drugs, alcohol, painkillers, etc., end up having to face the same old pain when their escapist strategies eventually prove to be not just useless, but self-harming!

And you have to face your unavoidable pain with a *moderate* degree of Stoic *endurance* (or willingness to suffer the unavoidable pain of life); a sensible degree of scientific enquiry into the *possibility of changing things* instead of endlessly enduring them; and *acceptance* of the need to *digest* whatever cannot be eliminated by controlling yourself or your environment.

Our emotive-cognitive (E-CENT) theory also sees adult relationships as being the acting out, in the present moment, of childhood experiences of relationship with parents and siblings, because some part of those earlier relationships have not been properly digested and completed. In other words, we internalize 'models' of how our parents related to us, and we take them to school. We modify some of our internal models of relationship in school and take them into the wider world. It may be that our *childhood script*, or *life-story*, is updated around puberty, to expand into a vision of our autonomous, adult future, coloured by the experiences of childhood. (See McAdams' view, on page 63 of McLeod, 1997/2006).

And we always relate to others in the present moment on the basis of those old models, (or *Working Models*), or templates, of "how *they* (e.g. parent figures and others) related to me; and how I *must* respond (to them)". (Byrne, 2009b). This, of course, all goes on at *non-conscious* levels of mind, while the conscious mind deludes itself – (like a kid with a plastic steering wheel, on the top deck of a bus, deludes himself into believing that he is steering the bus) – into thinking that it, the conscious 'me', is *choosing* relationships and *deciding* how to act within them.

Furthermore, there are significant disruptions that can occur at various stages in the early childhood experience of the individual which can produce specific forms of relationship dysfunction in later life. Most of these have to do with disruption of attachment relationships, which render the individual 'insecure' in future attachment relationships. (The lucky 'few' [which might actually be 50 – 60% of us!] end up with 'secure attachment styles' of relating to parents, and later to significant others, like lovers, spouses, etc. About 20+% acquire the *Avoidant Attachment Style*, and another 20+% acquire the *Anxious-Ambivalent [clinging] Attachment Style*).

And, because we are body-minds, and not floating heads, the state of our bodies affects our emotions and thoughts, and thereby our actions in the world. At the most basic level, we are either in a physically relaxed mode (with the parasympathetic nervous system activated) resulting in a feeling of emotional wellbeing; or we are in a physically tense mode (with the sympathetic nervous system activated) resulting in a feeling of anxious or angry over-arousal and a general state of unhappiness and dissatisfaction. This we normally call 'stress', or distress.

If we live like couch potatoes who eat junk food and subject our nervous systems to information overload; and/or struggle with economic insecurity and poor housing conditions; and/ or aim too high and are never satisfied with our material possessions; and/ or surround ourselves with relationship conflict, in a chaotic world; then we cannot hope to function well emotionally and mentally.

2.2: Basic description and origins

Emotive-Cognitive Embodied-Narrative Therapy (E-CENT) is a system of counselling and psychotherapy which integrates:

(1) A reformed and expanded version of the Stimulus-Organism-Response (Holistic-SOR) model (adapted from neobehaviourism and Behaviour Therapy);

(2) Freud's model of the 'it' (or body-brain-mind), the 'ego' (or socialized personality) and the 'superego' (or internalized conscience of significant others, like mother/father, etc.);

(3) Some elements of the mother-child relationship from Object Relations theory (Klein, Fairbairn, Guntrip);

(4) The Parent-Adult-Child (PAC) model from Transactional Analysis (TA);

(5) The concepts of the 'secure base', and 'attachment style', from Attachment theory; and the need for re-parenting of the insecure client;

(6) Some elements of moderate Zen Buddhist and moderate Stoic philosophy;

(7) Moral philosophy (especially the Golden Rule) and the importance of *egalitarian* relationships (especially in marriage):

(8) Plus several other elements of emotive, cognitive, narrative and psychodynamic therapies.

(And all of this is combined with an awareness of the importance of keeping the body-mind healthy through diet, exercise, sleep, self-talk - or inner dialogue - plus emotional self-management, and development of a capacity to conduct happy relationships).

The E-CENT counselling theory is **not** an eclectic system which has bolted elements of different counselling systems together. It is a *truly integrative system* which began by revisiting the basic model of the human personality developed by Sigmund Freud and asking: *How does this model link up with the ABC model used in REBT/CBT? What are the necessary implications of assuming that there is substantial truth in both models?* (When the **ABC model** outlived its usefulness to us, and became a liability, we replaced it with the Stimulus-Organism-Response (SOR) model, in which the organism is seen to be affected by a whole range of factors, like diet, exercise, self-talk, relaxation, meditation, hydration, sleep, relationships, personal history, and so on).

The same process was conducted with the **Parent-Adult-Child (PAC)** *model* from Transactional Analysis and aspects of cognitive science (for example: Hofstadter, 2007)[61]. The resulting *synthesis* (or synthetic model) was then compared with the implications of the British 'Object Relations' tradition. Moral philosophy and Zen Buddhism were also interrogated in this process of model building.

Before that system of integration of models was begun, I had studied thirteen different systems of counselling and therapy, including: Freud and Jung, Rogers and Perls, Behaviour Therapy theory and practice, Cognitive Therapy and REBT, Reality Therapy and Transactional Analysis, Existential Therapy and Logotherapy, Multimodal Therapy and Cognitive-Humanistic Therapy; and also committed myself to the proposition that all systems of counselling and therapy that are designed to be therapeutic are *broadly equivalent* in terms of the outcomes achieved, as argued by Wampold (2001)[62], and Messer and Wampold (2000)[63].

E-CENT theory and practice evolved in phases. 1968 to 1998 was a kind of incubation of some core ideas. 1999 to 2007 saw an intensification of thinking and learning about the core elements. Then, in the period 2007 to 2010 – after the death of Dr Albert Ellis, and my own 'post-mortem', designed to find out how REBT could have produced the mess that was the final three years of Ellis's life – I wrote the first version of this book. Over several years then - of developing and applying the emerging E-CENT model - a basic theory of human personality and psychological disturbance emerged. And I have continued to refine E-CENT with each passing year.

2.3: Basic theory of E-CENT

The basic theory of E-CENT begins with the relationship between the archetypal *new baby* and its *mother*. This is (for the baby) a *feeling* relationship. And the baby stores, in permanent memory, beyond conscious awareness, every emotionally significant event in that most fundamental relationship. This relationship between mother and baby gives rise (in the baby's body-mind) to emotionally-coloured expectations, attitudes, and ways of seeing itself and the world, which shape the later life of the child. The 'sea' in which the child swims is 'the sea of emotionally significant *experience* (which later includes *language*)' and the common currency of that language is the 'story'. (Of course, those stories are about 'something' – real, concrete – and not just sounds in the air. And one of those concrete forces that is reflected in our social stories is the question of power; physical power – the power to hurt or be hurt physically; and emotion power – the power to love or hate another, and to be loved or hated by another.

We grow up imbibing stories about 'the nature of reality' from our mothers, fathers, siblings, peers, family relatives, teachers, and so on. In most of the stage directions, we will tend to find lines for ourselves which put us in 'bit parts'; 'supporting cast'; or 'timid crowd-scene member'.

However, some of us, and perhaps most of us (at least some of the time), will find ourselves justifying the playing of **bullying roles** in some of our stories.

The key conception of the human individual which is held by E-CENT counsellors suggests that each of us is:

>(a) primarily a social body-mind;
>
>(b) which has innate potential to develop good and bad tendencies, and:
>
>(c) which accumulates interpretative, emotionally-significant experiences – in the form of schemas, scripts, stories and frames (or 'ways of seeing the world') and other narrativized and non-narrativized forms – which are stored in non-conscious, electro-chemical representations; and:
>
>(d) which manifest in Parent, Adult and Child forms of thinking/ feeling/ behaving (or perfinking/acting). And furthermore:
>
>(e) The 'emergent I' in each individual has internalized *'Working Models'* (or 'templates') of relationship (from their social encounters in their family of origin), which include *Attachment Styles* and *Personality Adaptations*, which dictate the patterns and limitations of relationships to which they will gravitate and be attracted in their adult lives.

~~~

Another way of saying this is that:

The social/emotional intelligence of the socialized individual is determined by their experience in their family of origin, and this sets the upper and lower limits of their ability to relate to others – all other things being equal.

Of course, it is possible to meet new 'curative' individuals, such as good friends, lovers, or counsellors, or others, who can begin to help the individual to reform and reshape their Internal Working Models of relationship, and to raise their social/emotional intelligence – but this involves hard work, and it is by no means guaranteed to happen!

2.4: The importance of emotion

In E-CENT counselling, I deal with the client's emotions. I offer them a 'safe harbour', and a 'secure base' from which to explore their life.

I look at the connection between their lifestyle and their feelings; their relationships and their moods; their thinking and their emotions; their physical state (in terms of diet, exercise, sleep, etc.); their experiences and their emotions; their meanings and their emotions; the links between emotions, goals and behaviours; and the emotional stories within which they live their lives.

I encourage them to change their self-talk; their habitual behaviours; to work on their bodily health (through diet and exercise; relaxation, sleep and meditation; vitamin and mineral supplementation); and to work on *the story of their lives*.

I try to provide the best possible analysis of the *potential reasons*, in the basement of their minds, for their current dysfunctional thoughts-feelings-behaviours. But I do not offer 'definitive analyses' characteristic of the Freudian approach.

I provide each client with 'a secure base', to re-grow or re-train their attachment style, from *insecure* to *secure*.

I work on their emotional intelligence by helping them to understand their own emotions, the emotions of those with whom they normally relate, and how to communicate their emotions to others.

And when I think diet may be a feature of their emotional problem, I refer them to information packs on some educational approaches to diet and nutrition. One of those was compiled by Renata Taylor-Byrne, my wife, who has a diploma in nutrition, and who has done a lot of research on this subject. (Please see Taylor-Byrne and Byrne, 2017, in the References list). I also have a lot of experience of managing my own diet, in order to control Candida Albicans, which is widely known to cause feelings of anxiety and depression. So this is not 'medical counselling' so much as it is *coaching in wellbeing!* And I always advise my clients to see a nutritional therapist before they make any significant changes to their diets. I also teach the importance of adequate sleep; and regular physical exercise.

~~~

2.5: Brief introduction to the E-CENT models of mind

From ancient Greece to modern Europe and America, philosophers and psychologists have struggled to understand the human mind. In the process they have developed many interesting models of the mind, to help us with our self-understanding.

After almost fifteen years of studying, exploring and developing models of the human mind (between 2001 and 2015), I concluded that tripartite (or three-part) models – like Freud's *'It'*, *'Ego' and 'Super-ego'* model, which we have adapted as shown here - have more *explanatory power* than 'binary (two-part) models'; and that both are preferable to the 'black box' model of behaviourism (and behaviour therapy).

Of course, the human brain-mind is the most complex entity in the known universe, and therefore any attempt to sum it up - to 'simplify it' - is fraught with difficulty and danger. However, in the interest of making the *management of mind* accessible to counselling clients, I have to take some risks in summing up what I have learned about the human brain-mind.

The most important and interesting (if incomplete) models seem to have come from the following sources:

1. Plato: Plato produced a model of the psyche (or soul, or mind) which had three parts: **The charioteer** (or *reason*) and **the two horses** which pull the chariot. The chariot represents the life of a person, and the two horses represent the *will* and *passion* which animate that person. When these elements of the individual mind are in unstable balance, problems emerge. If the *will* and *passion* are united against the *reasoning* of the *charioteer*, then the chariot runs out of control. Plato's solution was to advocate getting your *will* to support your *reason* against your *passions*. This model is contradicted by affective neuroscience, (Panksepp, 1998), which suggests that the charioteer is actually a set of innate emotional control systems, which are, of course, socialized by the family of origins. Reason (or cognition) depends upon emotion. And the will is a function of the socialized ego.

2. Sigmund Freud: One of Freud's main models has three parts to the psyche, or mind: **The 'it'** (or physical-emotional baby/person), **the 'superego'** (or internalized mother/other, as a social-regulator [the 'over-I']); and **the 'ego'** (or self-concept; self-identity; virtual self, or personality). We made good use of this model, in developing E-CENT theory, in a form which never occurred to Freud, because he overlooked the importance of the **bond** between mother and baby. And, although he had the concept of the super-ego, or over-I, he did not see how it *interacted* with the 'it' to promote the emergence of the ego.

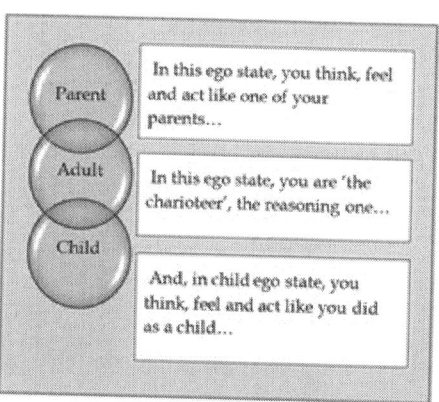

In this ego state, you think, feel and act like one of your parents...

In this ego state, you are 'the charioteer', the reasoning one...

And, in child ego state, you think, feel and act like you did as a child...

3. Eric Berne. Berne posited the existence of three states of the person's 'ego', or self-functioning: (The **'Parent'** ego state; the **'Adult'** ego state; and the **'Child'** ego state).

These are shown in the E-CENT model as emergent forms of the socialized ego. (See Figure 2.3, later in this chapter, for an illustration of how the PAC fits into the relationships between the mother and baby, as internalized).

The illustration above is a brief representation of the Parent-Adult-Child model developed by Berne and his associates.

And then there is:

4. Neo-behaviourism: The neo-Behaviourists (e.g. Tolman and Hull) rejected the black box view of the 'mind' of their research animals, which had been created by Pavlov, Watson and Skinner, and insisted that *goals* and *thoughts* were essential parts of animal behaviour. They overlooked the importance of *emotion*, or *affect*, however; and this omission was a central and enduring feature of the *entire* cognitive revolution. (Emotion was only ever given *a brief chapter* – and afterthought - at the end of textbooks on cognitive psychology).

But neo-behaviourism gave us the Stimulus-Organism-Response model, which we have modified in E-CENT, to include emotion, diet, exercise, and many other features apart from thoughts and goals.

This is how the S-O-R model works: A living organism (O) is conceptualized as being sandwiched between incoming stimuli (or signals) – which are appraised as good or bad - and outgoing emotional and behavioural responses. This model is central to the E-CENT approach, as mentioned above. But as we will show later, there are lots of determinants of the state of the Organism, and therefore lots of causes of emotional and behavioural responses – and not just thoughts and beliefs, which is asserted by REBT/CBT. The cognitive and rational therapy theorists (like Ellis and Beck) make the mistake of assuming that 'thoughts cause feelings'. Then, along comes the 'emotional revolution' (of Schore, Panksepp, Siegel and others) which assumes that emotions (or affects) are both regulated and regulating. To simplify this model, we would say that it's our feelings about situations that regulate our feelings about those situations. But this is to miss a crucial point: People perceive-feel-think in response to incoming stimuli. Our attention (A) is captured by an incoming stimulus (S). We respond to that stimulus from memory (M), which sets in train a process of Perfinking (or perceiving-feeling-thinking). And our perfinking capacities are both regulated and regulating. And we cannot separate out our 'thinking' from our 'feeling'. Typically, when we **perfink** that we are 'thinking', we are overlooking the *unavoidable fact* that we cannot 'think' *without the **feelings** which allow us to **evaluate** the objects of our **perfinking**!* (Damasio, 1994, on the case study of Eliot).

5. Other models: Some years after I developed the E-CENT tripartite model - (in which the mother and baby's minds overlap or interpenetrate each other, and give rise to an emergent ego or personality of the baby, as shown in Figure 1.2 in Chapter 1) - interpersonal neurobiology (IPNB) was announced by Dr Daniel Siegel, and I agree with his basic model of (1) the brain (of the baby) and (2) relationships (mainly with mother, initially), giving rise to (3) the mind of the individual child.

(However, the Hindu/Buddhist binary model – of *the Elephant and Rider* – is also helpful, up to a point. [It seems *the Elephant and Rider* model was first mentioned by Lord Krishna in the *Maharabhata*]. And Freud's other model, [the binary distinction between the Life urge {Eros} and the Death urge {Thanatos}] also needs to be taken into account]. These models are helpful in those situations where the client mainly seems to be split into two 'warring factions': one of which wants to be expansive or exploratory, and one of which wants to be cautious and withdrawn, for examples. We can related to those two elements as either the conscious Rider and the non-conscious Horse; place them on two chairs, and use Gestalt chair work to help the client to resolve the 'split'. [And those two elements could just as easily be labelled as the Life urge {expansive} and the Death urge {shrinking/ withdrawing}]).

From the main elements of the tripartite models of Plato, Freud and Eric Berne, I infer the following two conclusions:

Conclusion 1. That the most basic E-CENT model of the dialectical interaction of the mother and baby is the best way to conceptualize the origin of the child's 'personality' or 'self':

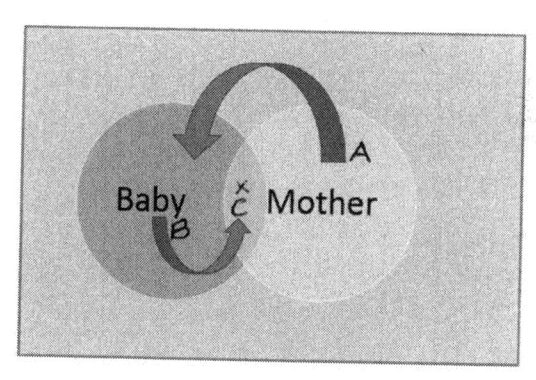

Figure 2.1: Interpenetrating minds of the mother-baby dyad

The three elements here are: (A) The mother's emotionally significant behaviour in relation to (B) her baby (and the baby's needs and desires), results in (C) a stored experience (in the overlapping space of their interpenetrating minds).

And these stored experiences build up over time into a sense of 'me' and 'you', and how I feel about 'me' and 'you' – and on into full-blown *personal identity*.

This is the best way to understand the *social nature* of the child (and later adult).

Figure 2.2, below, is how I presented this model originally (in Byrne, 2009a)[64] and in Byrne (2009b)[65]:

The ego is a product of relationship, and cannot exist without (external and/ or internalized) relationship.

The normal, 'good enough' mother has no real choice but to 'colonize' her new born baby, as it is totally helpless. She must 'march in', take over, and run the baby's life for 'it', otherwise (unless it is colonized by a mother substitute) it will surely die. The neonate, or baby, is also most likely wired up by evolutionary forces to 'seek' a connection with what must seem (physically and emotionally) to be 'another part' of itself: thus creating a 'natural symbiosis' which satisfies some innate needs of the baby, and some innate and socially shaped needs of the new mother. (The urge to seek a breast and suckle seems to be innate to all mammals).

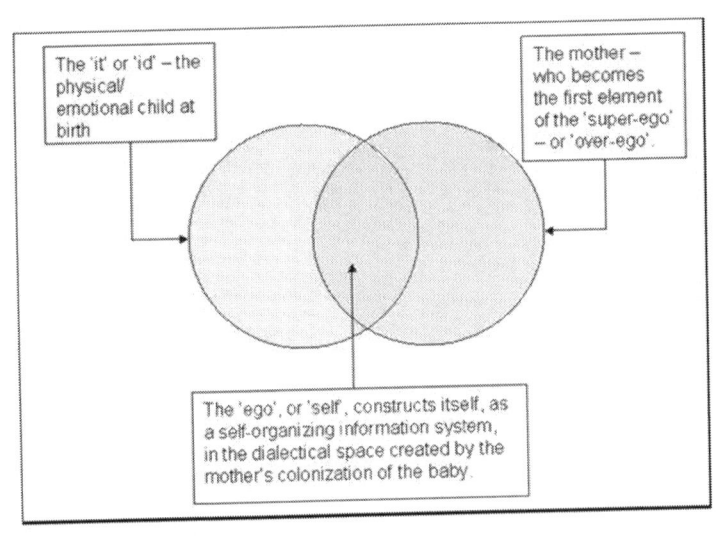

~~~

[Figure: Two overlapping circles. Left circle labelled "The 'it' or 'id' – the physical/ emotional child at birth". Right circle labelled "The mother – who becomes the first element of the 'super-ego' – or 'over-ego'". Overlap labelled "The 'ego', or 'self', constructs itself, as a self-organizing information system, in the dialectical space created by the mother's colonization of the baby."]

Figure 2.2: The most basic model of CENT:

The dialectical nature of the individual/ social ego.

~~~

Conclusion 2: That the best way to understand the socialized structures of the mind is to use another of the models I developed in 2009 (in Byrne 2009b), as shown in Figure 2.3, below. That image shows the mother and baby as overlapping circles; which are then split down the centre into a 'good side' and a 'bad side'. This echoes Freud's model of Eros and Thanatos – but also the Native American Cherokee view that there is a war going on inside each human being. A war between a 'Good Wolf' and a 'Bad Wolf'. The reason every society has a moral code that it teaches to its young is this: Moral behaviour, although innate, is not the *sole* innate tendency. We *also* have an innate tendency to seek self-advantage, and we will often lie and cheat

Or how to integrate nutritional insights, exercise and sleep coaching into talk therapy

and steal to pursue those self-advantages. Unless we are socialized into a strong moral code, wired into our conscience (or super-ego; or Over-I)!

The Ego element of Figure 2.3, below – the PAC in the middle – has ten subdivisions, as follows:

The 4P's are Good Nurturing Parent, Good Controlling Parent, Bad Nurturing Parent (e.g. Smother Mother, or 'Molly-Coddler'), and Bad Controlling Parent.

The 4C's are Good Free Child, Bad (anti-social or immoral) Free Child, Good Adapted/Rebellious Child, and Bad (anti-social or immoral) Adapted/Rebellious Child.

The Adult has just two subdivision: The Good (pro-social, moral) Adult, and the Bad (anti-social or immoral) Adult.

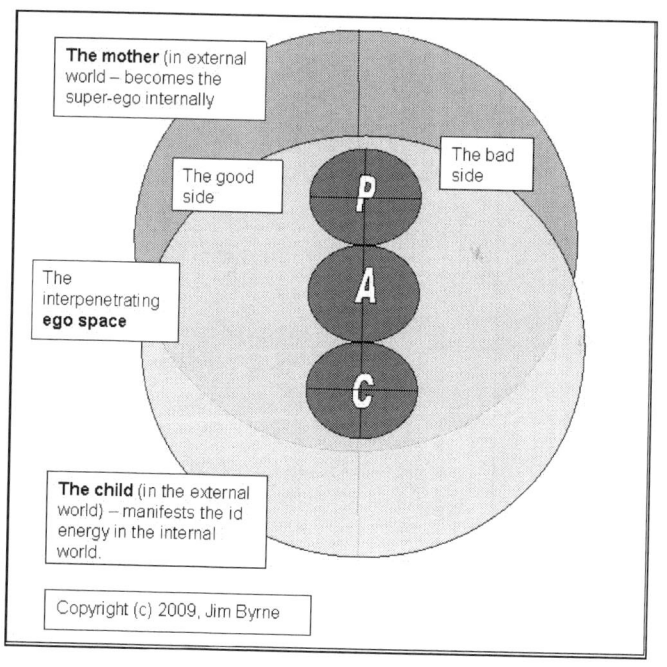

Figure 2.3: How the ten elements of the PAC model - (4 P's, 4 C's, 2 A's) - emerge within the dialectical ego space between the mother and child

The larger circles show that the psychic space, where the mind of the mother and child meet, and overlap, is divided into three elements: Mother; Child; and the Interpenetrating Ego space, or the element of socialized Child that emerges from the socialization process.

Furthermore, those two large overlapping circles have:

(a) A good side and a bad side;

(b) A Parent component; an Adult component; and a Child component. (See Byrne 2009b for a full explanation of this model). This is discussed further in sections 5.7 to 5.9 below.

So the client's ego (or personality) manifests in a range of states, from situation to situation. Sometimes s/he is 'in Child' (e.g. Playful Child, or Hurt Child, or Adapted Child, or Rebellious Child, or Destructive Child, and so on). Sometimes s/he is 'in Parent' ego state (e.g. Nurturing Parent, Controlling Parent, Critical Parent, Rescuing Parent, and so on). And sometimes s/he is in Adult ego state – the Charioteer; the Reasoning Information Processor; the Critical Thinker (with good or bad intentions. [Adult ego state can be used for various purposes. For examples: to plan a party; or to break into the local bank!]).

But in addition to those fluctuating states of the ego, there is also, woven into the overall ego-functioning, a set of Working Models of relationship, which were shaped by how mother related to baby; how father related to baby; and how baby learned to relate to them; and later to others: siblings, relatives, neighbours, school teachers, school peers, and so on. And the main Working Models are a guide to secure relationships, or insecure (avoidant or clinging) relationships. Or, in the worst case scenario, where the individual has been raised by frightening (or frightened) parents, the Working Models of relationship tend to be 'disorganized', and the individual is sometimes secure, sometimes avoidant, sometimes clinging, and sometimes they simply blank out, dissociate, or cease to be able to process what is going on in their relationships. These Working Models can also be reclassified into six Personality Adaptations; some of which produce people who lead with their thinking; others produce people who lead with their feelings; and some simply act without thinking/feeling. (Joines and Stewart, 2002).

2.6: The client's problems and tasks of counselling

The best way to understand the need for counselling and therapy is that, in the majority of cases, the client has most likely got one or more of the following problems.

(There may be some problems which cannot be subsumed under one of the following headings, but not many).

(a) They had a maladaptive relationship to mum and/or dad when they were a baby/infant/child, and this has not yet been fully resolved through subsequent corrective relationships.

(b) The individual's coping resources may be inadequate to cope with the various and very real external pressures bearing down upon them in their daily lives.

(c) They have repressed some significant emotional experiences – like traumas - out of conscious awareness, and they are now driven by those repressed experiences into acting dysfunctionally.

(d) They have poorly developed social/emotional intelligence, which causes them to mismanage their relationships, at home and/or in work.

(e) Their 'appetitive part' (or Child ego state [Berne]) is too powerful relative to the other two parts: which are, the Parent ego state and the Adult ego state. (Result: Too aggressive. Or narcissistic. They are too high on 'Bad Wolf'! [In E-CENT theory, every individual is assumed to have innate tendencies towards virtue and vice – good and evil – which I characterized using the Cherokee concept of 'Two wolves fighting inside']. See the tenth principle of E-CENT theory, in Chapter 3, below).

(f) Their 'Parent ego state' is too punitive in relation to their Child ego state, resulting in excessive and inappropriate guilt, shame and anxiety, and ego weaknesses. (They are too conformist, passive, victim-playing, and long-suffering; fearful, timid and/or paranoid. They lack self-confidence or show low self-esteem).

(g) They have experienced some loss or failure; or threat or danger; or insult or frustration; such that they have over-reacted emotionally, and they need to learn how to respond with a more appropriate emotion. They need 'external affect regulation' assistance from the counsellor, which they will, in time, internalize, so that can better self-regulate their own emotional responses. (Hill, 2015).

(h) They are trying to get from where they are to some new place in their life, but they have *no map* of the potential journey; and no idea how to construct such a map.

(i) They are neglecting their physical health needs, by failing to engage in regular physical exercise; eating a junk food diet; not drinking enough water; not getting adequate sleep; not taking essential nutritional supplements; and so on.

(j) They are socially isolated; or living in hostile surroundings; or cut off from work or other forms of useful activity.

(k) And, more generally, they tend to respond to stressful stimuli with either over-aroused emotions (of anger or anxiety), or under-aroused emotions (of sadness, grief, depression and hurt). (See item (g) above).

~~~

The role of the counsellor (from an E-CENT perspective) is then, to perform some or all of the following tasks:

(a) To act as a 'safe harbour' and a 'secure base' – or temporary, 'good enough' mother (and father) substitute – for the client; so they can learn to feel 'securely attached' to the counsellor. Once this secure attachment has been achieved – which is called 'earned security' – the client can generalize this new way of relating to include the significant other people in their life. (Wallin, 2007).

(b) To reflect the client back to themselves in a more realistic form - (not too big, not too small) - than was done for them by their mother/ father/ teachers.

(c) To speak to the client in a feeling language, providing them with a warm, helpful relationship, which is also educative and supportive. (Hobson, 2000).

(d) To explore the client's diet and physical exercise practices; self-talk (or 'inner dialogue'); relaxation practices; relationship skills; sleep pattern; and so on: with a view to helping them to improve their coping resources for dealing with daily stressors. (Taylor-Byrne and Byrne, 2017; and Chapters 4 and 5, below).

(e) To explore some of their **key stories** to see what kinds of painful experiences they need to reframe and digest from the past. (See Chapter 6 below). This involves integration of the left and right hemispheres of their brain, or "naming the emotions in order to tame them" (Siegel, 2015). This is how they learn to soothe their dysregulated emotions (or to *regulate their affects*).

(f) To help the client to develop an understanding of their own feelings, and the feelings of others; and how to communicate effectively about emotional matters. To provide some emotional education; and to help the client to update their map of their social and emotional world. To help them to understand social relationships.

(g) To help the client to grow their **Adult ego state**; to shrink their **Parent** and **Child ego states**; and to learn to *communicate assertively* rather than passively or aggressively. And to find ways of 'cutting the ties' from destructive parent figures (where appropriate).

~~~

Chapter 3: Core beliefs of the emotive-cognitive philosophy of counselling

In a broader sense than that outlined above, E-CENT counselling theory was developed by this author over twenty years of study and application, in private practice, with more than 1,000 clients. It was also developed through many conversations with Renata Taylor-Byrne about stress, meditation, relaxation, positive mental attitude, diet and nutrition, and various systems of physical exercise. In recent years, I set out to boil my learning down into a limited list of key principles. What I came up with was a list of twenty core principles of E-CENT theory, as follows:

The 20 core principles of human development

Firstly, I do not make the mistake of extrapolating from *adult functioning* in order to understand the psychology of human nature. Instead, *I begin with the baby* in the mother's womb (where the mother may be more or less stressed, and more or less well nourished, depending upon the actual circumstances of her life). I then move on to the baby post-birth, which is colonized by a carer (normally mother) who may be more or less sensitive to the baby's signals of comfort and discomfort; more or less responsive to the baby's needs; and more or less caring. And I also take account of how stressed the mother was, by her life circumstances, even *before* the baby was conceived. These are the *foundations* of human emotional and general psychological functioning.

~~~

Secondly, I accept the *Attachment theory* proposition, that the baby is born with an innate attachment drive, which causes it (after period of about twenty to twenty-four weeks of development) to seek to attach itself to a main carer. The attachment bond that is formed becomes either *secure* or *insecure*, depending upon whether the mother (or main carer) is "good enough" – meaning sensitive, responsive, and caring enough to soothe the *affective states*[66] of the baby. Later father and siblings become important attachment figures for the baby. And the baby forms a set of internal working models of relationship based upon those earliest relationships.

~~~

Third, the first five or six years of life are taken to be the *prime determinants* of what kind of life the individual will live. Very largely, the emotionally significant narratives (stories), scripts (maps) and frames (lenses) that the child learns and forms during this period – which manifest in the form of moods and emotional states, expectations, beliefs and habitual patterns of behaviour - will determine its trajectory through life, *all other things being equal*. There is, of course, some degree of malleability of the human brain-mind, and so what was once shaped badly (by negative relationship experiences) can *to some extent* be reshaped into a better form by subsequent 'curative experiences', with a love partner, or with a counsellor or psychotherapist. (Wallin, 2007; Doidge, 2008).

~~~

Fourth: With regard to the narratives, stories, schemas, scripts and frames that the individual learns and/or creates: these are, as J.S. Bruner said[67],

- *Enactive* (or experiences of *doing*);

- *Iconic* (or experiences of *seeing* or *visualizing*); and

- *Semantic* (or *language based* abstractions; verbal meanings; and spoken interpretations of events and objects).

In cognitive psychology, the development of the child and later adult is mapped through studies of *attention, perception, memory, language and thinking*. And *emotion* only gets a brief mention at the end of standard textbooks – as an afterthought. However, in E-CENT, I teach that a *human* being is **essentially** and **unavoidably** an *emotional* being.

It is *an emotional being* that pays attention, when a *human being* pays attention.

It is *an emotional being* that perceives. Perception is never 'purely cognitive'.

It is an *emotional being* that forms memories. We probably have no memories about which we have absolutely *no feelings* whatsoever!

It is an *emotional being* which uses language. The coolest languaging does not allow us to escape from our emotional foundations.

It is an *emotional being* that thinks: or should I say 'perfinks'; because we do not think *separately* and *apart* from our perceptions and feelings. *We apprehend the world in* **one** *perceiving-feeling-thinking (or perfinking)* **grasp** *of the body-brain-mind!*

And even the most abstract of academic thinking cannot be *totally separated* from the (strong or weak) emotionality of the person engaging in it.

In other words, ***the human brain-mind is an emotional brain-mind***. Human beings are emotional beings, at their very foundations, and they can also think (to some limited extent! Thought it is perhaps better to always stick to the concept that we 'perfink'!) They are not 'cognitive beings', if by *cognitive beings* we mean 'computer like'. Computers do *not* have emotions. And humans are not computers! (This is why I developed *emotive-cognitive* therapy, because cognition and emotion cannot ever be separated!)

Indeed, we could say that human beings are not thinking beings at all. They are, as suggested above, actually *perfinking* beings (Glasersfeld, 1989): or beings who *perceive-feel-and-think* all in one grasp of the mind. And the feeling component never sleeps! You cannot leave it at the door on your way into school or work.

~~~

Fifth: We accept that temperamental differences are detectable in new born babies; that an individual may be born with a tendency towards introversion or extraversion; and that a particular new born baby may also be *more* emotionally disturbable, or *less* emotionally disturbable than average. We accept that there are fundamental differences (emotionally and behaviourally) between boys and girls. (For example, the case of John Money and David Reimer)[68]. We accept that the innate nature of the baby will influence and impact the mother in how she relates to the baby; and the mother's personality and character and temperament will also influence and impact the baby.

But in general the mother has much more influence than the baby. "Genetic determinism" has been replaced by "epigenetics", which accepts that genes have to be "switched on" by an environment, and that the genes of identical twins can be changed – as often as not - by placing them in two different home environments. And even where identical twins are raised in the same home, they may well develop different personalities. (See the case of Ladan and Laleh, who were monozygotic [single egg] twin sisters, with significant personality differences: [Spector, 2013)][69].

Returning to the dialectical (or interactional) cross-influence between mother and baby: this will eventually settle down into a stable pattern of relating, which will be experienced by the baby (and the mother) as more, or less, satisfactory.

Depending upon whether or not the mother can function as a 'good enough' mother (in terms of being sensitive, caring, responsive and in good communication with her baby), the child may develop either a *secure* or an *insecure* 'attachment style'. And these attachment styles play out in all significant future relationships.

~~~

Sixth: E-CENT theory takes into account that we are bodies as well as minds, and so diet, exercise, sleep, relaxation/ stress, social connection and relatedness, meditation/ mindfulness/ detachment, personal history, drugs and other physical inputs and stimuli, are seen as important factors in determining the *emotional-thinking-perceiving state* of the individual client. That is to say we are body-minds, and our body-mind has needs – both physical and emotional. It is *wrong* to assume, as the CBT and REBT theorists assume, that *the only factor* which intervenes between a noxious stimulus (or a negative experience) and a negative emotional or behaviour reaction, is the client's thoughts and beliefs, attitudes and values. The whole body-brain-mind of the client plays a role in the processing of significant incoming stimuli, or feedback from the environment.

~~~

Seventh: We need to be loved, liked and accepted by some significant others, if we are to live fulfilling lives. (This need is very strong when we are babies, and it continues to be strong throughout our lives. However, it is not as strong as our need for oxygen or food. If we fail to get oxygen, we will die in seconds; if we fail to get food, we will die within days; and if we fail to give and get love, we will wither and die more quickly than those individuals who do learn how to give and get love. This fundamental reality was denied by Dr Albert Ellis, who had a very severe *insecure attachment style*, which caused him to deny his own need for love, and then to generalize that to all other adults! (Byrne, 2013; and Byrne, 2017).

~~~

Eighth: E-CENT starts from the assumption that we are primarily social animals, and not solitary individuals. We are social to our very roots, especially from the moment of birth, when we are handed into the arms of our mothers. Everything that happens from that point onwards - and also including the original birth trauma - is significant for the development of the so-called 'individual' (who is really a psychological amalgam of significant other 'individuals' with whom the baby is related from birth onwards, and who we [the baby] 'internalize' as 'models'). In particular, our mothers and fathers are electro-chemically braided into the very foundations of our personality and character (in networks of neurons): Byrne (2009b).

~~~

Ninth: From the Object Relations school, E-CENT takes the view that the first three phases of development of childhood can be disrupted, between birth and about the age of six years - or the first four sub-phases from birth to age three - resulting in specific forms of relationship dysfunction in later life. (Mahler, Pine and Bergman, 1975/1987). The solution to these problems tends to include a mixture of:

- 'being with' the client in relationship;

- 'holding' the relationship in a suitable, warm dialogue;

- teaching the client how to re-frame their difficult problems and challenges;

- helping the client to make conscious, and then to process, their un-experienced or resisted emotions;

- providing analysis and models as feeling-thinking ways forward; and:

- providing a 'safe harbour' and a 'secure base' for the client, so they can learn how to have a secure relationship, perhaps for the first time.

~~~

Tenth: E-CENT theory represents the new born baby as containing two fundamental potentials: to develop pro-social and caring attitudes (or virtues); and to develop anti-social and destructive egotistical attitudes (or vices). One of the functions of the process of socialization is to ensure that the new person mainly develops their 'good side' (or what the Native American Cherokee people called the 'good wolf') through the moral teachings of their parents, teachers and others; and that their 'bad wolf' is constrained and contained. (It cannot ever be totally or permanently eliminated. We each contain the capacity for significant levels of evil [or immoral and criminal acts] to the ends of our days!) But the happy functioning of social animals depends upon the extent to which we develop our pro-social, moral virtues, and resist our anti-social, immoral or amoral vices. Some clients are clearly operating mainly from 'good wolf' and some are significantly operating from 'bad wolf'. That latter client group often needs direct or indirect coaching in moral philosophy; and encouragement to operate mainly from 'good wolf', for both the sake of their community and the sake of their own happiness.

~~~

Eleventh: E-CENT theory sees humans as ***primary*** *non-conscious beings*, who operate tacitly, automatically, from layers of cumulative, interpretative experience - stored in the form of schemas and stories, and non-narrativized experience, in long-term memory - and permanently beyond ***direct*** conscious inspection. At least 95% of all of our daily actions are executed non-consciously and automatically[70]. So change is not easy; delusion is our normal state (i.e. our perceptions of ourselves, others and the world are not 'snapshots of reality')[71]; and we project our own 'stories' onto our environments, and judge them accordingly[72]. To wake up to a more accurate understanding of life - with our Adult-functioning in the driving seat - is not easy, but it is possible, at least to some degree.

~~~

Twelfth: We mainly operate from one of three so-called 'ego states', or 'ways of being' (as described in Transactional Analysis [TA])[73]. These are:

(P) **Parent** ego state: When we are operating from this ego state - where we think, feel and behave just like some parent figure from our past experience - we are said to be *'in' Parent ego state*;

(A) **Adult** ego state: This is the logical, reasonably cool and rational, or language-based, 'computing' part of the personality - (but still *somewhat* emotive/evaluative). Most of us strive to be 'in Adult ego state' when we are studying, and/or teaching, and or trying to be reasonable. But our Adult ego state always has a contribution from the emotional centres of our brain. And, finally:

(C) **Child** ego state: This state of being is characterized by our thinking, feeling and acting just like we once did as a young child. We are said to be 'in Child ego state' when we are playful, rebellious, creative, or (more controversially) amorous.

The aim of E-CENT counselling, in this area of ego state functioning, is to try to help the client to get their Adult ego state into the Executive position of their personality; aided and abetted by their Nurturing Parent ego state; and their Free Child. But we also need some elements of Adapted Child, for good manners and social responsibility; and some Rebellious Child, for the sake of self-assertion and self-defence.

~~~

Thirteenth: We seem to be emotional story tellers in a world of stories. Language is the sea in which we swim, unknowingly; as fish swim in water without ever 'spotting' the water. And so our neurotic reactions *often* tend to be outgrowths of old, illogical, unreasonable and unhelpful narratives and stories, scripts, schemas, beliefs and attitudes – all of which have feeling components.

The exceptions to 'narrative disturbances' tend to be:

1. When our neurotic feelings are a result of **unprocessed** *experiences* from the past; or:

2. When we are trying to *control the uncontrollable*; or:

3. We are *rejecting the truth* of our situation. Or:

4. When we are sleep deprived; or:

5. Stressed by **low** or **high** *blood sugar* (from dietary mistakes or transgressions); or:

6. We are deficient in particular nutrients which affect our moods; or our brains are being affected negatively by particular food toxins; or:

7. We have not done enough physical exercise to move our lymph around and to eliminate stress hormones from our body. Or:

8. We are stuck in a high stress situation, such as an unworkable relationship; or financial difficulty; or homelessness; or the threat of any of those kinds of serious problems.

~~~

Fourteenth: One of the major sources of emotional disturbance among humans is *unmanageable* stress and strain. Throughout the whole of the life of the individual, the external environment will continue to exert an impact on the moods and emotions of that individual. Only the most highly trained and committed Stoic or Zen practitioner could ever come *anywhere near* to ignoring (or being largely unaffected by) their external environment! Indeed, only a **rock**, or lump of **wood**, or other inanimate object, ever achieves *complete indifference* to its environment. (And the more extreme statements of the Stoics – such as "Nobody can harm me!" - are *easy to utter* but largely **impossible** to live!)

~~~

Fifteenth: It may be that we each have a (socially induced) vulnerability towards angering, panicking or depressing ourselves when we are stressed by external events or objects; and E-CENT tries to help the client to work on curing those vulnerabilities, by:

> 1. Re-parenting the client, so they *rewire their orbitofrontal cortex*, which is where they have stored their 'personality adaptations' and attachment styles in response to their childhood parenting experiences;
>
> 2. Encouraging them to change elements of their beliefs, attitudes, schemas and stories (about themselves, other people and the world); or:
>
> 3. By learning to reframe problematical activating stimuli; or by *'completing their (unprocessed, or traumatic) experiences'* from the past; or:
>
> 4. By integrating the feeling and thinking sides of the brain.

Significant stories, which we explore with clients, include: The story of origins, including birth and birth-family; The story of personal identity; The story of key relationships (mother/ father); Stories of transitions; The story of career/ wealth/ success/ poverty/ failure; The story of present problems; The connections between the story of origins, the story of relationships, and the story of present problems; and so on.

~~~

Sixteenth: Our clients may be distressed because of their illogical, unreasonable, unrealistic or insupportable beliefs and attitudes about themselves, other people and the world, and we try to get them to reframe those beliefs and attitudes, using the Six Windows model. (See Chapter 6). From the (moderate) teaching of the Buddha and (moderate) Stoicism we learned that people often disturb themselves by having *unrealistic desires*; *goals* that cannot be achieved; and those goals might be about self, other people, or the wider world. For examples:

"I want to be more like this; I wish I could be less like that; and the world should be different from the way it is!"

But we do not make the simplistic mistake of thinking that the problem here is the word "should". The problem is *desire or appetite, taken to unachievable levels*. And *we need the word 'should'* to define our moral rules! So we do not fetishize the world 'should', or any other word. We mainly focus on *meanings* and *emotions*! And on *concrete realities!*

~~~

Seventeenth: Our clients may be distressed because they have failed to process some earlier emotional experience, which is now stuck in the basement of their mind, causing neurotic symptoms to emerge in the form of distorted thoughts, feelings, behaviours, relationship conflict, or physical symptoms. In this kind of situation, the E-CENT therapist's role is to help the client to dig up that part of their past; to process the unprocessed experience - which we call *'completing your experience' of what happened*, or what *failed* to happen. In order to do this successfully, we have found that they need to be able, simultaneously, or concurrently, to **reframe** *those previously unprocessed experiences*, so they do not merely re-stimulate the distressing feelings which caused those felt experiences to be denied, rejected and buried in the first instance, all those years ago. In practice, we teach our clients to reframe their problems before we ask them to engage in digesting old traumatic experiences. (See Chapter 6; and Byrne, [2016]).

~~~

Eighteenth: Our adult relationships (such as marriage and living together) are strongly coloured, shaped and driven by the original drama between our babyhood-self and our mother and father, and sometimes key siblings. We repeatedly re-enact our family drama, until we work on it and resolve it. We have to 'complete' our relationships with our parents (and sometimes key siblings) before we can grow up and move on. And completing those relationships means *allowing them to be, exactly as they were* - accepting them, feeling the related feelings, and getting over our judgemental attitudes and hurt feelings about our parents, who were just 'blokes and birds doing their (highly imperfect) jobs'. And our *most oppressive* siblings were little, ignorant kids! (But it can take a lot of processing time to get to the stage of *forgiving* them all). A further complication arises from the fact that our definition of relationship comes from what we saw our parents do to and with each other, when we were less than five years old; and somewhat beyond that age, say up to the age of ten years. Unfortunately, that 'relationship modelling' means we copy one of our parents as our Adult Role Model; and we go out and seek a life partner on the basis of the parent who was our Mate Model! (In E-CENT practice, we now help clients to revise those old 'movies' of inadequate relationship skill; and to replace them with healthier modelling. This involves revising the client's Adult Role Model and their Mate Model).

~~~

Nineteenth: When the relationship between the client and his/her parents is too damaged, E-CENT offers the client the option to engage in a 'puberty rite', in which they 'cut their ties' to their parents – *divorce them*, as it were – and in this way clean up their psychological baggage about their parents. (This is a fourteen day process of visualization of cutting the ties with the parent(s) – one parent at a time – and allowing both the client and the parent(s) to be free to live their own lives). The client then feels much freer to run their own lives from their *Adult ego state*, based on present time realities, instead of constantly wrestling with emotional ties from the past. And the relationship with the parent from whom the client has cut the ties – if they are still alive - often becomes much better and more satisfactory in the present moment. (But even if the parent or parents are dead, it is still *possible*, and often *necessary*, to cut the ties in the case of relationship damage).

~~~

Twentieth: When the client is very distressed about their early childhood experiences, we deploy a process of **'*externalizing' the inner child***, so the client can nurture and heal their own childhood self in the present – in the form of a *physical referent* or *symbolic self*. This process gradually changes the perceptions-feelings-thoughts of the client, as the inner child gradually 'grows up' and becomes more content with its lot.

~~~

These twenty principles are the bare bones of E-CENT theory. We could probably identify a few sub-principles or supplementary processes within each of those main principles/processes. We could also identify some intermediate principles, processes or propositions that reside between those core principles/ processes/ propositions. And we may well keep expanding this list as the theory unfolds. However, we also recognize the value, in terms of human memory, of keeping lists as short as possible, and no shorter. As lengthy as necessary, and no longer.

~~~

Lifestyle Counselling and Coaching for the Whole Person:

Or how to integrate nutritional insights, exercise and sleep coaching into talk therapy

Chapter 4: Overview of diet and exercise impacts upon mental health

By Renata Taylor-Byrne and Jim Byrne

4.1: Introduction

The core of this chapter was originally published as *Part 5: Summing Up* – of our book on diet and exercise - (Taylor-Byrne and Byrne, 2017) – and was written by Renata Taylor-Byrne. This current version of this chapter has been updated and revised and expanded with the co-authorship of Dr Jim Byrne.

Part 1 of that earlier book (Taylor-Byrne and Byrne, 2017) looked at a number of questions about the ways in which nutrition affects our body-brain-mind and emotions.

One point that we did *not* cover is this: *How do the effects of diet and exercise fit into a psychological model – or psychobiological model - of the human body-brain-mind of the counselling client?* So let us explore that question here and now.

4.2: The psychobiological model of E-CENT and the impact of diet and exercise

Briefly, the system works like this: Firstly, Figure 4.1 represents a person (B1-3 + Y) subjected to an environmental stressor (A1) who is showing signs of anger (for example) as their outputted emotional Consequence (C2). Y represents the body, and B the brain-mind; and also note the overlap, which stores *lived experiences*, as little y's.

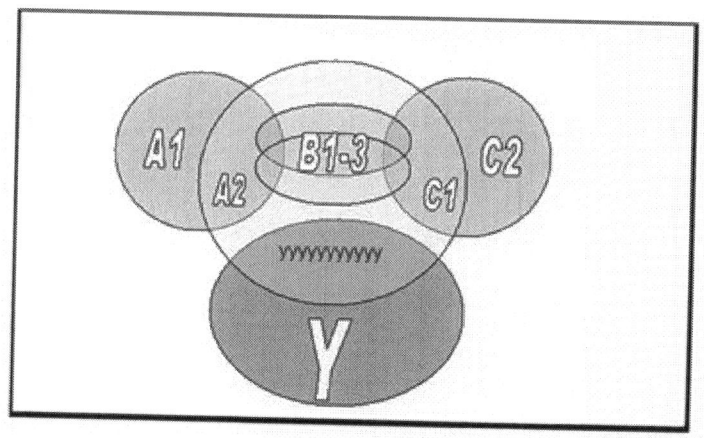

Figure 4.1: The A>B1-3>Y>yyy>C Model of body-brain-mind

A1 is the external stimulus (or what happened) and C2 is the outputted angry response.

Secondly, the elements of *causation* of the emotional Consequence (C2) amount to at least six, or eight, in our view (depending on how you count the B's)! (See Chapter 7 of Byrne, 2017).

By contrast with our view, Albert Ellis (1962) asserted that there was **only one cause** of any emotional response, and that was the **B** (or **Belief**) of the client about some *noxious stimulus* or *stressor* (at point A – which is also called the 'Activating Event'). However, by contrast with Ellis, and very much in support of our perspective, Aristotle considered that every event had *several* causative factors involved, which he listed as: (1) The *material* cause; (2) the *efficient* cause; (3) the *formal* cause; and (4) the *final* cause. We do not follow Aristotle into using this four-part system of causation, but instead, consider the elements which arise out of our consideration of the client as a whole, complex, open system: or body-brain-mind-environment complexity. For example, the 'environment' aspect includes lots of stress and strain: like time pressure; noise; interpersonal stressors (like conflict, or loneliness, or isolation, or overcrowding); financial stressors (related to debts, job security or insecurity); performance demands; and so on. And the body-brain is supported or undermined, in handling those stressors, by the quality and quantity of the foods the person eats; what they drink; how much sleep they get, and the quality of that sleep; how much they exercise; the quality of their social connections and social supports; and so on.

As shown in Figure 4.1 above, the factors which *cause* the C2 (or outputted emotional response) include the following:

The A1 (external Activating Event): The *physical* or *immediate* cause. Something happens which is picked up by the senses of the counselling client.

The A2 (internal Activating Event): The *evaluative* cause: The client automatically 'evaluates' (habitually, non-consciously, and non-linguistically) the significance of this A1 (stimulus). (This could be seen as the *habit-based* cause).

The B1-2-3 (Biological emotive-cognitive processing): This is *the socially shaped* cause. The innate emotions of the client – managed from the limbic system – have been shaped, socially, by mother, father, teachers and others (in the past, including childhood), which has resulted in a particular kind of 'affect (or emotion) regulation compromise' (Hill, 2015), stored in the **orbitofrontal cortex** (OFC) of the client's brain. Therefore, the B1-2-3 is *a habit-based, automatic, socially shaped, evaluation of the stimulus* at A1.

The Little yyyyy's: The *historical body-state* cause. These are stored *states of the body*, (stored in the body-brain-mind) in response to similar A1's in the past, which caused particular kinds of responses in the guts, heart, lungs, facial muscles, and major muscles (like legs and arms) of the client. These are linked to a particular kind of stimulus, and are 'matched' – or 'pattern matched' – and ready to be triggered whenever *that A1* (or something very similar) is experienced in the future.

The Big Y: This is a representation of the body of the client. It's capacity to cope with the A1 (or *external* or *physical* or *initiating* cause) is affected by many factors, including the quality and quantity of recent sleep; the level of blood glucose in the body-brain, delivered by particular kinds of foods; the level of cell hydration, delivered by regular supplies of (good or bad) water sources (filtered; from the tap; or from a [plastic or glass] bottle). And also by the state of the gut bacteria of the client. Some bacteria promote healthy functioning of the body-brain-mind; and some promote unhealthy functioning of the body-brain-mind. (See Enders, 2015; Kaplan and Rucklidge, et al, 2015).

The C1: This can be thought of as those aspects of emotive-cognitive processing that integrate the signals coming from the B1-2-3 (OFC), the little yyyyy's (body memories), and the Big Y (general health-state of the body, including effects of diet and exercise, sleep, etc.), and this C1 processing (rapidly) selects an appropriate (or *apparently* appropriate) output (without too much time-wasting 'cogitation').

The C2: This is the *outputted emotional and behavioural response* to the A1 - (which was dictated by the C1 summation of the earlier processing).

It is obvious from this model (and the research quoted in this book) that a well exercised body will handle greater stress (from the A1) than a body that has not been exercised. (Blumenthal, et al., 2012; Ratey and Hagerman, 2009; Taylor-Byrne and Byrne, 2017; and Sapolsky, 2010).

A client who sleeps at least eight hours each night will handle greater stress from the A1 than a person whose sleep pattern is broken, or is too short, or is in some other way inadequate. (Walker, 2017; and Van der Helm and Walker, 2009).

And, the quality of the food that the client consumes will either support or undermine their capacity to withstand stressors at A1. (Korn, 2016; Perlmutter, 2015; Greger, 2016).

~~~

In the main body of this chapter, we now want to turn our attention to some of the key points that emerged from our consideration of the impact of (historical and current) diet and exercise practices upon the body-brain-mind of the counselling client.

4.3: The importance of food for the body-brain-mind

Firstly, we can't function properly without food, because food provides the energy for physical and mental activity, and the material to rebuild our cells. Inadequate nutrition impacts our ability to live, work, communicate, heal, and fight off all the viruses and germs which are present in the atmosphere. We need to have a diet which has all the essential amino acids, vitamins and minerals, complex carbohydrate, fats, and fibre. These should come from healthy sources of *unprocessed* food, plus some nutritional supplements. The Mediterranean diet is highly rated, plus the Nordic diet, as potential models to follow; or rather to build upon and to personalize.

Some others were also commended, for short-term use; such as (aspects of) the Paleo, Atkins, and Ketogenic diets – which might, unfortunately, be too high in meat content, which causes inflammation; and inflammation is linked to mood disorders. For example, the 25-year *China Study* – Campbell and Campbell (2006) -found that the people who ate the most vegetables were the healthiest, while the people who at the most meat suffered the most ill health.

Some of the evidence in favour of the high-fat, low carb diets – like the Paleo and Atkins diets - may be misinterpreting the findings (e.g. Elliott, 2014). Although Elliott goes along with the idea that it is the high-protein, high-fat content of the Atkins/Paleo-type diets that reduces depression; Mozes (2015), looking at the effect of carbohydrates on the incidence of depression, shows a better understanding.

Alan Mozes reports that:

> "The study (under consideration) involved 70,000 women aged 50 to 79. The findings, the investigators said, only show an association between 'refined' carbs and elevated depression risk, rather than a direct cause-and-effect relationship".

But could it not be the case that the Atkins/Paleo diets work, not because of the high fat, high protein end of the equation, but because of the 'low carb' end of the equation; which must (most often) also be 'low *refined* carbs', as opposed to 'low *wholegrains* and *vegetables*'?

Certainly the research cited by Mozes (2015) seems to suggest this view as a valid interpretation, where he writes that "*...the women who consumed diets higher in vegetables, fruits and whole grains had a lower incidence of depression*". (However, this does not prove that *everybody* can tolerate grains!)

Complex carbs, in the form of vegetables, and whole (gluten free and gliadin free) grains, seem to be okay (for many people, much of the time), and are not at all in need of being replaced by proteins and fats!

By eliminating *refined carbs*, in the form of junk foods and highly processed foods, the Atkins/ Paleo diets make it impossible to evaluate the impact of protein and fats *per se*!

Some new research is clearly needed to separate out these competing interpretations.

(And some people may need to avoid all grains, at least some of the time; and some will have to permanently exclude them. But they should do this by experimentation, under the guidance of a qualified nutritional therapist!)

4.4: Balanced diet and toxic foods…

What is a balanced diet?

Firstly, at the moment, there is no universal agreement about the definition or content of an ideal, balanced diet; and national guidelines vary considerably between, say, Britain and the USA; and both of those guidelines differ significantly from the Mediterranean and Nordic diets. However, we know (some of) what is bad for us, and we have some clues as to what may often be good for people, but we also have to allow for individualized diet and nutrition plans.

The official British guide to nutrition suggests that we should eat about 30% grains; 30% vegetables and fruit. And about 40% split equally between (a) dairy products, (b) meat and fish, and (c) nuts and seeds.

We recommend that you experiment with that kind of guideline; perhaps moving the proportion of vegetables up to 40% or higher; but also consider the elements of the Mediterranean diet and the Nordic diet, both of which have high levels of oily fish and vegetables. Oily fish (which is high in omega-3 fatty acids) is important for brain and heart health, and also for preventing depression, anger and anxiety. So it is probably a good idea to have oily fish once or twice each week. Also, if you have problems with grains, increase your vegetable consumption; reduce your grains; and keep your meat consumption low (because it tends to boost your omega-6 levels, which promote inflammation, which is linked to both depression and physical illness). For a more detailed set of dietary guideline, please see Part 1 (sections 3[a] and [b]) of Taylor-Byrne and Byrne [2017]). And bear in mind that you can always consult a nutritional therapist for confirmation of your own conclusions about your dietary needs.

~~~

However, in practice, most people do not follow official nutritional guidelines. For example, on average, the British population is currently eating more than half of its food from *ultra-processed sources*. To state that more precisely:

"Half of all the food bought by families in Britain is now 'ultra-processed', made in a factory with industrial ingredients and additives invented by food technologists and bearing little resemblance to the fruit, vegetables, meat and fish used to cook a fresh meal at home". (Boseley, 2018)[74].

What this could mean is that poorer people are eating a lot more than 50, or 60, or perhaps more than 70% junk food, while richer people eat less than 50%, or 40, or 30% junk food. And there are very serious health implications – including mental health implications – of eating more than a very small amount of junk food. (Brogan, 2016; Perlmutter, 2015; Holford, 2010).

And over the years of counselling individuals, we have found that people who eat sugary, yeasty foods, like breads, cakes, biscuits, sweets and puddings – which is to say, high sugar, high grains and high dairy diets - are prone to develop a form of *gut dysbiosis* called *systemic Candidiasis* – or generalized *overgrowth* of Candida Albicans in the large intestine – which shows up as *unaccountable* anxiety or depression, combined with low levels of energy or chronic fatigue. (See Taylor-Byrne and Byrne, 2017).

~~~

Personalized diet

The safest way to follow healthy diets seems to us to be this: Get a couple of good recipe books which emphasize the kinds of foods found in elements of the Mediterranean, Nordic, and Vegetarian diets; and Chapter 11 of the China Study, which emphasizes eight principles of food and health. And, if you can afford it, consult a good nutritional therapist.

According to Leslie Korn:

"No single diet is right for everyone. Each person has a different cultural-genetic heritage and therefore a different metabolism. Some people, like the Inuit, require mostly meat and fish, whereas people from India do well on a predominance of legumes, vegetables, fruits, and grains. Most people require a mix. However, that mix of food can vary greatly. Know your ancestral and genetic heritage and try to eat for your individual metabolic type". (Page 14, Korn, 2016).

But one thing we can safely predict, based upon scientific studies which are cited in this book: No race of people will ever exist, who can, for long, remain physically and mentally healthy on a junk food diet; or an inadequate diet in terms of nutrients![75], [76].

Invest time and effort in shopping for raw ingredients, and spend time in the kitchen engaging in food preparation. This can become a highly enjoyable way to spend your time, and it's a great way to express *love* for our nearest and dearest!

Make more than fifty percent of your meals raw salads, combined with nuts and seeds. (And some theorists think we should always eat fruits at a time separate from our main meals, unless our main meal is just fruit!).

Eat lots of plant based proteins: such as, vegetables (avocado, broccoli, spinach, kale, peas, and sweet potato); legumes (such as lentils and beans); nuts and seeds (including sesame, sunflower, almonds, walnuts, and hazelnuts); non-dairy milk (such as almond, coconut, and/or oat milk); gluten-free grains (quinoa, amaranth, and buckwheat [if you can tolerate them] and brown rice). And take Spirulina and Chlorella for their nutrient and protein content.

Supplement with: Vitamins B, C and E (at the very least!); plus omega-3 fatty acids (as in fish oils), Co-enzyme-Q10 (Footnote[77]), and live acidophilus and other live bacteria[78].

Eat some fermented foods, like Miso, Kimchi and sauerkraut. Chew your food well, and use a squat-toilet (if at all possible) to optimize elimination. (And if you don't have a squat toilet, use a foot stool – sit on the toilet with your feet on the stool [of 6-9 inches in height] - to simulate the traditional squatting position).

Drink eight glasses of filter water per day. Do the reading, and find out for yourself.

Monitor the effects of dietary changes on your moods, emotions and energy levels, and adjust accordingly. The best way to do that is to keep a food diary for a few weeks, and record everything you eat and drink. And also record your exercise and sleep patterns.

And check each day to see how you feel: *Is your energy up or down since yesterday? Is your mood up or down since yesterday? Do you feel physically better or worse than yesterday? Any sign of skin allergies?* And if any of those indicators is negative, that should be linked back to what you ate 24 to 30 hours earlier [approximately]. Plus what has been happening during those 24 to 30 hours: like sleep disturbance; lack of physical exercise; increased stress from any source; the emergence of a problem that you feel you cannot handle; and so on. (If you can't track it back on your own, see a professional helper to support you).

And consult a suitable nutritionist, medical expert or health coach, when and if necessary. (And also read Part 1 of Taylor-Byrne and Byrne, 2017).

~~~

Beware toxic foods

Secondly, beyond sensitivity to grains and dairy products, there are foods whose *toxicity* is very *high*, and it is only in the last twenty years or so that people have been able to gain access to research studies and investigations which have looked at those 'foods' which, though always on sale in the supermarket and shops, are really bad for our bodies and brains.

Let us briefly review the top six toxic foods:

1. The **first** culprit is ***trans-fats*** (also called hydrogenated fat, and nicknamed "Frankenfats"). They begin life as harmless vegetable oils, which are then industrially processed by superheating processes which add hydrogen atoms to the oils.

Why are these vegetable oils put through this damaging process?

Because it makes the fat much easier to use in the manufacturing of bread, cakes, biscuits; snack bars; ready meals; and it is preferred by fast food shops and restaurants. It is much cheaper than real butter or natural vegetable oils. These trans-fats last longer than healthier fats, which means processed foods can last longer on supermarket shelves – but the effects on the body are grim!

Because the trans-fat is created by being boiled at very high temperatures, this affects its chemical structure. This type of fat is thus unnatural and (wo)man-made, and causes chaos in our body and brain on a cellular level. For examples: it affects the enzymes that our body needs to fight cancer; and it has been implicated in a major study which showed a connection between rage and the consumption of trans-fats. Trans-fats also interfere with the insulin receptors on the body's cell membranes, which promotes obesity. And they cause major blocking of the arteries! Recent studies have linked trans-fats to both depression and anger management problems. (See Taylor-Byrne and Byrne, 2017).

2. The **second** enemy of our body-brain-mind is *sugar*. It's described as the enemy of the immune system, because it takes four hours for our immune response to recover from the effects of consuming sugar. Sugar reduces the ability of the immune system to protect us properly; increases inflammation in the body (which is linked to the causation or triggering of depression); interferes with the proper functioning of our brain cells; and makes our blood sugar levels fluctuate wildly (which causes stress symptoms, including anxiety). Sugar creates fat around our internal organs; causes obesity and diabetes; attacks the collagen in our skin; stiffens our skin and causes wrinkles; and increases blood pressure! It is also implicated in heightening the stress response, when we face any difficulty in life.

3. The **third** enemy? It's *alcohol*, described by Patrick Holford as 'the brain's worst enemy'. Its effects include: unhelpfully dissolving essential fatty acids[79] in the brain; negatively impacting the way our memory works; draining certain B vitamins, vitamin D and calcium from our body; and damaging our ability to get a good night's sleep. It leaches water from the cells of our body, creating dehydration and producing large amount of 'free radicals', which increase the risk of hormonal cancers, particularly breast cancer. It is also implicated in depression and suicide ideation, suicide completion, and self-harm.

4. **Caffeine** is next in line in terms of its harmful effects: it overstimulates the heart, stomach, pancreas and intestines. And it reduces calcium, potassium, zinc, vitamin C and the B vitamins. It also alters the acid/alkaline balance in the body in a negative direction; plays a part in premature ageing; and affects our sleep. Its main negative effect on our emotions is to simulate anxiety, and to trigger panic attacks.

5. **Processed food** is the next problem (and much processed food is also 'junk food'). When people are short of time, they are very tempted to get processed food for meals, because of the convenience. Processed foods are normally faster to prepare, but if they have been altered in any way, apart from being washed and packaged, then they normally become suspected of being 'junk foods'. Junk food (which is most processed food) is food which has been altered from its raw, natural state by chemical or physical means. It is sold in jars, tin cans, bottles, and boxes. And it has very dodgy add-ons, like excessive amounts of salt, sugar and transfats, and artificial

flavours and colours. They also often have constituents that are low in nutrition. Because there can be so much fat, sugar and salt in processed food, this increases the risk of high blood pressure; and the increase in sodium increases the risk of stroke. Furthermore, processed foods create constipation due to lack of fibre. And they can increase the risk of depression, according to a research study by Akbaraly et al (2009), which compared the level of depressive symptoms of middle-aged people on diets which were *either:* (1) high in processed food; or (2) high in wholefoods. Those on a diet high in processed foods had a 58% increased risk for depression over a five year period, according to the research findings. (Wholefoods are normally bought in the state in which they came out of the ground or off the trees and bushes [fruits and vegetables]; or they have remained minimally changed post-harvesting, and essentially left in their natural state [like wholegrains, legumes, etc.]).

6. What about *gluten*? This is an enemy for our bodies because of the way gluten behaves when it's in our intestines. Gluten is actually the name of the mixture which is formed (or expanded) when cereal flours (like wheat, rye or barley [or contaminate oats]) are mixed with water. When these two substances are mixed together they expand the chains of proteins called gliadins and glutenins. These substances tend to create inflammation, and to pull the cells of the gut walls apart, producing a condition called 'leaky gut'. This allows whole molecules of food to escape into the blood stream, and travel to the brain. And, according to Dr Giulia Enders' (2015) book on the guts, this also tends to break down the blood-brain barrier, and allow food particles to affect the brain, causing inflammation. (Inflammation is now recognized as the main cause of all the major diseases, including the emotional problem of depression, and possibly other emotional problems, like anxiety).

Many people are *gluten intolerant*. This is called **Celiac disease**, and people with this condition have to avoid all forms of gluten, otherwise they will further damage their guts. Some other people (perhaps 26% of us) have non-Celiac gluten sensitivity (NCGS), which damages our brains, but not our guts. And people with neurological damage of unknown origin should therefore always be tested for NCGS. There may be other people who have a form of non-Celiac gluten sensitivity which causes abdominal discomfort, pain, and gas. And there may be people who think they have gluten sensitivity, but who actually have gut problems resulting from the Fructans in fruits and vegetables, or other food stuffs. (These people can be helped by the Low FodMaps diet. See Taylor-Byrne and Byrne, 2017).

Because of this situation, many people are now opting to avoid gluten. The official advice to those people is to get themselves tested, for both Celiac disease and Non-Celiac Gluten Sensitivity (NCGS), to make sure they are treating the right condition!

Technically, the gliadin within gluten draws apart the 'tight junctions' between the cells that form the walls of our intestines. This leads to an increase in the space between the cells, allowing toxins and larger molecules of food, (which would normally pass fully through the intestines, and be eliminated), to be released into the blood transmitting system of our bodies, causing havoc in the form of bowel problems, celiac disease, headaches, brain inflammation, anxiety and depression. Apparently many people are unknowingly suffering from the side-effects of gluten, according to Julia Ross (2002); and researchers have found that symptoms of depression tend to disappear when wheat and other grains have been taken out of the diet. (But we can always use gluten-free whole grains, if we find, by experimentation, that we can tolerate them in our diet. On the other hand, many people find they have little or no tolerance for any form of grains).

4.5: The importance of nutritional supplements for mental health

Having looked at toxic foods, we then went on to look at nutritional supplements, like vitamins, minerals, Co-Q-10, gut bacteria, and so on (in Taylor-Byrne and Byrne, 2017).

The question as to whether nutritional supplements actually help us improve our physical and emotional well-being was addressed.

The findings show a range of opinions on their effectiveness, which we have reviewed and resolved.

The NHS Direct UK, considers that nutritional supplements are *unnecessary* unless there are specific *reasons* why someone may need extra nutrients, such as pregnant women; and women who may be breastfeeding; and young children who may have a lack of variety in their diets.

Also, doctors may prescribe specific nutrients e.g. the recommendation to take iron supplements when a patient has iron deficiency anaemia.

We reject this view, of the *limited* need for nutritional supplements, as being ill-informed. This NHS viewpoint is based on the flawed assumption that everybody either does, or could, eat a balanced diet, which would give them all the nutrients they need. This is a false premise, because most people do *not* eat a balanced diet; would not know what a balanced diet *looked* like; and would also find it hard to get *all the nutrients they **need*** from modern, processed, *denatured* foods!

There are also contrasting views on this subject, held by the following experts: a professor at the Yale School of Public Health's Division of Chronic Disease Epidemiology; Patrick Holford; and Dr David Perlmutter.

Susan Taylor-Maine considers nutritional supplements to be inappropriate because: 'They deliver vitamins out of context' (Ballantyne, 2007);

And Patrick Holford, a British nutritional expert, considers them to be *essential* as we need good nutrition for the creation of optimum mental health.

(See Part 1, section 5, of Taylor-Byrne and Byrne, 2017)

~~~

For us, the most powerful arguments are these:

(1) Much of our food is now denatured, and low in nutritional value.

(2) Most people would not know how to put together a balanced diet for a day, not to say a week, so they tend to miss out on many nutrients.

(3) Therefore, nutritional deficiencies are highly likely to be widespread and serious.

(4) Furthermore, nutritional deficiencies are definitely implicated in the causation of not just physical diseases, but also emotional problems and mental illnesses. Therefore it makes sense to take multivitamins and minerals, plus vitamin C and vitamin B complex, and a strong, natural source vitamin E (400 iu), even if it could be shown that *some proportion* of those supplements are then urinated out of the body. Depressed individuals have been found to be deficient in Magnesium, so it makes sense to supplement with Magnesium citrate. (Deans, 2018).

This approach – of using nutritional supplements, *in combination with* the best wholefood diet you can devise for yourself - is a safer option than relying on an *inadequate diet* for our full range of nutritional needs.

Furthermore, Dr David Perlmutter considers that we need to use probiotics (or live, friendly bacteria, like Acidophilus Bifidus), as supplements, if we want to have a healthy gut and brain. He was inspired by the views of Nobel Laureate Elie Mechnikov, who considered that a proper balance of good and bad bacteria in the gut was an essential factor in making sure human beings live a long and healthy life.

Since Mechnikov has put this theory forward his views have been confirmed by many scientific studies. Perlmutter states the view that the research results confirm that '*Up to 90% of all known human illness can be traced back to an unhealthy gut.*'

4.6: The link between food and anger, anxiety and depression

Our experience of anxiety, anger and depression is affected by the nutrients in our bodies. This is the core subject of our book on diet and exercise: (Taylor-Byrne and Byrne, 2017).

Firstly, let us look at **_anxiety_**. Our book on diet and exercise examined how nutrients can affect the experience of anxiety, which is defined by the Oxford dictionary as a '*Feeling of unease or concern*'. It can be an invaluable warning signal, part of our physiological/psychological make-up that can alert us to danger in our immediate environment, but which can also send false alarms! We can experience anxiety because of false fears; a build-up of stress hormones in our bodies; and also due to the condition of our guts, and the nature of the foods and drinks that we consume.

Dr Perlmutter (a board-certified neurologist and fellow of the American College of Nutrition, and President of the Perlmutter Health Centre), has done extensive research on this subject. In Perlmutter (2014, 2015), he presents compelling evidence that the condition of the gut; its ability to process food; and the bacteria which is present in the gut; all have a role to play in the creation of anxiety disorders.

Our guts apparently contain 70-80% of our immune system and they exert control over the production of cortisol and adrenaline (which are the main stress hormones secreted when we are under great pressure).

Perlmutter (2015) cites evidence from two research studies:

- One conducted in 2011 - (Published in the Proceedings of the National Academy of Sciences, and conducted by J.A. Bravo et al., 2011);

- And one conducted at Oxford University in 2014 (by K. Schmidt et al., 2014).

Both experiments confirm that the use of 'prebiotics' (like certain fibrous foods), and 'probiotics' (like Acidophilus and other *friendly* bacteria), lower the levels of corticosterone and cortisol in the guts of animals and humans, thus reducing the stress response. (Prebiotics are foods that promote the growth of good [or 'friendly'] bacteria in the gut; and probiotics are microorganism which, when eaten [normally in capsule form], maintain or reinstate beneficial bacteria in the digestive tract).

In his book titled 'Brainmaker' (2015), Dr Perlmutter describes a client called Martina who started a regime of gluten free food, an oral probiotic programme with prebiotic foods, vitamin supplementation, and changes in her lifestyle, such as aerobic exercise and more sleep. After six weeks, when she came back to see him, "She was transformed….she looked radiant". She had no more chronic anxiety, and was off all her medication (anti-depressant and non-steroid anti-inflammatory drugs). Dr Perlmutter and his colleagues always take pictures of their clients at the start of their treatment and at the end. If you would like to see the "Before" and "After" pictures of Martina then they are on his website. The web address is as follows: https://www.DrPerlmutter.com.

Jenny Sansouci, a nutritional researcher, found that the top offenders for the creation of anxiety in the human body are caffeine, sugar, artificial sweeteners and alcohol.

~~~

Secondly, let us consider the connection between **_anger_** and diet: This emotional state is also affected by nutrition to a surprising extent, which is confirmed by the research findings of Dr Julia Ross (2003).

Ross is a psychotherapist and director of Recovery Systems, a clinic in California that treats mood, eating and addiction problems with nutritional therapy and biochemical rebalancing. And her findings are mirrored by the research findings of Patrick Holford (Chief Executive of the Food for the Brain Foundation, in the UK, and a leading nutrition expert).

Both of these experts quote research results which show that angry, aggressive behaviour can originate from chemical imbalances in the body, and they give examples of aggressive behaviour being transformed when nutrients were given to people suffering from low levels of serotonin or who were suffering from hypoglycaemia. For example, there were some astonishing results from the work done by Professor Stephen Schoenthaler, with 3,000 prison inmates in California in 1983. There was a massive reduction in aggressive behaviour when the research study participants, the inmates, were given a diet which was stripped of refined food and sugar.

Schoenthaler's research findings were later replicated in a double-blind study of 1,482 juveniles and several follow-up studies confirmed his findings, which revealed strong, unequivocal evidence of the link between anger and aggression, on the one hand, and the consumption of sugar, processed food and transfats, on the other.

And in the UK, between 1995 and 1997, at Aylesbury Young Offenders Institution, a placebo-controlled, randomised trial, was conducted by Dr Bernard Gesch (2002), in which young offenders were given food supplements (including vitamins, minerals and essential fatty acids), and it was found that they committed 37% fewer violent offences, while the inmates who received the placebo showed no such reduction; thus demonstrating that improved nutrition reduces angry outbursts (which were being fuelled by vitamin and mineral and fatty acid deficiencies).

The whole range of research studies, described in Taylor-Byrne and Byrne (2017), point out the relationship between the body and its reaction to:

(1) Toxins in the diet - like alcohol, caffeine and trans-fats – and also:

(2) The negative effects of nutritional deficiencies (such as lack of omega-3 fatty acids, vitamins and minerals), and/or:

(3) Blood-sugar regulation...

...in these cases resulting in anger and anti-social behaviour; but also potentially playing a role in anxiety and depression.

~~~

Thirdly, what about _**depression**_? Can the foods that we eat cause depression, or is it purely down to our life circumstances?

There are many factors to take into account in understanding depression, (which are all considered in Taylor-Byrne and Byrne 2017).

For example: People can easily confuse depression with grief, and if someone has a bereavement, and they are still suffering from deep feelings of loss and sadness after eighteen months have elapsed, then this is a sign that their grief may be stuck. They may be resisting feeling their grief, and this becomes stuck depression

Dr Kelly Brogan, a practising psychiatrist in America, considers depression to be a grossly misunderstood state. She explains that having one in four American women in their 40's and 50's using psychiatric drugs shows that medication is being given without a proper understanding of the role of lifestyle factors, including dietary habits, and the physiological state of the client's body, especially their guts.

"If you think a chemical pill can save, cure or 'correct' you, you're dead wrong. This is about as misguided as taking aspirin for a nail stuck in your foot", she states. She considers it to be essential to get a full picture of her client's biological make-up and their lifestyle, dietary habits, level of sugar consumption, the state of their guts, hormone levels, genetic variations in their DNA, and their beliefs about their own health.

Both Dr Kelly Brogan and Dr David Perlmutter consider that the state of our guts is a very important determinant of our well-being, and that our guts play a role in the experience of depression. For example Perlmutter cites a research study in which scientists gave people, who had no signs of depression whatsoever, an infusion to precipitate inflammation, which would begin in the guts. And apparently classic depression symptoms developed immediately, in response to that physical inflammation.

As 70-80% of our immune system is in our guts, we need to keep our guts in a good state of health. Our guts play a crucial role in keeping our levels of cortisol and adrenaline in check. Those stress hormones can cause mayhem in the body when they are continually stimulated. So taking care of your intestines is very important, and being aware of the effects on our guts of the food and drink that we consume is part of that process.

Finally, Robert Redfern (2016), who is a nutritionist, author and broadcaster, has publicised the findings from research done at the University of Eastern Finland, in the publication 'Naturally Healthy News'. A study examined the diets of 2,000 men and when the participants ate a diet free of processed food, and instead ate a healthy selection of food, there were fewer symptoms of depression. They also discovered that eating processed food (or 'junk' food), and sugar, increased the symptoms of depression.

4.7: The conclusion regarding diet and mental health

The take away message from this examination of the links between anxiety, anger and depression, on the one hand, and diet and nutrition, on the other, is this: the state of our bodies, our lifestyle, and the food and drink that we consume, all contribute a great deal to the creation of emotional distress.

And these insights about nutrition need to be taken into account in the understanding and treatment of emotional and mental problems in counselling, psychotherapy, psychiatry, health coaching, lifestyle coaching, and alternative health advice and support services.

In particular, we should avoid sugary foods; caffeine; alcohol; gluten; and junk foods. We should drink six to eight glasses of filtered water per day. We should mainly eat vegetables - with small amounts of fruit (between meals, with at least one hour of a gap between fruit and other meals). Keep meat consumption super-low – like once each week, for example – and keep oily fish high – at twice each week. Mainly eat salads, as cooking destroys nutrients. Use grains (in the form of breads and cereals) sparingly, assuming you can tolerate them at all; but avoid wheat, rye, non-organic oats, and barley completely – because of their gluten content. Take vitamin and mineral supplements, like a full spectrum B-Complex; a multivitamin and mineral supplement; at least one gram of vitamin C powder each day (and possibly two or three). For more specific guidance on foods and supplements for particular emotional states, please see Taylor-Byrne and Byrne (2017).

4.8: Physical exercise and emotional wellbeing

Part 2 of Taylor-Byrne and Byrne (2017) was about the relationship between physical exercise and emotional well-being; and the power of exercise to reduce the incidence of anxiety, anger and depression.

Sitting down for long periods of time is now recognized as being linked to both physical disease and emotional disorders.

When we get up and move around, we force our lungs to draw in more oxygen, which is good for us; and we force our lymphatic drainage system to work, which eliminates toxins from our bodies.

Thirty minutes of brisk walking per day is the minimum that we recommend to list our mood and reduce your feelings of anxiety or anger. And walking near trees and/or a body of water is also very good for health and mood.

Exercise and the stress response

In Taylor-Byrne and Byrne (2017), the effectiveness of exercise in reducing stress, in all its forms, was explored. The opinions of the NHS in the UK and the Mayo Clinic in America were cited; and two forms of exercise which are highly rated (Chinese and Indian), were examined.

Normally, when we experience stressful events in our daily lives, if we also have an *active* lifestyle, this physical activity can burn off the stress hormones which would otherwise accumulate in our bodies.

In an emergency (or an apparent emergency), our internal protective mechanism, called the *'fight or flight response'*, will normally mobilise our body-brain-mind, by pouring very powerful stress hormones into our system to empower us to get moving and to resolve the problem we are faced with, in a physical way. This is called *activation of the **sympathetic** system*. The *sympathetic system* gets us into action!

We automatically either fight our way out, or flee; or sometimes freeze.

When we get to a safe place, or have resolved the emergency, and can breathe more easily, the *'rest and digest'* system kicks in and our bodies slowly return to a relaxed state and our digestion returns to normal.

This is called *activation of the* **parasympathetic** *system*. The *parasympathetic system* calms us down!

4.9: Anxiety and physical activity

But if we don't give our bodies a chance to work off the stress hormones, with physical activity, then tension can build up, which can trigger anxiety; and this can accumulate and become a habitual anxiety problem (which some would call 'an anxiety disorder'. But it should not be given such an apparently 'medical' label!) This habitual state of anxiety means that we can feel stressed even when there is no danger in our immediate environment.

How is this problem of excess anxiety solved?

Partly the answer is to adjust the client's diet. (For example, remove stimulants, like caffeine and sugar). Partly it involves helping them to **rethink** their *perceptions* of danger. And partly it has to do with *keeping* **physically** *fit*. Sometimes one of these approaches will do the trick; sometimes it takes two; and sometimes we need to address all three aspects (the dietary, the exercise program, and the self-talk, or inner dialogue). And, of course, if it is possible to change the environmental stressors, they should also do that! Or move to a new environment!

Research evidence

How effective is the exercise component on its own?

This question was answered by the research findings from Joshua Broman-Fulks who recruited two groups of students, 54 in total, and got them exercising.

Both sets of students had generalised anxiety disorder and high levels of anxiety, and they exercised less than once a week.

One group ran on treadmills (at 60–90% of their maximum heart rates) and the second group walked on treadmills at a rate that was equal to 50% of their maximum heart rates. Each of these two groups had six sessions of the exercise (twenty minutes in length) spread over two weeks.

As a result of the exercise sessions, both groups of students became less sensitive to anxiety, and the more physically demanding exercise produced beneficial results in a shorter period of time.

But why did the exercising work?

In a nutshell, the exercise reduces the tension levels in your muscles (stopping the *anxiety feedback loop* going to your brain). So you stop feeling anxious about feeling anxious! Or, you stop having psychological feeling about your physical sensations.

4.10: Exercise and anger

Can anger be reduced by exercise? How about taking easily-angered people and seeing if exercising has any effect on their levels of annoyance and irritation?

This is exactly what was done by Reynolds (2010), at the University of Georgia, and presented at the Annual Conference of the American College of Sports Medicine. It was described in the *New York Times* Sunday Magazine, as follows:

Research evidence

Sixteen University of Georgia students were selected on the basis of their responses to a questionnaire on their moods. The questionnaire results revealed that the students were easily enraged or hypersensitive.

These easily-angered students were shown a sequence of slides which were deliberately designed to really annoy them. But they were in fact shown them at two different time intervals. One group of students had exercised *before* viewing the second set of slides, and the other group **hadn't**.

The group of students *who hadn't exercised* became angry when viewing the slides for a second time.

In contrast, the students who *had* exercised, before seeing the slides for a second time, kept the same level of emotional arousal and annoyance, and there was *no increase in their level of anger* when seeing the slides for a second time. The lead researcher, Nathaniel Thom, stated that: *"Exercise, even a single bout of it, can have a robust, prophylactic (therapeutic) effect against the build-up of anger."*

Thom reported that, when the students (meaning the study participants) didn't exercise, they were weak in the face of emotional provocation, and were unable to manage their anger. But after the exercise, the students were able to show calm self-assurance when confronted with the provocative, anger-arousing slides used in the experiment.

4.11: Depression and physical exercise

Finally, let us take a look at the effect of physical exercise on depression. It has long been a part of European common sense, and the philosophy of some major philosophers, that walking is a great cure for low moods and depressed feelings. But what about modern studies on this subject?

In relation to what is often called 'clinical depression', or 'major depression', it's apparent from the research findings reviewed in Taylor-Byrne and Byrne (2017) that exercise has an invaluable part to play in reducing and controlling these serious emotional disturbances. (We define 'clinical' or 'major' depression like this:

significantly debilitating levels of low mood and loss of pleasure in life, combined with low energy and often disrupted sleep, the effects of which can be devastating).

Research evidence

A key research study was undertaken by Blumenthal et al. (1999 and 2012).

The goal of the research project was to compare the effectiveness of exercise against an anti-depressant called Sertraline (which is called Lustral in the UK and Zoloft in the US). Sertraline is one of a group of drugs known as selective serotonin reuptake inhibitors (SSRI's).

Three groups of participants (156 people in total) were randomly assigned to three different research conditions.

- Group 1 received Zoloft for their depression.

- The second group were given exercise activities to do.

- And Group 3 was given a combination of Zoloft and exercise.

The results showed that all of the three groups showed a distinct lowering of their depression, and approximately half of each group had recovered from their depression by the time the research project had finished. (Thirteen percent had reduced symptoms but didn't completely recover).

Then six months later Blumenthal and colleagues examined the health of the research participants and found that, over the long haul:

#1. 30% of the exercise group remained depressed,

#2. 52% on medication remained depressed,

#3. while 55% in the combined treatment group remained depressed.

These three results mean that:

- *70% of the exercise group got over their symptoms of depression,*

- compared with *only 48% of the medication group,*

- and 45% of the combined group.

Let us repeat the most important part of that result:

70% of participants got over major depression through exercise alone!

A year later there was a second study, identical to the first one, and when the participants were reassessed a year later (by Hoffman and his colleagues), they found that, regardless of the treatment group the participants had been in, the participants who described doing regular exercise, after the research project had finished, were the least likely to be depressed a year later. And this study was about major depression – not mild depression!

The NHS in the UK, on their website, support the view that exercise is good for mild or moderate depression, but they don't clarify that it can also be invaluable for *major depression*, which was demonstrated by Blumenthal's 1999 and 2012 research findings.

In a very interesting book, *'Spark'*, (2009) - on the science of exercise and the brain – the authors, Ratey and Hagerman, comment upon the findings of Blumenthal's and Hoffman's research, like this:

> *"The results (of this research, showing the effectiveness of exercise in reducing depression) should be taught in medical schools and driven home with health insurance companies and posted on the bulletin boards of every nursing home in the country, where nearly half of the residents have depression"* (page 122).

However, this is not currently done, because the drug companies dominate the medical profession, with their delusion that antidepressants are highly effective, which they are not! Indeed, there is research evidence to support the view that most antidepressants tested against placebos are no more effective than the placebo (or sugary pill!)

4.12: Exercise for stress reduction

Dr Robert Sapolsky, who is a professor of biology, neuroscience and neurosurgery at Stanford University in America, has been studying stress management for many years and uses exercise as his favourite way to manage stress.

He points out that the value of keeping to an exercise regime, in addition to reducing your stress level, is this:

> *Whatever the type of exercise might be, when it is regularly practiced, it is very good for providing individuals with a sense of achievement and self-efficacy.*

In addition, he makes two key points:

> (1) The stress reducing benefits of exercise will **wear off** if they are not repeated; and:

> (2) If you do not want to exercise, but are **forced** to do it, then it won't help your health. It has to be **voluntary**, and **personally enjoyable**!

Sapolsky (2010) writes: *"Let rats run voluntarily on a running wheel and their health improves in all sorts of ways. Force them, even when playing great dance music, and their health worsens."* (Page 491)

Finally he recommends that you have a consistent, regular pattern for a prolonged period of time (a minimum of twenty to thirty minutes per session, several times a week) and that you don't overdo it (because it is possible to harm yourself while exercising. For example, by pulling a muscle. this is a particular problem with 'hard' [Western] exercise; and much less of a problem with 'soft' [Eastern] exercises, like yoga and Chi Kung).

4.13: Yoga and Chi Kung for emotional self-management

We wanted to look at specific approaches to physical exercise in our earlier book – (Taylor-Byrne and Byrne, 2017). Although brisk walking has been shown to reduce depression and anxiety symptoms, we wanted to look at some of the more formal systems which claim to help with emotional problems.

Therefore, we examined evidence about the value of Qigong (Chi Kung) and yoga, and found that they both have lots of evidence supporting their ability to help people manage anxiety, anger and depression. (See Taylor-Byrne and Byrne, 2017).

We also advocate the use of brisk walking, because it is so easy to do, and does not cost anything. We advise against jogging, especially on hard surfaces, because of the damage it does to knee joints.

Press ups and sit backs are a good way to strengthen arms and core muscles; and also to lift your mood. Swimming is a good form of general workout, which is good for body and mind.

Competitive sports tend to push up stress levels; but friendly games and sports can be fun and mood enhancing.

But in general, Eastern 'soft' exercise systems (like yoga and Chi Kung) have bigger up-side advantages, and smaller down-side disadvantages, than Western 'hard' exercise.

4.14: Summary of research on diet and exercise for mental health

Food for health and emotional well-being

In this summary, I have reviewed the reasons why food is vitally important for our physical and mental health. The evidence is clear: without a balanced range of nutritious foods of decent quality, our bodies and brains can't function properly in the long term. Some foods are toxic to the body-brain-mind, and some are enhancing of physical and mental health.

There are particular body and mind toxins being sold to us, as if there is nothing wrong with them: transfats, sugar, alcohol, caffeine, processed (junk) foods, and gluten, to take a few examples. Becoming aware of the effects of these toxins is crucially important, if we are to protect our physical health and emotional wellbeing. For example, anxiety, anger and depression are affected by the types of food we eat, and the liquids we consume.

The take away message from this examination of the causes of anxiety, anger and depression, is that the state of our bodies, our lifestyle, and the food and drink that we consume, contributes a great deal to our emotional state – positive or negative.

All those contributing factors need to be taken into account in the understanding and treatment of emotional and mental problems.

Exercise for health and emotional well-being

Part 2 of Taylor-Byrne and Byrne (2017) was about the relationship between physical exercise and emotional well-being and the power of exercise to reduce the incidence of anxiety, anger and depression. The effectiveness of exercise is demonstrated; the opinions of the NHS in the UK and the Mayo Clinic in America are referred to; and two forms of exercise which are highly rated (Chinese and Indian), are examined, and found to be beneficial.

Finally the recommendations of Robert Sapolsky (2010) are mentioned: the personal benefits to be gained from creating an exercise plan and sticking to it, (which includes a feeling of achievement and self-efficacy); the importance of a lack of outside coercion in relation to doing exercise (otherwise our health will deteriorate); and not to do too much of it.

The crucial well-being messages for you, the reader, are these:

1. Do not eat, drink and be merry; for tomorrow we may all be very much alive, but very, very ill!

2. Eat for health and happiness! Nutritious food, freshly prepared at home, can be very pleasurable, compared to processed junk foods.

3. To overcome anger, anxiety and depression: eat well; exercise often; and develop a good, calm, mindful philosophy of life. Get at least eight hours of sleep each night. And, take extremely good care of yourself!

4.15: Dr Jim's Stress and Anxiety Diet

In Part 3 of Taylor-Byrne and Byrne (2017), Dr Jim Byrne introduced his stress and anxiety diet. This came out of his years of struggling with the side-effects of *Candida Albicans* overgrowth, which include low energy and low mood, plus anxiety. He described how he used supplements and a particular diet to overcome those side effects, and to boost his mood and stabilize his emotions. The anti-Candida diet eliminates most sugar, yeast and fermented foods: (see Chaitow, 2003; Jacobs, 1994; and Trowbridge and Walker, 1989). But you still have to find a way to balance your consumption of protein, carbohydrates and fats.

From this experience of managing his own gut-brain-mind interactions, he was sensitized to any new research he came across, on any aspect of the body-brain-mind and emotions, and he passed this learning on to any of his counselling clients who showed an interest, or a need to know about it.

He then describes certain pieces of advice, from the Stress Management Society, and other authors; and from the Paleo, Nordic and Mediterranean diets; which can normally be expected to have a positive effect upon mood and emotions; but watch out for the down side of the Paleo diet, which may be too high in animal fats.

Some of his key recommendations included:

Don't skip breakfast; eat a balanced diet (which has to be established by trial and error); avoid sugar, caffeine, alcohol, gluten, and dairy products. (One cup of real coffee per day is probably okay; and one glass of wine every other day; but sugar and gluten should be avoided completely! Some theorists think we can get away with one or two junk food meals per week, but no more than that!)

Close to 70% percent of your diet should be in the form of low-sugar vegetables (and [gluten free] grains, and legumes, if you can tolerate them), with fibre intact; plus 10% in fats; 10% nuts and seeds; plus the remainder (of approximately 10%) in the form of meat, fish and alternative forms of protein (like tofu).

Try to eliminate all *processed* grains (e.g. white bread, white pasta, etc.), but keep whole grains (if you can healthily tolerate them!) at about 20% of your diet (and make sure they are gluten free). He also talks about the importance of adequate water consumption, meaning six to eight glasses per day of filtered tap water, or glass-bottled mineral water. Eating snacks (like nuts and seeds) mid-morning and mid-afternoon is also an important form of blood-sugar management.

Raw food is very important, because cooking kills so many nutrients. And organic vegetable are best, and should be emphasized ahead of fruit, because fruit sugars, taken in excess, can cause physical and emotional health problems. For some people, who are particularly sensitive to sugar, even vegetables have to be selected for low-sugar content (as described in the **Low FodMaps** diet). (Some people are fructose *intolerant*, and have to avoid it completely. While some are fructose *sensitive*, and have to *reduce its consumption*).

Jim recommends various supplements, especially vitamin B, C and E, for stress management; plus a good strong multivitamin supplement, with the full range of minerals.

The body needs every single nutrient known to science (according to Dr Leslie Korn, 2016).

One of the best ways to proceed is probably to take a good, complex multivitamin and mineral supplement every morning; plus magnesium, (400 iu's); plus a yeast-free B-complex tablet; and a couple or more grams of vitamin C powder in water per day.

Plus a natural source vitamin E capsule (400 iu's); plus omega-3 fatty acids (in the form of foods and supplements). Plus a *friendly bacteria* supplement, like **Acidophilus**, or preferably a multi-strain variety, in capsule form.

4.16: The science of nutritional deficiency and mental health

In Part 4 of Taylor-Byrne and Byrne (2017), Jim writes about old and new research on nutritional deficiencies, and what those studies have taught us about the effect of even single nutrient deficits on our physical health and our emotional states. (See also Kaplan and Crawford, et al [2007]; Kaplan and Rucklidge, et al [2015]; and Baker and Keramidas [2013]).

The most stunning findings were that, just as vitamin B3 deficiency causes the *psychosis of Pellagra*, more general nutritional deficiency causes a range of emotional problems, including depression, irritability, apathy, social withdrawal, hysteria and self-harm: (Baker and Keramidas, 2013).

Furthermore, depression is (or can be) linked to (meaning *caused by*) inflammation, which is also the main cause of most chronic physical diseases: (Kaplan, et al. 2015). And according to the Paleo diet theorists, all grains and dairy products, and legumes, cause inflammation.

Of course, a person on the Paleo diet - or other form of *grains and dairy exclusion*; who has little or no inflammation in their body - could still experience depression for psychological reasons, such as the loss of a child, a marriage partner, or a significant material loss, like a job. Or even a symbolic loss, like a sense of loss of *assumed* social status.

But much of the modern explosion of depression and anxiety may well be caused by inflammation in the guts, coming from junk food and other dietary mistakes!

And a lot of depression and anxiety is triggered specifically by *Candida Albicans* overgrowth in the large intestine. Dr Jeffrey McCombs (2014) recommends that people suffering from Candida overgrowth should eliminate all grains and dairy for a period of about eight weeks, and then add them back slowly and check the effects of both elimination and reintroduction. (But please make sure you get the help of a nutritional therapist with this task, to avoid subjecting yourself to the possibility of nutritional deficiencies, which could worsen your moods and emotional states!)

In addition, Dr Michael Greger (2016) has highlighted the problem with diets which contain too much omega-6 and too little omega-3 fatty acids. It seems omega-6 fatty acids cause inflammation, and a common source of this problem in America is too much grain-fed meat consumption. (This may also be on the increase in the UK).

Much of the current explosion in depression may be a result of over-consumption of omega-6 through red and white meaty diets. So largely vegetarian diets, with small amounts of Wild Alaskan salmon, plus nuts, seeds and perhaps organic eggs, might be a good way to go.

According to Dr Michael Greger, "*Higher consumption of vegetables may cut the odds of developing depression by as much as 62 percent*"[80].

And the China Study established that *people who ate the most vegetables were the healthiest*, while the people who ate the most meat were the least healthy. (Campbell and Campbell, 2006).

However, you have to find out for yourself, through trial and error, which foods suit your body-brain-mind; and perhaps you can get some help from a nutritional expert. (But always preserve your own judgement!)

The best way to do that is to try a new food, and write a food diary. Check one hour later for symptoms of the new food – mood changes; energy level changes; skin reactions. Check again 24 hours later, for the same symptoms. And again after 36 hours.

Or you can exclude a suspect food for a while, and keep a diary of any changes in symptoms whilst that food is excluded from your diet. Add it back after a couple of weeks, and monitor the results in your food diary. (And always check with a qualified nutritional therapist to make sure you do not harm yourself!)

~~~

Chapter 5: The impact of sleep on mental health and emotional wellbeing

By Renata Taylor-Byrne and Jim Byrne

~~~

5.1 Introduction

If you want to be able to stay in control of your anger, anxiety and depressive tendencies, under pressure, then you have to give a high priority to your sleep patterns, on a nightly basis.

What do the experts say about the impact of sleep disturbance, sleep loss, deprivation, or sleep insufficiency?

Firstly, according to Dr James Maas (1998), an early expert on sleep science, if you are getting less than eight hours of sleep each night, including at weekends, then you are one of the millions of chronically sleep-deprived individuals, who normally are unaware of how sleepy and ineffective they are, or how much more effective they could be, including emotionally, if they got enough sleep.

Later, Shawn Stevenson (2016) argued that every aspect of your mental, emotional and physical performance is affected by the quality of your sleep.

And just last year, Matthew Walker (2017) wrote that if you sleep less than six or seven hours a night as a regular habit-pattern, then this will destroy your immune system and double the likelihood of you developing cancer. It would make you more susceptible to the development of Alzheimer's disease, and if you had just one week of such reduced sleep, it would destabilise your blood sugar level to the extent that you could be diagnosed as pre-diabetic.

And of course, most sleep science commentators refer to the negative impact of sleep insufficiency on mood and emotions, including depression, anxiety and anger causation.

Indeed, Walker (2017) considers that sleep is the foundation upon which diet and exercise need to stand, if the whole system is to work well.

If you have an inadequate sleep pattern, this cannot be compensated for by good dietary and exercise practices!

~~~

In this chapter, we will look at the following subjects:

    Common sense ideas about sleep;

    Distractions from sleep;

    Problems caused by sleep insufficiency;

The benefits of sleep; and:

Insomnia and sleep insufficiency; as well as science-based, researched remedies for sleep problems.

5.2: The primary importance of sleep

In our earlier book on diet and exercise - Taylor-Byrne and Byrne (2017) - we presented a range of studies which show that human emotional disturbances are caused, or affected, for better or worse, by what we eat, and fail to eat; how we exercise, or fail to exercise; and we also referred in passing to sleep as another major factor in determining our mental health and emotional well-being.

This range of three major sources of good or poor mental health, and high or low levels of emotional well-being, are well documented in the scientific literature. (Lopresti, 2013).

And many theorists would say that sleep is *the most important* of these; followed by diet; and then exercise.

For example, as Walker (2017) points out, although it's not good for us to go without food and/or liquid for one day, we can fairly easily recover from that deprivation.

However, on the other hand, if we were to go without sleep for *one night*, it would have a significantly damaging effect on us, both mentally and physically. So this shows *the relatively greater need* for sleep sufficiency.

Walker goes on to say that: "I was once fond of saying, 'Sleep is the third pillar of good health, alongside diet and exercise'. I have changed my tune. Sleep is more than a pillar. It is the foundation on which the other two health bastions sit." (Walker, 2017. Page 164).

This lines up with the views of Professor Colin Espie[81], who wrote that:

> "Alongside eating and breathing, sleep is one of the fundamentals of life, and arguably the most important – you could survive for three times as long without food as you could without sleep, and 17 hours without sleep produces performance impairments equivalent to 2 alcoholic drinks."

If you do not sort out your sleep hygiene, it is unlikely you will be able to greatly improve your sense of emotional wellbeing, and mental health, by diet and exercise alone.

If you fix your sleep, but fail to improve your diet and nutrition, it is unlikely you will be able to make up the deficit via exercise alone.

So we have to take sleep very seriously, followed by diet and exercise, if we want to be happy, healthy and emotionally well.

5.3: Common sense views of sleep

William Shakespeare, in his play, *Macbeth*, expressed a profound truth when he declared that, "'Tis sleep that knits the ravelled sleeve of care!'" And we have always taken this to mean that the cares and worries of the day are resolved by a good night's sleep, as a *sleeve* is fixed by *darning* or re-knitting. Some people have contested this simple interpretation, and insisted that the word intended here was 'sleave' of care, and not 'sleeve' of care; where 'sleave' is a bunch of silk filaments as worked by silkworkers. (McGuinness, 2013).

Macbeth's mind is not just unravelled, but knotted and tangled, with a web of difficult emotions, like a tangled knot of silk filaments, and it's a good night's sleep, according to Shakespeare, which will help to unknot those emotions, and sort them out in order to present a viable resolution.

"Sleep brings to order this bundle of emotions as the hand of a silkworker unravels a tangled sheaf of sleave-silk." (McGuinness, 2013).

To be clear, a 'sleave', in silk work, as a noun, is defined like this: "...a filament of silk obtained by separating a thicker thread." Hence, sleep is represented as untangling the strands of our day which have become tangled, and especially those which are emotionally charged, stressful and difficult to process. Thus Shakespeare is saying that sleep helps to sort out our stresses and strains, and makes sense of our days.

Surprisingly, as we will see later, sleep is not just about sorting out thoughts and feelings, but includes a physical and hormonal tidying up of the brain's structure. Indeed, as Matthew Walker (2017) points out, Shakespeare knew that sleep "...is 'the chief nourisher in life's feast'." (Page 108 of Walker, 2017).

Shakespeare was not the only great artist who studied the effects of sleep on the mind.

According to John Steinbeck, the American author of the novel, *The Grapes of Wrath*:

> "It is a common experience that a problem difficult at night is resolved in the morning after the committee of sleep has worked on it."

The sleeping brain has an enormous capacity to resolve the stresses and strains of competing demands of a too-busy day. And, as it turns out, it also helps to prepare the brain-mind for the day ahead.

Another famous American author, Ernest Hemingway found that sleep was the best time of his life, and his waking hours were more difficult:

> "I love sleep", he wrote. "My life has the tendency to fall apart when I'm awake, you know?"

Of course, we are not advocating 'escape into sleep'. Rather, we advise our clients to make sure they get at least eight or nine hours sleep, of good quality, every night, so that they have the best chance of processing the experiences of the preceding day, and preparing for the stresses and strains of the following day.

And this recommendation is backed up by scientific studies, as well as common sense, as we will see below.

5.4: Distractions from sleep

Many people allow themselves to become distracted from the need to sleep. They may be ambitious, and spend too many hours working. To them, we give the advice that they should follow the 8-8-8 rule:

- Do eight hours work;

- have eight hours rest (sleep);

- and divide the remaining eight hours between play and self-care activities, like shopping, cooking, dining, conversing with family and friends, and so on.

This balance will ensure that their working hours are *optimally productive*, and that their health will be sustained for *long-term productivity*.

Over-working may seem productive in the short-term, but will most often prove to undermine physical health and emotional wellbeing in the longer term; and it is *actually* less productive in the here and now (because our 'saw blade' of mind becomes dulled; and needs rest and sleep to sharpen it!)

When people of the authors' generation were growing up (in the 1950's and '60's), there were very few distractions from going to bed when it got dark. The public houses closed at an early hour (about 10.30 pm on a week night). The three available TV stations (in the UK) closed down at about 11.00 pm. And there was still a residual awareness that it is important to get eight hours sleep, if you wanted to feel well and fit and happy the next morning. This was also an era of (relatively) full employment, and so most people needed to get up early each morning, to go to work in factories, offices, transport systems, hospitals, and, to a lesser extent, shops.

Today, all of this has changed.

Now we have 24-hour cities, where the bars never close.

TV stations broadcast around the clock. And, even if there is nothing worth watching on TV, the Internet narrow-casts lots of seductive material in the form of videos and blogs, and chat rooms.

And then there's the *ping* of incoming emails. And the *ping* of instant messages to mobile phones.

And the TV screen and the computer screen and the mobile phone screen have all found their way into too many bedrooms; distracting people from sleep. Indeed, the *blue light* from those devices – which is short-wavelength light – is twice at powerful at suppressing the release of melatonin as ordinary incandescent light bulbs. And when melatonin levels are too low, it is very difficult or near impossible to sleep.

So, at the very least, people who are overexposed to blue light before bedtime, or who have blue light devices in their bedrooms at bedtime, lie awake in their beds for a long time before getting to sleep. This is called 'sleep onset insomnia'.

Melatonin is a hormone which is secreted in response to the failing daylight, and normally switches on around 9.00 pm. But is can be delayed by over-exposure to artificial lighting, especially blue light from LED's. Simply reading an iPad at night can inhibit the release of melatonin by 50%. The consequences? It takes much longer to fall asleep, (because our body-brain-mind has to wait while the melatonin level is built up again); and this sleep disruption affects your level of energy, your mood, and alertness, the following day; as well as your longer term biologically-programmed sleep rhythms.

Furthermore, consuming alcohol or sugary foods before bed tends to produce a feeling of tiredness, initially; but a few hours later it causes a surge of stress hormones, which wakes the sleeper up, to a night of insomnia, or broken sleep.

And too much caffeine (more than one or two cups of coffee) during the day, can rob us of the capacity to easily fall asleep when we do go to bed.

5.5: Problems of sleep insufficency

Why we need sleep

The science of sleep suggests that, while you are asleep, your body is busy:

- detoxifying itself, including getting rid of waste products, resulting from stress and strain during your waking hours;

- repairing tissues;

- and also balancing or rebalancing your hormones.

These various biochemical processes are so complex that it is not difficult to see how things might go badly wrong if the body does not have enough time to do this repair and maintenance work.

Insufficient repair and recovery work could "...impact emotional regulation, memory, mood, and other factors..." (Osmun, 2015).

And, according to Mauss, Troy, and LeBourgeois (2013), who tested hypotheses linking poor quality sleep and poor quality of emotional self-regulation, in a laboratory setting:

> "Participants with poorer self-reported sleep quality exhibited lower CRA (or cognitive reappraisal ability [or ability to *re-think* or *emotionally reframe* a problem – Eds.]), even after controlling for fourteen potential key

confounds (e.g., age, negative affect, mood disorder symptoms, stress). This finding is consistent with the idea that *poorer sleep quality impairs individuals' ability to engage in the crucial task of **regulating negative emotions**.*"

According to Strine and Chapman (2005), about 26% of (American) adults get insufficient sleep, on at least 14 days out of 30.

This lack of sleep has a negative impact on "...general health, frequent physical distress, frequent mental distress, activity limitations, depressive symptoms, anxiety, and pain": (Strine and Chapman, 2005).

These authors also found that once sleep had been lost in this way, this led on to a higher likelihood of use of tobacco, lack of physical exercise, obesity, and (among men) heavy drinking of alcohol.

And Osmun (2015), having reviewed a significant slice of the scientific research on sleep, concluded that

"...the research makes a strong case for getting a good night's sleep on a regular basis, but particularly before reacting to emotional events or making difficult decisions."

~~~

How much we need, and the effects of not getting it

So, people often get insufficient sleep because of all the *distractions* (which encourage them to stay up too late); *pressures* to over-work, which come from the poor state of the Anglo-American economic system, and over-ambition; and *disruptions* like caffeine, alcohol, and computers, phones, TVs and so on, in the bedroom.

Furthermore, as James Maas (1998) pointed out, people tend to overestimate the amount of sleep they are getting, and many who think they are getting seven hours - (which is one or two full hours less than their [normal] minimum need for healthy living) – are actually getting closer to six hours, which is woefully inadequate.

Most adults need between 7.5 and 9 hours of sleep per night to be happy, healthy, emotionally well and successful, according to Dr Maas (1998).

Matthew Walker (2017) whose scientific research is more up to date, would put that figure higher, at 8 to 9 hours. And people in the 16-24 age range need nine or more hours of sleep each night to ensure reasonable cognitive functioning during the following day.

Daytime exhaustion, cognitive fog, physically illness, irritability, anxiety and depression can be expected to follow from repeated episodes of sleep deprivation. (Sources: Walker, 2017; Maas, 1998; and Stevenson, 2016).

~~~

Seven major negative results of sleep insufficiency

What are some of the effects of not getting enough sleep? According to Strine and Chapman (2005):

> "Sleep-related problems, which affect 50-70 million Americans, involve all areas of life, including cognitive performance, emotional well-being, work and leisure-time activities, and general physical and mental well-being".

And the range of research studies that we have reviewed suggest that you can expect some or all of the following:

1. Your emotional intelligence will be reduced. Here are three studies that support this conclusion:

Firstly, Walker (2017) conducted an experiment in his sleep lab, to show how the lack of sleep affects people's emotional intelligence.

He took two groups of people and placed them under two different experimental conditions:

- One group had a full night's sleep, and

- the other group had insufficient sleep.

Both groups were then were then (separately) shown a range of pictures of individual human faces, which displayed a wide range of emotions, varying from friendliness through to intense dislike and anger. The participants had to individually assess this range of facial expressions, to decide if they were displaying threatening or friendly messages. While they were engaged in this activity, their brains were being scanned in a Magnetic Resonance Imaging (MRI) machine.[82]

The results of Walker's experiments were as follows:

- If participants had had a good night's sleep beforehand, then they had no difficulty in distinguishing facial expressions ranging from hostility through to benevolence. Their assessments (spoken, and neurological, confirmed by the MRI scans) – unlike those of the sleep deprived condition - were accurate, showing that the quality of their sleep had helped them in their reading of facial expressions.

- But in the sleep deprived condition, participants found it much harder to differentiate between the facial expressions displayed on the faces in the range of pictures shown to them. This clearly has huge implications for emotionally intelligent function in our personal and professional lives.

Secondly, Gordon (2013) states that

> "...people who are more sleep deprived report feeling *less friendly, elated, empathic,* and report a *generally lower positive mood*".

This report shows that one bad night of sleep can have a negative effect upon moods and emotions. Again, this will affect that aspect of emotional intelligence which allows you to read and manage your own emotions. And when we fail to manage our emotions well, there is often damage done to our relationships at home and in work or business.

And, ***third***, (and finally), inadequate sleep, in terms of quality and/or quantity, was found to reduce research participants' ability (in laboratory experiments) to regulate their negative emotions (Osmun, 2015; and Mauss, Troy, and LeBourgeois, 2013).

This occurs because lack of sleep reduces our ability to brush off intrusive negative thoughts, which then become worry and preoccupation, which interfere with our ability to manage our emotional encounters with others.

~~~

2. Your concentration will be negatively affected. In an online blog, Dr Simon Kyle summarizes several research studies that show a definite link between inadequate sleep and problems concentrating on essential tasks. He summarises the results like this: "...increased sleepiness and fatigue are associated with the inability to concentrate or 'think clearly'. Indeed, along with impaired energy/fatigue and mood, concentration is one of the most common daytime issues reported by patients with insomnia disorder – this is what was found in *the recent Great British Sleep Survey*. This inability to concentrate might reflect an issue with sustained attention or shifting attention. In studies where sleep-deprived subjects have been tested after sleep loss, it is commonly the case that they will take longer to respond to a stimulus that appears on the screen (and experience more attentional lapses; failing to respond within a certain time interval). A study in insomnia patients found that a complex attention task – where subjects had to respond on a computer screen to the letter 'p' but not the letter 'd' – revealed impairments in reaction time to making this judgment." (Kyle, 2018).

~~~

3. Lack of sleep can lead to depression, sometimes as the main cause, but often combined with other causes, such as lack of physical activity, and/or poor diet. (Strine and Chapman, 2005; Kyle, 2018).

According to Asp (2015):

"Not getting enough restful sleep can affect your emotional health. In other words, a chronic lack of sleep can cause depression. Although it is unlikely that lack of sleep alone can be the sole cause of depression, it combined with other factors can trigger depression in some people. Links between depression and lack of sleep have been commonly found in studies".

Other studies have linked lack of sleep to depression and anxiety, via the mechanism of intrusive, repetitive thoughts, and a lack of ability to disengage from negative stimuli. (Coles, 2018).

Dr Simon Kyle draws attention to the Great British Sleep Survey's conclusion that lack of sleep leads to low mood: "Emotionally, we may find ourselves more irritable and lower in mood, as a result of poor or insufficient sleep. Research has consistently found that sleep deprived people show less stable patterns of behaviour and are more likely to be emotionally labile. Indeed, the Great British Sleep Survey revealed those suffering from insufficient sleep *were **twice** as likely to suffer from low mood* as those who sleep well."

Of course, the other side of the equation is this: When you become depressed, this can further disrupt your sleep. You may find you have difficulty getting to sleep; staying asleep; or that you wake up in the early morning feeling tired.

~~~

4. Sleep loss can lead to anxiety: According to researchers at the University of California, at Berkley, sleep loss increases feelings of anxiety, especially among individuals who are prone to worry. (Nauert, 2018). The Berkley research report begins like this:

> "UC Berkeley researchers have found that a lack of sleep, which is common in anxiety disorders, may play a key role in ramping up the brain regions that contribute to excessive worrying."

> "Neuroscientists have found that sleep deprivation amplifies anticipatory anxiety by firing up the brain's amygdala and insular cortex, regions associated with emotional processing. The resulting pattern mimics the abnormal neural activity seen in anxiety disorders." (Anwar, 2013).

The researchers also suggest that if you can fix your sleep problems, you can also reduce your anxiety conditions.

~~~

5. Anger problems can also be linked to inadequate sleep. According to Gordon (2013):

> "Both correlational and experimental ... evidence suggest that when people are sleep deprived, they feel more ***irritable, angry*** and ***hostile***".

Like other emotional problems, the causation of anger tends to be multi-factorial; it comes from many supplementary sources; like diet, exercise, sleep deprivation; and poor stress management in general. A blog post by 'My-Sahana' cites nine sources of anger-including problems, of which lack of sleep is one:

> "Not sleeping enough can result in feeling edgy and easily irritable. Chronic insomnia, sleep apnoea or other sleep disorders can be linked to recurrent bouts of anger". My-Sahana (2012).

~~~

6. **Inadequate sleep is linked to physical illnesses**, including heart disease, cancer and other physical illnesses.

According to the NHS Choices (UK) website, lack of sleep affects physical health as much as emotional wellbeing:

> "Many effects of a lack of sleep, such as feeling grumpy and not working at your best, are well known. But did you know that sleep deprivation can also have profound consequences on your physical health?"

The bottom line of their statement was this:

> "Regular poor sleep puts you at risk of serious medical conditions, including obesity, heart disease and diabetes – and it shortens your life expectancy." (See NHS Choices, 2015)[83].

~~~

7. **Insufficient sleep can also cause early death**, as suggested above by NHS Choices (2015). This finding is corroborated by one meta-analysis, in the UK and Italy, which analysed 16 studies involving a total of 1.3 million people, before reaching this conclusion:

> *"People who sleep fewer than six hours a night are more likely to die early"*. (Cited in an article by Rebecca Smith, medical editor of *The Telegraph*. See Smith, 2010).

5.6: Famous cases of sleep-deprived individuals and the negative consequences

We spent a little time exploring famous cases of sleep-deprived individuals who, as a consequence, did not manage their emotional lives very well; or who damaged their brains in the process.

The first possibility that came to mind was Sylvia Plath. She famously wrote this:

> *"I wonder why I don't go to bed and go to sleep. But then it would be tomorrow, so I decide that no matter how tired, no matter how incoherent I am, I can skip one hour more of sleep and live."* (The Unabridged Journals of Sylvia Plath).

Perhaps the fact that she did not live beyond the age of **thirty years** was, to some degree, linked to her skipping of 'one more hour of sleep'!?!

Rihanna - the famous pop singer – made public statements about her difficulty resting after touring in 2011, mentioning getting less than 3 hours a night for several weeks. And then again, she has great difficulty controlling her body weight, which swings up and down dramatically. She may be *comfort eating* to compensate for her lack of sleep.

A famous American baseball player - David Ortiz – who plays for the *Boston Red Sox* - reported difficulty turning his mind off and getting to sleep. Later, this lack of sleep was blamed for a massive slide in his sporting performance.

Jay Leno – the host of the American TV hit, 'The Late Show' - broadcast the news in 2007 that he sleeps about five hours per night. And he got away with it for years. But then, in 2009, he suddenly missed two shows. He admitted suffering from *exhaustion*. (Surprise, surprise!) And now (in 2018) Leno is 67 years old, and just as committed to *overworking* as always. But the scientific research shows that he will have shortened his life expectancy, reduced his happiness and emotional intelligence, reduced his capacity to concentrate, risked physical disease, and lowered his quality of life by skimping on sleep in order to overwork.

Then there are the cases of Margaret Thatcher and Ronald Reagan, both of whom skimped on their sleep, and both of whom ended up *losing their brain-minds to Alzheimer's disease!*

And now, Donald Trump announces that his long-term success is based on the fact that he only sleeps for five hours per night! Enough said! But is it actually true that his sleeplessness made him successful? This is a highly questionable assertion, given the number of *business failures* he has experienced. One of the most famous was Trump Airlines. According to Jacob Koffler, on the *Time* blog:

"**Trump Airlines:** In 1988, Trump bought Eastern Air Shuttle, an airline service that ran hourly flights between Boston, NYC and DC for 27 years prior, for $365 million. He turned the airline, once a no frills operation, into a luxury experience, adding maple-wood veneer to the floor and gold-coloured bathroom fixtures. The company never turned a profit and the high debt forced him to default on his loans. Ownership of the company was turned over to creditors. It ceased to exist in 1992". (Koffler, 2015).

Looking through the blog post by Koffler (2015), it looks to us as though the following businesses were Trump failures:

- Trump Airlines; Trump Vodka; Trump Casinos (which apparently filed for bankruptcy four times!);

- Trump: The Game (a board game, which lasted one year);

- Trump Steaks (Lasted a few years. According to Koffler: "The company has since been discontinued — maybe it had something to do with the Trump Steakhouse in Las Vegas being closed down in 2012 for 51 health code violations, including serving five-month old duck.").

- Trump Magazine (lasted just 18 months);

- GoTrump.com, a travel search engine (lasted one year);

- Trump University (ended badly);

- Trump Mortgage (lasted one and a half years).

That makes 9 major failures.

And what about the successes:

+ The Grand Hyatt Hotel;

+ Trump Tower;

+ Wollman Rink;

+ No. 40 Wall Street;

+ Trump Place;

+ The Apprentice (TV show);

+ Trump International Tower Chicago.

That makes seven impressive successes.

So **nine** major failures, and **seven** impressive successes.

Not a great balance to achieve by somebody who goes for just 5 hours sleep per night!

A bit more sleep might have helped his business decisions. And his lack of sleep will have caused him a loss of longevity, poor mood control, and reduced emotional intelligence! (Who would have guessed it?!)

5.7: The benefits of sleep

Scientific research and traditional wisdom confirm the following benefits of a good night's sleep:

Benefit # 1. Increased capacity to cope with stress and strain.

One report concluded:

"...consistent sleep may serve as an effective strain intervention, thereby preventing negative acute and chronic health effects." (Barber and colleagues, 2009).

And Osmun (2015) reports on scientific research which shows that subjects responded to emotional experiences less reactively after a good night's sleep (Van der Helm, et al. 2011).

Osmun (2015) also argues that "sleep plays a protective role in emotional processing", based on research by Van der Helm and Walker, (2009); in which they "...survey an array of diverse findings across basic and clinical research domains, resulting in *a convergent view of sleep-dependent emotional brain processing*."

And it is not without significance that Van der Helm and Walker (2009) titled their article: *Overnight Therapy? The Role of Sleep in Emotional Brain Processing*. For it seems sleep had significant therapeutic effects upon the emotional centres of the brain.

~~~

Benefit #2. Deep sleep improves emotional intelligence, making it easier for us to read other people and to manage our own emotions. One significant study, in which Matthew Walker was the lead researcher, found that "...quality sleep matters. The deeper the sleep, particularly REM sleep, the better you'll be able to assess the emotions of those around you." (Source: The Brain Flux blog, 2008).

~~~

Benefit #3. Willpower and self-control are also affected by quality of sleep, though the research in this area is not as well developed as we would like. One significant study - by Pilcher, Morris, Donnelly and Feigl (2015) - at Clemson University, Department of Psychology, came up with this conclusion:

> "Good sleep habits and effective self-control are important components of successful functioning. Unfortunately chronic sleep loss and impaired self-control are common occurrences for many individuals which can lead to difficulty with daily self-control issues such as resisting impulses and maintaining attentive behaviour. Understanding how self-control is depleted and how good sleep habits may help replenish and maintain the capacity for self-control is an important issue. A sleep-deprived individual who has expended the necessary resources for self-control is at an increased risk for succumbing to impulsive desires, poor attentional capacity, and compromised decision making." (Pilcher and colleagues, 2015).

~~~

Benefit #4. Better mood control, through the capacity to read social situations, and to manage repetitive thoughts, and to change significant appraisals of distracting concerns.

~~~

Benefit #5. Reduced tendencies towards anxiety and depression.

- **Firstly**, let's look at anxiety. According to Calm-Clinic online:

> "It's said so often it has become cliché, but the truth is that the mind and body are genuinely connected. The way your body feels affects the way your mind feels, and vice versa. ... That's why *one of the most important tools for fighting anxiety is sleep*, and that's also why not getting enough sleep for multiple days in a row also known as 'sleep debt' can be a serious problem for those living with anxiety and anxiety disorders". (Calm-Clinic, 2018)[84].

- **Secondly**, on the link between sleep-debt (or cumulative sleep loss or insufficiency), according to the National Sleep Foundation (USA):

> "The relationship between sleep and depressive illness is complex – depression may cause sleep problems and sleep problems may cause or contribute to depressive disorders. For some people, symptoms of depression occur before the onset of sleep problems. For others, sleep problems appear first. Sleep problems and depression may also share risk factors and biological features and the two conditions may respond to some of the same treatment strategies. Sleep problems are also associated with more severe depressive illness." (NSF, 2018)[85]

~~~

Benefit #6. Better physical health. As argued by NHS choices (2015), better health is linked to good quality and quantity of sleep; and inadequate sleep leads to major physical diseases.

~~~

Benefit #7. More enjoyment of life. In her blog, titled **Happier**, Nataly Kogan writes about, 'The magic of a good night's sleep: Because an exhausted person is never a happy person'.

Here are two brief extracts:

> "Even though most of us don't get nearly enough sleep these days, everyone knows that sleep is important: human beings need sleep to live and function. But what a lot of people don't know or misunderstand about sleep is how important it is to our overall sense of happiness and wellbeing.
>
> ...
>
> "Even when people describe their own levels of happiness, being well-rested comes out on top. Researchers Daniel Kahneman and Alan B. Krueger found in their research on life satisfaction a direct correlation between sleep quality and overall happiness. In fact, they found sleep quality was the single most influential factor in rating daily mood, too. A recent Gallup poll got the same results: people who get adequate sleep are more likely to rate their lives as happier." (Kogan, 2018)[86].

5.8: Insomnia: the curse of sleeplessness, and how to treat it

Some people, who know that sleep is a wonderful part of life, still have difficulty achieving it. For example, in David Benioff's novel, *City of Thieves*, we read this:

> "I've always envied people who sleep easily. Their brains must be cleaner,

the floorboards of the skull well swept, all the little monsters closed up in a steamer trunk at the foot of the bed."

And traditional Irish wisdom teaches us that "A good laugh and a long sleep are the two best cures for any problem."

Insomnia is a growing problem in the Anglo-American world, due to the pressures of neoliberal economic policy, and growing inequality, and intensified exploitation of workers at every level. Insomnia is defined at the inability to fall asleep, in the first ten or twenty minutes of being in bed. It can also include the tendency to wake up again, a couple of hours after going to bed.

Sleeplessness is a horrible place to be. Not only will it rob you of the peace and happiness of a gentle tomorrow; but it's torture to endure.

As Emil Cioran writes: "Insomnia is a vertiginous lucidity that can convert paradise itself into a place of torture."

Or, as Jessamyn West expresses it: "Sleeplessness is a desert without vegetation or inhabitants."

As early as 1998, Dr James Maas, an American sleep expert, wrote that

> "About 70% of the (American) people are not sleeping well for at least one or two nights each week".

Similar statements have been made about the British population, and sleep problems have most likely worsened on both sides of the Atlantic since that time.

Why is this a problem? As we saw above, at the very least, lack of adequate sleep will reduce your emotional intelligence, reduce your effectiveness in the world, and render you less dynamic than you could be. And you will be less happy, and prone to depression and other emotional disorders. It is widely recognized that, unless you get enough rest and sleep, you will tend to be irritable and anxious. (Wagner, 1996).

In working with insomnia, and general sleep hygiene, with our counselling clients, we tend to offer the following advice:

1. Make sure you get plenty of physical exercise and you breathe in good quality air during each day. And make sure you get out in direct sunlight for at least one full hour each day during the summer time, and two or more hours in the winter.

2. Eat a healthy diet, which omits most caffeine, all gluten, and keep your sugar and processed carb consumption low. Eat complex carbs, as in vegetables and gluten-free grains, with a small amount of protein.

3. Avoid stimulants, like caffeine, nicotine, chocolate, or sugary foods, from 12.00 noon onwards. These stimulants are likely to keep you awake. Also, do not eat large meals before bedtime. You should breakfast like a king (or queen); lunch like a prince

(or princess); and have a modest evening meal. Some experts recommend mixing protein and carbs at breakfast time (such as eggs on toast); lunch based on protein and salad (or cooked) vegetables; and evening meal based on carbohydrate with salad (or cooked) vegetables. The carbohydrate will tend to make you feel relaxed and tired enough to sleep.

4. Manage your bedroom sleeping space, so it is calm, cool (but not cold), private, and relatively dark.

5. Pick a time for bed which is at least nine hours before you have to get up for work; and strive to always go to bed at that time, even at the weekends (with a few, rare exceptions!)

6. Invest in a good quality mattress, which should be firm enough to support you, but not so hard as to be uncomfortable.

7. Wind down in preparation for bed. Do not do any vigorous activity in the hour before your bedtime. But do make sure you do vigorous exercise most days of the week, well before bedtime: such as first thing in the morning; or walk home after work; or go swimming in your lunch break.

8. If your insomnia is particularly bad, take a warm bath before bedtime. And/or meditate about an hour before bedtime. And/or have an audio relaxation CD on an audio machine by your bed, and listen to it while you fall asleep. We recommend some of the relaxation CDs by Paul McKenna and/or Glenn Harrold.

9. Get in the habit of writing out your problems in a diary, journal or notebook, about one hour before bedtime: (as described by Hubbard, 2018, reporting on the research report by Scullin, and Krueger et al, 2018). Our advice, based on this research, and earlier research, is this: Make a written plan to fix your problems, and then let them go. Before bedtime tonight, write down the main activities you need to engage in tomorrow, and then your mind will be cleared of those things you could have ended up mulling over in bed.

10. If you can't get to sleep, after 30 minutes in bed, get up and read something relaxing, until you feel tired enough to sleep.

11. Do not get up early just because you wake up early. Aim to get at least eight or nine hours of restful sleep every night. Stay in bed until you've got your healthy allocation of sleep.

~~~

Additionally, Wagner (1996) recommends that you pay attention to your consumption of vitamins B complex and vitamin C. B6 is particularly important, it seems, because it is implicated in converting tryptophan to serotonin, the neurotransmitter that many theorists believe promotes normal sleep. We teach our clients that they need to take regular supplements of particular vitamins to control their stress level. These include:

- Vitamin B complex.

- Vitamin E, natural source – 400 iu strength.

- Vitamin C powder – 2,000 to 3,000 mgs per day, minimum.

(You can always check these recommendations with a nutritional therapist, or your preferred medical practitioner).

You may also benefit from an extra strong magnesium supplement, of 500 mg, three times per day. (Wagner, 1996).

You could also drink camomile tea from lunchtime onwards; and have an infusion of valerian and hops before bedtime; or *kava kava*.

Do not take sleeping pills, as they will destroy the quality of whatever sleep you do get, by disrupting your REM sleep. And in any case, drinking tart cherry juice, from the Montmorency cherry, is much more effective at boosting your melatonin levels, which are necessary for sleep to occur. (See Howatson *et al*, 2012).

Finally, develop a good, positive, flexible philosophy of life, which includes the idea that there are only certain things you can control; and you have to give up trying to control the uncontrollable. (See the *Six Windows Model* in Chapter 6, below).

~~~

Or how to integrate nutritional insights, exercise and sleep coaching into talk therapy

Chapter 6: Reframing experiences with the Six Windows Model

6.1: Introduction

We begin from the position that our counselling clients are largely *feeling* beings; and indeed, *habit-based feeling beings*; who mainly operate from the emotional, non-conscious right side of their brain. We therefore set out to provide a warm, accepting relationship for our clients, in which we help them to regulate their feelings and moods, by a mixture of emotive and cognitive strategies.

In this chapter, I want to present one of the main *cognitive strategies* that we use to help clients to *rethink* their problems in a way which will empower them.

We emotive-cognitive (E-CENT) counsellors normally utilize a range of models to conceptualize and manage various stages in the counselling process. (See Chapter 8 below).

For example, the simplest model is the EFR model, which looks like this:

E = Event = What happened (or what happens)?

F = Framing = The client has a non-conscious, habitual way of 'framing' that Event, so that it shows up in some predictable form: (good or bad; manageable or overwhelming; etc.)

R = Response = The client feels and acts upon a characteristic emotional response to the framed-event (which could be with anger, fear, sadness, depression, etc.)

(A frame may be thought of as being like a *tinted lens*, which tints whatever is perceived through it. A frame is a predisposing way of seeing things).

The EFR model differs from the ABC model of rational and cognitive therapy (REBT/CBT) in that the F (or framing) is *always* non-conscious, spontaneous, habit-based, and emotional. The client is not assumed to 'chose' the frame they use; nor are they blamed (implicitly or explicitly) for being wired up (currently) with their particular range of frames. Those frames which colour their perceptions:

(1) are *products of their* **socialization**;

(2) can be changed, with effort, over time;

(3) but cannot be other than they are right now!

The EFR model is normally used in conjunction with the Holistic-SOR model which is shown in Figure 6.1(a) on the next page. This Holistic-SOR model is used to teach the client that *everything* that affects them as an organism (O) – like sleep, diet, exercise, stress and strain - also affects their emotional and behaviour responses (R) to noxious stimuli (S - or negative experiences).

However, in this chapter I mainly want to introduce *the Six Windows Model*. This is our most original model, though it is not as central as the Holistic-SOR model. Although it is not as central as the Holistic-SOR model, the Six Windows model requires more space and time to explain and illustrate the six key perspectives involved. Hence the need for its own chapter.

6.1(a) Context:

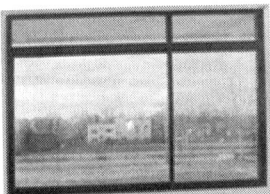

The Six Windows Model is applied in the context of having assessed the client's overall state of body-mind, (using the Holistic-SOR checklist, in Column 2 below). It is only used when it has been decided that it would be *most helpful* to focus upon re-thinking, or re-framing, at this time (as opposed to diet, sleep, exercise, etc., which would be dealt with later, or which have already been dealt with). The concept of *'re-framing'* is defined as meaning *'changing the lens through which the client views the problem'*. And this can often (though not always, or easily) help the client to reduce the intensity of their felt emotional response to a noxious stimulus.

The Holistic Stimulus-Organism-Response Model (H-SOR)		
Column 1	Column 2	Column 3
S = Stimulus	O = Organism	R = Response
When something significant happens, which is apprehended by the organism's (or person's) nervous system, the organism is activated or aroused (positively or negatively)	The organism responds, well or badly. The incoming stimulus may activate or interact with: (1) Innate needs and tendencies; (2) Family history and attachment style; (3) Recent personal history; (4) Emotive-cognitive schemas (as guides to action); (5) Narratives, stories, frames and other storied elements (which may be hyper-activating, hypo-activating, or affect regulating); (6) Character and temperament; (7) Need satisfaction; goals and values; (8) Diet and supplementation, medication, exercise regime, sleep and relaxation histories; (9) Ongoing environmental stressors, state of current relationship(s), and satisfaction with life stages, etc., etc.	The organism outputs a response, in the form of visible behaviour and inferable emotional reactions, like anger, anxiety, depression, embarrassment, etc.

Figure 6.1(a): The E-CENT holistic SOR model

However, for us, there is a tension here between *two* processes, which are labelled (1) 'completion', and (2) 'reframing'.

The first of these processes calls for a 'digestion', or 'completion', of a previously denied, repressed or rejected experience. This involves the client being taught that experiences which **they could not tolerate (emotionally)** when they were younger, including those experienced when they were a small child, can **most likely** now be tolerated and faced up to, with the support of their therapist: (Byrne, 2011)[87].

However, having looked at the *ethics* of this situation, we decided that it is important to teach the client how to **re-frame** their experiences, in general, **before** we help them to dig up and confront particularly difficult material which was previously denied!

The rationale for this approach is that the client only needs a brief exposure to traumatic memories in order to complete the experience, but then they need to quickly re-frame it as being less traumatic than it previously seemed. Otherwise they are in danger of simply *re-traumatizing themselves*, by re-living the original experience *with the old,* **child-created** *emotional-interpretations*. This would almost certainly seem devastating and over-whelming, alarming and panicking, or deeply depressing to the client.

However, with a (previously established) good working knowledge of the Six Windows model, the client can *quickly re-frame* the old, painful experience as being *less significant* than it once seemed.

6.1(b) Elaboration of the theory:

In E-CENT theory, we see the limbic system – or emotional centres of the brain-mind - (including the orbitofrontal cortex) - as the central controller and integrator of the information flows from

(1) the neo-cortex (or higher order mentation in the outer brain);

(2) the body (muscles, heart, guts, face, etc. – coming up through the brainstem); and

(3) socio-emotional incoming information (through sight and sound, touch, etc. (Hill, 2015).

Much of our work is involved in helping to integrate right-brain emotional states with left-brain language-derived mentation.

And the Six Windows Model is one of our best tools for this job of integration.

6.1(c) Re-framing:

Human beings are largely delusional beings, who think they are looking out through their eyes, and seeing what is "there to be seen". This is called "naïve realism", because it ignores the extent to which we *construct* what we see.

We do not see with our eyes so much as with our brains. (Of course, this does not mean that 'everything is relative' to our individual viewpoint. We are *social* animals, *socialized into family and communal stories*; and 'official' stories via the TV, schools, books, newspapers, plays, and daily conversations).

Eyes are part of the machinery of perception, but the decisions - about 'what it is' that we see - are not made by our eyes. Those decisions are made by our *stored social experiences* driving our *interpretations* and *judgements*; followed by *feelings and behaviours*; followed by *thoughts*.

We look at the world through (emotive/evaluative) interpretive lenses, all of which are non-conscious, and permanently beyond direct, conscious inspection. We can infer what they might be. But we can never be sure.

However, without knowing what a client's *non-conscious frames* might be, we can help them to *over-write them* with new, more self-supporting frames, like the following six, and many others:

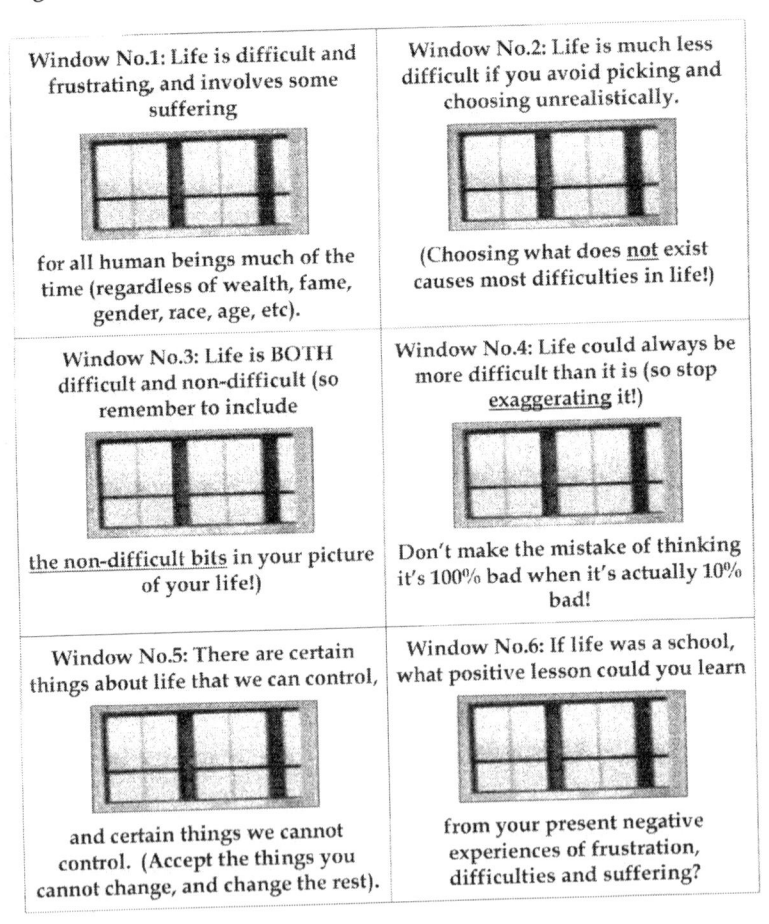

Window No.1: Life is difficult and frustrating, and involves some suffering	Window No.2: Life is much less difficult if you avoid picking and choosing unrealistically.
for all human beings much of the time (regardless of wealth, fame, gender, race, age, etc).	(Choosing what does <u>not</u> exist causes most difficulties in life!)
Window No.3: Life is BOTH difficult and non-difficult (so remember to include	Window No.4: Life could always be more difficult than it is (so stop <u>exaggerating</u> it!)
the non-difficult bits in your picture of your life!)	Don't make the mistake of thinking it's 100% bad when it's actually 10% bad!
Window No.5: There are certain things about life that we can control,	Window No.6: If life was a school, what positive lesson could you learn
and certain things we cannot control. (Accept the things you cannot change, and change the rest).	from your present negative experiences of frustration, difficulties and suffering?

Figure 6.1(b): The Six Windows Model of E-CENT

We do not see 'external events' so much with our eyes, then, as we see them through *'frames of reference and interpretation'*, which were created (socially) in the past, and which we now implement as habit-based, non-conscious, stimulus-response pairings. (This does not mean that Epictetus was right to say that "people are not upset by the things that happen to them". They are! But the extent of our emotional distress can be **reduced** by *moderating* our *expectations* and our *judgements* – at least to some degree!) Epictetus was an advocate of **both** moderate and extreme Stoical ideas. And the idea that *we are not upset by what happens to us* is one of his *most extreme* ideas; and one that *nobody* can live by; and nobody should be *expected* to live by such an inhuman standard.

As Shakespeare wrote: *"If you cut us, do we not bleed?"* And the people who, on average, experience the most traumatic experiences – like war, rape, destitution, economic stress, employment redundancy, business failure, and so on – also show *the highest degree of emotional distress* – all other things being equal!

Because we are socialized animals, *we see what we have been trained by our social experiences to see.* And because we are fleshy bodies (with innate affects) and fragile emotional egos (or virtual personalities), we fear being hurt, physically or emotionally; or abandoned by our significant others; or subjected to unusual deprivations or cruelties. We are born with innate emotional control systems, including anxiety; and we learn *what to fear* from our culture.

A **lot** of what we see/ perceive/ interpret is okay, good, and helpful! That is to say, many of our *socialized perceptions* are helpful in allowing us to know *what to think* and *what to do* in relatively standardized, predictable, routine situations. We could call these *socialized 'seeing' responses* our *non-conscious 'pattern matching' processes*. (Griffin and Tyrell, 2004[88]).

To put this as Jonathan Haidt put it, in a different context: If you had a good moral education, then you can trust your moral intuitions. (Haidt, 2006). And from this perspective, I would also say that if you have had *a good socialization process*, in general, then you can most often trust your *automatic thoughts and feelings.*

This is how the perceptual process works: The incoming stimulus or experience – (which is seen, and/or heard, and/or felt [and/or recalled]) - triggers the lens, or frame, (or schema), through which we view and interpret it.

It is **as if** the automatic, non-conscious processing part of our body-brain-mind is concluding:

"I've seen this stimulus (or 'external event') before. This (remembered interpretation) is the sense I made of it last time. So that is how I will relate to it this time".

However, most often, this pattern matching goes on wordlessly, and non-consciously.

So we never get to know what tint of lens, or what form of frame, we are using, non-consciously, to interpret and respond to our moment to moment social experiences.

Figure 6.1(b) above presents the six perspectives, or 'slogans', or 'captions', related to each of the re-framing windows. Please read through those slogans to get a feel for the re-framings that we promote.

We teach our clients the six perspectives of the Windows Model, in order to overwrite whatever unhelpful frames they normally (*non-consciously, and habitually*) use in the basement of their minds, when interpreting difficult incoming information. (Of course, they have to review these six new perspectives **many times** to get them into their long-term memory, in an emotive, automatic form of response to adversity).

Let us go back and look at the normal process of 'perfinking', or perceiving-feeling-thinking:

We humans react and respond *automatically* on the basis of well-established habits, (probably on the basis of right-brain and limbic system processing of signals), and *we make sense of our responses afterwards* in the form of left-brain, language based rationalizations. (Or some 'quick and dirty' electro-chemical *equivalent* of language based rationalizations!)

The Windows Model is predicated upon 'frame theory', which includes the idea that all of our perceptions are *interpretative*. Furthermore, our interpretations are driven by habit-based 'framings' of incoming stimuli, picked up by our senses.

~~~

6.1(d) Frame theory

So an individual who had a particular kind of childhood may normally respond, when he sees a strange man coming towards him, as if he were concluding (non-consciously, and on the basis of automatic habit,) that: "This is a threat to my happiness!" Or that, "This is a threat to my survival!" He will therefore feel anxious, and be avoidant of contact (because this is his habitual way of responding to threats and dangers).

The main frame through which this person is (non-consciously) 'looking' – we may *guess* – is something like this: "Strange men are dangerous". And this may be an *overgeneralization* from a particular life- or happiness-threatening experience he had in his childhood, or in later years.

The 'frames' that we use to interpret incoming stimuli are **nested sets of inferences**, or hunches, which are derived from past, cumulative, interpretive, social/ emotional experiences.

Depending upon the negativity or positivity of the frame through which you are perceiving an incoming stimulus, you will produce a correspondingly negative or positive emotional/ behavioural response.

I developed this model over a period of three or more years (probably around 2007-2010), beginning with a Four Windows model, and gradually expanding it to Six Windows. It could be expanded further, but then it would lose its obvious ease of use and memorability.

The key philosophical ideas that went into the construction of the Windows Model came from moderate Buddhism and moderate Stoicism; combined with ideas from 'social constructionism' and 'phenomenology'.

These insights about framing and interpretation also underpin **the EFR model** of E-CENT. The EFR model, as described above, is structured like this:

> **E** = An Event or Experience (which is impinging on the consciousness of a person).
>
> **F** = Framing or interpretation – by that person - (of this event or experience), based on past experience.
>
> **R** = A Response – by that person - (which is emotional and behavioural, and which perhaps subsequently could involve reflective thinking, or afterthoughts).

To change undesirable (emotional and behavioural) responses (R's), we need to change the way we frame (F) our experiences (E's).

And the main educational tool that we use to help our clients to reframe their experiences is the Six Windows Model itself.

6.2: Defining, describing and justifying this approach

The Six Windows Model of E-CENT is a way of drawing attention to the fact that you have already _framed_[89] some stimulus (or object or event) in an unhelpful way, *if* you are suffering emotionally, or overreacting behaviourally. However, our frames are ***mostly non-conscious*** and difficult to identify and change. A racist does not realize that s/he is looking at *another human being* through a ***distorting*** lens. They think they are clearly and unambiguously *looking out through their eyes* – like a car driver looking out through their windscreen – and seeing what is 'objectively wrong' with their victim!

One way to conceptualize 'framing' is to imagine you are looking out through a window on which is written **the ideal attitude for you to adopt towards what you *are seeing*** outside. For example, you look out through a house window at some teenagers playing football in a street. If the 'slogan' on the frame says: 'They are up to no good', and you buy into that attitude/belief/frame, you will feel much more negatively towards them than if the 'slogan' on the frame says: 'Playing football with friends is fun', and you subscribe to that belief or frame.

In cognitive science and cognitive psychology, 'Frame theory' uses the concept of 'Frames' to describe the format of **stored experiences** *in long term memory*. So when I say you are looking at a stimulus through a frame, I am saying that *you* – by which I mean *some parts of your body-brain-mind* - are looking at something in the present moment *through a **past** experience, or **cumulative** past experiences*. (This is also sometimes called using a 'schema' from the past, where schema means 'packet of information', like the key features of a situation which allow you to identify it).

One way to clarify the concept of frames and framing of experiences is to look at some common, recurring upsets that appear in Christian and post-Christian communities at Christmas time. Many people disturb themselves every Christmas, because

(1) somebody has not come to visit them; and/or

(2) because they did not get the present they desired; and/or

(3) because they could not afford to give impressive presents to their loved ones; and/or

(4) because their Christmas, which "should" have been the final transformation of their life from *manure* to *magic* did not happen quite as they had hoped and expected; and so on.

The stresses and strains of the holiday season, in November and December and into January tend to push up rates of anxiety and depression, and to cause feelings of isolation, frustration and lack of fulfilment. Anger also leads to conflict within families, and this is a bad time for domestic violence flare-ups.

Some of those stresses and strains are objective and unavoidable, but some are largely a result of how the individual frames their difficult situations.

Clients often come to me with these kinds of holiday upsets. And in the next section, I will describe how I address their problem (or any other problem for that matter, which involves distorted frames).

6.3: The Mind Hut Model

The first thing I set out to do is to teach people *the **Mind Hut** model*. It begins like this:

Imagine you are standing outside a special kind of garden shed – which I call ***the Mind Hut*** - on a piece of lawn. You are looking at some upset about Christmas - either in the run-up to the holiday, or during the festivities, or after it's all over.

You think you are looking out through your eyes at "the reality"; "the truth"; but in fact you are looking through a non-conscious 'filter', 'lens', or 'interpreting frame'.

So your upset feelings about Christmas are really a result of a *distorted perception or interpretation*, but you cannot see that, because you, like all humans, take your interpretations to be a "reality". (I am **not** saying there is *nothing bad* or difficult about your problematical situations. There most likely is something very bad here: but you can learn to *accept the inevitable*, and only try to change what is realistically changeable).

So now, come with me into the Mind Hut, and let me walk you, one by one, through the six windows, or frames, through which you had better learn to view your upset, if you want to be calmer and happier.

The Mind Hut has, as mentioned above, six windows - one in each wall, plus two in the sloping roof: one on each side.

Each window frame has a 'view of life' (perspective, or caption) written around it. Each view of life is like a *slogan* which **claims to be true**.

Here, one by one, are the slogans from the six windows, and the aim of the game is to *assume they are true*, and check to see how believing them changes the intensity of your feelings about your problem:

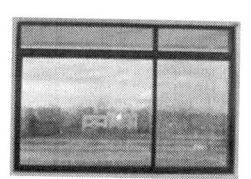

Window No.1

has a frame that says:

Life is pretty difficult and frustrating for all people at least some of the time, and often much of the time.

It does not matter how wealthy or famous a person becomes, they still suffer. Indeed wealthy and famous people may often suffer even more than most! Take a look through Window No.1 at *your* Christmas problem (or other problem) of unhappiness, and recognize that it is happening in the context that *life is pretty **difficult** and **frustrating** for **all** humans much of the time.*

Does that make your problems seem any smaller? Any less distressing? Normally it will!

If it does not, then you are most likely looking at this window frame through an *additional* unconscious frame that 'says' something equivalent to this: '*Life should not be this way!*'

But the frame around Window No.1 is telling you the truth; and *your additional frame* is completely *unreasonable, unrealistic*, and ultimately *unachievable*!

(It may be that your problem should not [morally] have happened; but please bear in mind that immoral things often do happen, and it is futile to demand that the world should never deliver an injustice against you. Life should, again morally, be just; but in practice it often fails to be so! And, in my experience, most people are not struggling with moral problems, but rather with *desires and preferences, and likes and dislikes,* which cannot be achieved or satisfied).

Indeed, all of us do suffer somewhat, from frustrations, difficulties and thwarted ambitions, much of the time. And this applies whether it is "Christmas time" or not.

"Christmas time", of course, is a "cultural creation", which mainly has *commercial* drivers these days.

(And consider this: In December 1978, in the days before 24th and 25th, I was living in Bangkok. I was eating crabs' legs - or was it frogs' legs? - and drinking Chinese beer. I was still thinking about the weeks remaining to Chinese New Year (in early February). It was **not** Christmas in Bangkok! "Christmas" is a *social construct*! It is no more "real" than "Yogi Bear"! Can you "feel it in your bones" when Chinese New Year arrives, or is arriving? No? Well in Bangkok *the locals **can***! Because they have been *trained* to think and feel that way; just as you have been *socialized* into having some *childish fantasies* about Christmas. [Just how realistic are your expectations of Christmas? How old were you when you learned to *fantasize* about Christmas 'magic'?]).

If you realize that it is perfectly possible to suffer at "Christmas time", just as it is at any other time of year, then what is so wrong with the fact that you are suffering "this Christmas time"?

And where did you get the idea that Christmas time would be "magical"? Who told you that your life would inevitably *get better* in this period of time?

If you have suffered a tragic loss, then, of course, you should grieve it. And we should all feel sympathy for you. But disappointment of *unrealistic expectations* is a different matter.

Why must your Christmas disappointment **not** be happening, if it is? Since all humans suffer somewhat, much of the time, why *exactly* must you not be suffering somewhat this Christmas?

It would be *nice* if it could be different, but is there an absolute rule that says you *must get* what is nice? And since suffering is *commonplace*, should you not *expect* to do some suffering, some but not all of the time?

Of course, I am not saying that we should not *empathize* with you in your suffering. If you are sad or grieving, then we *should* accept that.

If you are upset about things going wrong, we need to *feel for you*.

And once you understand that *we really do care about your suffering*, you are still left with the problem of 'what to do about it'.

If you **stay with** your *negative feelings*, without any *conscious* thoughts or *deliberate* ruminations about them, they will eventually burn out.

But you might want a quicker solution, which is what the Windows Model can facilitate.

If you quickly *reframe your problem*, the pain will be diminished *sooner* than it otherwise would be!

When you look at your Christmas frustrations and disappointments through the frame of Window No.1, you should feel the relief of knowing that *you are suffering because humans suffer under particular kinds of circumstances!*

And it is only by being willing to stay with your suffering - to complete *your experience of that suffering - that you can then make it disappear; and you can grow as a person.*

Most humans like to run away from their suffering – to 'jump over it' – through the use of alcohol, marijuana, cocaine, sugary foods, sex addiction, exercise addiction, overloading their lives with busy-work to distract themselves. But, most often, the attempt to jump over your suffering will only postpone it for a later date! You cannot make it disappear without *completing it, digesting it, chewing it up!*

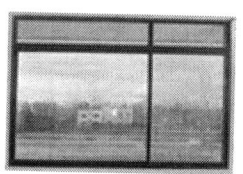

~~~

Window No.2

has a frame with this slogan:

Life is much less difficult, provided you learn to pick and choose sensibly, realistically, and non-magically.

In other words, if you look out through Window 2 at your problem and you feel there is any *insurmountable* difficulty involved here, then you need to know that this is *because you are picking and choosing* that it **should** be significantly different from the way it is!

If you *give up choosing what is* **not** *available*, and learn to accept that (to begin with) reality is real and has to be accepted, does that feel better? (Normally it will!)

I am not saying you have to like it being the way it is; just to accept that it is the way it is (for now). If you want it to (*magically*, and *immediately*) change into being the way you would like it to be, doesn't that make it feel intolerable?

We have found in practice that it is best to begin by accepting reality as it is; and to leave change for a later date.

If you did not like the Christmas present that you got, then you are implicitly *choosing* (or *preferring*) to have got a different present - *the one you did not get*. Is that sensible?

In Buddhism they say: "S/he who *wants nothing* **has everything!**" And: "Desire is the *cause* of all human suffering".

So, do try to *moderate* your wants and desires. It seems to be unrealistic for us humans to abandon all wants and desires. Indeed, once we acquire something, we want more of it, and more of it; and there really is no end to our appetites!

Try to keep your expectations in line with reality. This is not always perfectly easy, because humans have great difficulty identifying what is real and what is unreal. My map of reality looks like this:

We live in a world of *limited* resources (despite Rhonda Byrne's fantasies about the 'law of attraction'). We are born into circumstances of greater or lesser endowment – depending upon our family of origin. Some families can give their children lots of material resources, and some cannot give their children enough to eat healthily! That is the reality of our unequal world. It is okay (and important) to campaign to change that reality, but you have to *begin* by *accepting* that it is the way it is! It is unequal; it is unfair; it is unjust; and it got that way because of the *crazy emotional wiring* of previous generations of humans, battling for personal and familial advantages. It got that way because of innate human greed, envy, jealousy, pride, covetousness, lust, excessive anger (of a sadistic variety), cowardice (and masochistic surrender to threats), and the variable physical endowments of the actors in those wars and battles.

But sometimes it's easy to distinguish what is real from what is unreal.

For example, if you are upset because the person you wanted to come home for Christmas did not come; and it is the case that that person *often* does not turn up (or has *recently* failed to turn up more than once); then strongly expecting them to arrive is *unrealistic*. Your expectation was out of line with reality.

If you ended up in the company of somebody other than the person you would have preferred, aren't you *choosing* to have been with the one you were **not** with?

Aren't you *choosing* that it be Sunday on Monday, and evening time in the morning!

Aren't you foolishly saying: *"What is happening **should not** be happening; and what is not happening **definitely should** be?"* Instead of this kind of crazy **picking and choosing** of what is **not** available, why not focus on some **positive aspect** of what **is** available?

However, please not that, in order to become seriously upset, it not *essential* to *demand* that something has to be different from the way it is. Simply *choosing* that things be different from the way they are will upset you significantly, according to the insights of the Buddha. "One hair's breadth difference between what you want and what you've got and Heaven and Earth are set apart!" In other words, *to the degree that you **refuse** to acknowledge that things are **precisely** the way they are, you are likely to be **upset**;* and your upset is *normally* going to feel **pretty bad**, even if the deviation between what you want and what you have got is **not vast!**

Back to the Christmas examples: If you could not afford to buy the presents you would like to have bought, for your significant others, aren't you really saying: *"I live in this reality, but **I want to be** living in another reality"*. And doesn't this often lead on to: *"**I have to** be able to change the world to make it be the way I want it to be!"*

How realistic is that?

Of course, we have to also point out that you do not go around *articulating statements* of the type illustrated above. These are really the *guesses* of external observers.

Those statements are really *translations into language* of what, in reality, are normally *non-conscious, habit-based attitudes of body-mind*. They are knee-jerk reactions to external stimuli.

They are created through *years and years of experience* of encountering our parents and their pre-existing values and attitudes. And, although lots of *language* – words, phrases, sentences - gets braided into those *years and years of experience*, language is *not* the most abundant or most important component of the way those experiences wired up our brains for emotional reactions. For a start, we were emotional before we had any of those experiences. And the *experiences* shaped our emotions to make them more socially acceptable (within our family of origin).

And with each experience, we had to *perfink* (or perceive-feel-think) our *interpretation* of the experience, and store it in long-term memory. And the bulk of our childhood perfinking was normally automatic, emotional, habit-based, and cumulative-interpretive. (We might *occasionally* have 'thought' our way through a situation, using language and logic – but *not very often!*)

So, your particular craziness about Christmas (and everything else!) was *shaped* by *your particular family of origin*, which had its own particular crazinesses (mum's and dad's) which were shaped by their parents; and back and back through the generations, to some *unknowable original festival* where some appetites were disappointed!

To be really kind and considerate towards yourself, you have to become more realistic. When you find yourself in a situation which cannot be changed, you have to begin by accepting that, at the moment it cannot be changed! It is the disappointing way that it is! Then, I would encourage you to think of some re-framing phrases, such as these:

'If this is the way things are this Christmas, then this is the way things are this Christmas'.
And/or:
'It's tough stuff that my life happens to be the way it happens to be!'
And/or: *'I am willing to accept that life is the way it is!'*

Try these phrases out, and see if they help you to feel better.

In our experience, if you review those kinds of statements over and over again – and *really try to feel that they are true* – then **eventually** you can rewire your body-brain-mind for a less disturbable way of dealing with disappointments.

To revisit Plato's model of the charioteer and the horses: Your ***Passion Horse*** is upset about some Christmas disappointment. Your ***Charioteer*** is being drawn into that upset, and your ***Wilful Horse*** is just going along for the ride. So, your ***Charioteer*** can be trained to use the *re-framing phrases* above; to teach them to your ***Wilful Horse***; and then, between your ***Charioteer*** and your ***Wilful Horse***, you can *overpower* your very emotional ***Passion Horse***! Given enough time and effort, you can tame your ***Passion Horse***: or **teach yourself** to *regulate your affects (or emotions)!*

~~~

Window No.3

has this slogan:

Life is <u>both</u> difficult and non-difficult.

When you look out through this window at your Christmas problem, do you notice anything? Where in this vista are ***the non-difficult bits*** of your Christmas? *Isn't it the case that you have **filtered them out** of the picture?*

In other words: although your mono-focal[90] (or single lens) angle of orientation towards your problem *makes it look as if* the world is "all bad", there are lots of really **good things** about your life right now, which you are filtering out of your awareness.

Before I pointed this out to you, you had no choice but to look at your Christmas disappointments through *a deeply non-conscious frame of perception*, through which you *filtered* your experiences. But now you have the possibility of choice.

And doesn't it make sense to make a list of ***all the things that went well*** over Christmas; and all those things that ***did not go wrong!***

If you write up those good things into a Gratitude List, it will lift your spirits and make your Christmas look much happier and fulfilled. (Seligman, 2002)[91].

~~~

When you have finished that task, of writing up a Gratitude List, there is another activity you can do to help 'tame your Passion horse'.

You can try "negative visualization". This is a moderate Stoic technique which involves imagining all of your current 'possessions' - things and people alike - have been taken from you, including your own health, wealth and sustenance[92]. Eventually life will take everything from us, in death.

So think of all the things you will lose in the future *which you are actually able to enjoy today.*

Normally you do not even notice these 'blessings', because of a psychological phenomenon called 'hedonic adjustment', or 'hedonic adaptation', whereby, as soon as we get something we once valued getting, we now downgrade its significance and value, and we ask the world/life: *"What else ya got for me?"*

And then we feel bad if there is not much 'new stuff' coming our way!

Negative visualization is a way to wake up to all the 'goodies' we have in our lives, and to enjoy them now. Try to focus on *what you've* **got**; and *not what you* **want**. If you train yourself do that – to focus on what you've got, and not what you lack - you will tend to be much happier, at 'Christmas time', and all through the year.

Write down the things you've got in your life, for which you can be grateful, and go over them many times, to remind yourself to be thankful for your blessings; to enjoy what you have, right now.

Suppose you burned the turkey; the person you were hoping would turn up for the festivities decided not to come; you got crummy presents; and somebody did not like the present you gave to them.

So what? That is *disappointing*, but these are *not* the only things that *happened*!

Were there any good moments? Did you eat anything that was nice?

Did you drink anything you appreciated?

Did you have any little conversation with anybody that was positive?

And what kinds of things - which *could* have gone wrong - actually did *not* go wrong?

Make a list of the things you can appreciate about this Christmas, and then go over it many times until you overbalance your pessimistic 'frame' of mind.

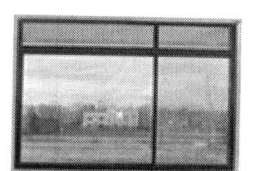

~~~

Window No.4

has these words written around the frame:

Your life could always be a whole lot worse than it is right now.

If you look at your problem and think it is totally bad, then know that you are being unrealistic. Imagine how much worse it would be if, in addition to having the problem that you can see through Window No. 4, you **also had** an alligator eating your rear end off at a terrifying rate of knots!

Be realistic in the way you rate the badness of your problems! Your Christmas could have been a whole lot worse than it was.

For examples: *Did you die of starvation?*

Did a civil war occur in your hometown, resulting in your home being torched?

Were you driven from your home by enemies; or kidnapped by pirates?

No. None of those kinds of bad things happened to you!

Then many good things did happen, and many bad things that could (theoretically) have happened, did not happen.

Be grateful for small mercies. Don't focus on the negative events to the exclusion of the positive. And don't forget that things could always be a whole lot worse than they are!

Recognize that your situation is not now, and never will be, 100% bad! It might be 20% bad; or 40%; or even (sometimes) 60% bad. (See Appendix D, of Byrne, 2016).

But it is not now, and (probably) never will be, 100% bad.

So be grateful for that fact! And remind yourself that your situation could always be *very much worse* than it actually is!

~~~

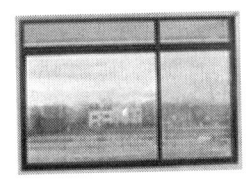

Window No.5

(which is a skylight in the left side of the roof of the Mind Hut) has this slogan on the frame:

There are certain things you can control and certain things you cannot control.

(Although this is Window No. 5, it is often best to begin with this window, before proceeding to Window No. 1).

If you are upset because it is raining - instead of snowing, (for a 'white Christmas') - then that is crazy. You cannot control the rain; or how other people have already behaved; or how Christmas turned out in terms of guests and presents, etc.

What aspect of your current problem is controllable? Look for it. Clarify it. Then make a commitment to *change only* that *bit* which is changeable.

Which bit of your current problem is uncontrollable? If the turkey is burned, it's burned. There is nothing you can do to control that!

If you got the wrong present, you got the wrong present. The outcome is cut and dried! It cannot be changed.

If you got the 'unwanted' outcome, you got the unwanted outcome! If it cannot be changed, it cannot be changed!

*Learn to **accept** the bits that cannot be changed.* That does not mean becoming a victim of anybody.

Let's take the example of difficulties in relationships:

If you cannot *change* your partner, give up trying. But *relocate* if it's too unpleasant being with them! (For example, if they treat you disrespectfully, or engage in domestic violence!)

The first bit (how they are) is beyond your control. But the second bit (where you choose to live, and with whom) is (normally) entirely (or at least somewhat) within your control - ultimately!

~~~

At the start of the Christmas holidays, it is a good idea to decide how you want to proceed. Do you want to be Zen-like, and allow whatever happens to happen? Or are you going to be more 'intentional', and establish a vision of the festive season, including meals, and invitations to guests, etc.

If you decide to go down the 'intentional' route – recognize that intentions are just goals and targets, and not 'actualities'. It is a big mistake to assume that your *intentions* will always and only become *realities*! Sometimes they do, and sometimes they don't!

So, produce a list of your goals for the season (if you are choosing the intentionality route!); and an action list to try to bring them about. Divide a sheet of paper into two columns, with the following headings:

(1) What I can control	(2) What I cannot control.
1.	1. ......
2.	2. ....
3.	3. ....

Table 6.1: The controllable and the uncontrollable

Begin by putting all your goals and planned actions in column one.

Then try to achieve them. When it becomes obvious that there are some things in column one that you *cannot* control, move them into column two.

For example, if some of your planned guests have other, more compelling plans, then they cannot be present at your celebrations also.

You now know you cannot control that - like somebody special turning up on Christmas Eve. So you had better let it go, feel the sense of loss, and then move back into the present moment.

Focus on what is controllable:

What do I have? Or what can I bring about?

What can I do with what I have, where I actually am?

Who is here? And who else could be invited?

Let's see what fun I can have with what I actually have here and now?

And if there's nobody here, go out and find somebody.

~~~

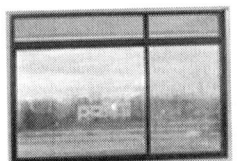

Window No.6

bears the slogan:

If life was a school, what valuable, positive lesson could you learn from your present problems and adversities?[93]

Instead of seeing only the difficult or frustrating aspects of problems, try to see that *problems can teach us valuable lessons*.

In particular, they can teach us *how to solve problems, and/or how to live with them unless and until we can solve them.*

If you had never encountered *any problems*, you would not have any experiential knowledge or skill in *problem solving*.

Although the concept of thinking has its limitations – because we never engage in *pure thinking*, since we always engage in *perfinking* (or *perceiving-feeling-thinking*, all in one grasp of the mind [meaning body-brain-mind!]).

Without losing sight of this definition of perfinking, let us assume that we can 'think'. There are two main operational definitions of the process of thinking:

(1) Asking and answering questions; and:

(2) Finding, defining, analysing and solving problems.

The way to deal with problems, in order to learn from them, is to *think!* (By which I really mean: to *consciously perfink*, or, more specifically, to perfink on paper). Stop *automatically emoting* about the fact that you have difficulties.

Ask yourself (preferably on a written page):

What can I do to solve this problem?

If this problem is not solvable in itself, what action can I take to counterbalance that outcome?

How can I minimize the negative impact of this problem?

How can I try to avoid this problem in the future?

And on and on.

If you will only **perfink in writing** about your problems, you can learn valuable (school of life) lessons from them.

You could say, problems are 'sent' to educate you in the refinements of effective living! So welcome them; embrace them; and learn how to work on them and profit from them!

The problem wakes you up to an intractable aspect of current reality. Can you change it, or do you need to adapt to it?

Your **'Passion Horse'** will want to emote automatically, using its historically shaped set of emotions, from your family of origin.

Your **'Wilful horse'** may be in the habit of *passively* going along with your **'Passion horse'**.

From the **'Charioteer'** part of your brain-mind – your **Adult** ego state – it is possible to **write out** *the details of the problem*; *evaluate them* **logically** and **realistically**, and to come up with *a 'new attitude'* towards the problem.

But you have to get the **'Wilful horse'** on the side of that new attitude, and to teach it to your **'Passion horse'** over and over again, until it becomes the automatic wiring of your **'Passion horse'**!

~~~

6.4: Case illustration

Rita was a woman in her mid-thirties who was angry and depressed because of all the problems in her life. She had lots of debts; an ex-husband who gave her a hard time; children at school who were too often bringing home problems and difficulties; and many other such common problems of daily living.

I introduced Rita to the Six Windows Model, and asked her to look at her cluster of real problems through *Window No. 1: Life is difficult and frustrating for all human beings at least some of the time, and often much of the time.*

I then asked her if she felt any better about having her set of real problems, knowing that this is *normal* for all humans, much of the time. She replied that ***she did not***.

I then suggested that she was most likely looking at Window No. 1 through another (non-conscious) window, and she suddenly blurted out that: *"Window No.1 should not be the reality of life. I don't want it to be this way! Life **may be** suffering, but it **should not** be like that, and I don't accept it being like that".*

And so I said: "And **that** is the window that is preventing you getting some relief by looking through Window No. 1. If it is *true* that 'life **is** suffering for all humans much of the time', then how can you say 'It ***should not*** be like this, because I don't want it to be'?"

I told her that many of the things that I don't like; that I don't want; also happen to be realities; and so I have to accept that they are real, otherwise I would go mad. I don't like racism, but it is all around me. I don't like domestic violence, but it keeps occurring. I don't like having a Roman nose, but it's the only nose I've got!

I then asked her: "What are the premises of your argument? And how exactly is it going to help you in life – this habit that you have of **resisting** reality?"

"No. You're right", she said then. *"There is no way to justify the view that Window No. 1 **should** not be how it is. Life is difficult, and I have to accept that fact!".*

"So look through Window No.1 again, without any reservation", I said, *"and see if that reduces your upset feelings about your cluster of real problems".*

She was quiet for a moment, and then said, *"Yes. It's not the worst situation imaginable. I have some big problems. So do most other humans. And everybody will suffer to some extent over the next few hours and days".*

"That's great", I said. *"So, take the sheet of paper with the Six Windows on it away with you, and learn them over and over again, until you know them off by heart. Then use all six of them each time you feel upset. This process of repeatedly learning (or over-learning) the window-frame slogans will slowly over-write and replace your old, **unhelpful frames**, and produce **more helpful frames** which will keep you **reasonably** calm and accepting when things go wrong in your life".*

This is my story about Rita (not her real name), based on my recollections.

~~~

Chapter 7: Understanding and managing human emotions - including the integration of talk therapy and dietary and exercise guidelines

7.1: Introduction

Because counsellors and psychotherapists deal with their clients' *emotions* - (as well as their behaviours, goals, relationships; plus their environmental stressors, and so on) – every system of counselling and therapy has to have *a theory of emotion*. This, however, is a significant problem, for three reasons:

1. **Firstly**: Human emotion is hugely complex. For example, Stephen Pinker, in his book on how the mind works, draws attention to a quotation from G.K. Chesterton about the *unutterable complexity* of human emotional tones and moods and shades, which begins like this:

"Man knows that there are in the soul tints more bewildering, more numberless, and more nameless than the colours of an autumn forest". (Page 367)[94].

Therefore, at the very least, we should show some humility in developing our systemic models of such complexity.

2. **Secondly**: As one psychotherapist has pointed out:

"The terms 'feeling' and 'emotion', and 'affect' are used in many different senses in psychology. A review of more than twenty theories of emotion reveals a plethora of widely diverging technical definitions. These vary with the technique of investigation, the general theoretical framework, and the value-judgements of the psychologist. Often, they are so diverse as to defy comparison let alone synthesis".[95]

So we are not going to arrive at a universal definition of emotion in this book; though we have to come to some working hypotheses, in the form of practical conclusions, which allow us to understand and help our clients.

3. **Third**: There is a good deal of confusion regarding whether emotions are innate, or socially imposed; and whether they exist 'inside the client' or 'outside' in social relationships.

With regard to point 3, which is the most fundamental question we face, we should resolve that issue up front:

In E-CENT counselling, we use the insight from Dylan Evans' (2003) book on emotion, about 'degrees of innateness or learned emotions'. This means that we accept the conclusion that some basic emotional wiring is innate, at birth. However, those basic emotions (or feelings, or affects) are inevitably shaped by the culture of the mother (and father [normally]) into *acceptable* and *unacceptable* expressions of affect – or observable manifestations of feelings - over time. The main concepts we use are:

(1) Innate emotional wiring (Panksepp 1998) like, anger, fear, disgust, sadness, etc.; which are also seen as basic emotions[96] – (Siegel, 2015);

(2) Higher cognitive emotions (like pride, confidence, guilt and shame, jealous, trust and so on – (as in Panksepp and Biven, 2012); and:

(3) Culturally specific emotions: (For example: the ways in which various universal emotions are *manifested* *differently* in different cultures; e.g. the more restrained Japanese versus the more expressive Americans – (Evans, 2003).

Somewhere between the universal, higher cognitive emotions and the culturally specific emotions, I would place the "family variations" in the range and mode of expression of the basic emotions and higher cognitive emotions.

So, individuals have some of the 'universal shape' implied by Plato, Freud, Albert Ellis, Eric Berne, etc.; but also quite a lot of 'family shaping' which is idiosyncratic and unique. Plus national (and class) variations in how those emotions are expressed.

In evolving our theory of emotion, we went back as far as it is possible to go in developing knowledge of our ancestors, and what we inherited from them. For example, we have been influenced by the perspective of Jonathan Turner (2000)[97], which can be summarized like this: "...our ability to use a wide array of emotions evolved long before spoken language and, in fact, constituted a preadaptation for the speech and culture that developed among later hominids. Long before humans could speak with words, they communicated through body language their emotional dispositions; and it is the neurological wiring of the brain for these emotional languages that represented the key evolutionary breakthrough for our species".

And according to Panksepp (1998), those emotional systems are located in the most primitive parts of the brain: the limbic system and brainstem. (These are the neurological substrates (or foundations) underpinning what Freud called the 'It' – the *physical baby*, and the *primary (emotive) processes* of its mental life. Those primary, sub-cortical (limbic) processes inform our secondary, more culturally shaped emotions, which modulate our capacities for cognition: which means that our *attention, perception, memory,* and *thinking* can never be **separated** from our feelings. As Damasio (1994) demonstrated with his patient, Elliot, *we* **cannot** *make choices and decisions* **without** *the emotional capacity to* **evaluate** *options!* (We are *perfinkers*, (perceivers-feelers-thinkers) and not pure thinkers! [Glasersfeld, 1989]) .

Finally, in E-CENT counselling theory, we would never go along with a list of categories of emotional disturbances like that displayed in the *Diagnostic and Statistical Manual 5* (or any other *DSM*), or any other equivalent manual, such as the European's International Statistical Classification of Diseases.

Humans are too complex to be classified into 'disease boxes' or 'personality disorders'. And we will argue elsewhere in this book that much of the modern explosion of emotional disorders are a result of *lifestyle* *distortions*, especially in the areas of sleep deprivation, poor diet, lack of physical exercise, and rising levels of externally imposed socioeconomic stress. (See in particular, Chapters 4 and 5).

~~~

Afterthought: However, despite the fact that we in E-CENT have clarified our own understanding of human emotions, there are lots of disagreements within the field of counselling and psychotherapy on this subject. Since there is no universal agreement regarding the nature of human emotions in counselling and therapy, we, in E-CENT counselling theory, have to account for our own theory of emotion: to justify it, as well as defining and elaborating its elements. So let us begin with some of the older theories of emotion.

7.2: Buddhism and Stoicism on emotion

E-CENT counselling has been influenced by moderate Buddhist ideas and moderate Stoic ideas, including some of their ideas about human emotions. This is obvious from a reading of Chapter 6, on the Six Windows Model.

With regard to Buddhism, it seems from The Dhammapada[98], that the Buddha taught that all human disturbance arises out of *desire*; and this idea is shared with Stoicism.

In E-CENT theory we have taken some of these ideas as points of departure, but we have also found serious flaws in both of those philosophies.

For examples:

7.2(a). Regarding Buddhist theory:

The opening lines of the Dhammapada are as follows:

"What we are today comes from *our **thoughts** of yesterday*, and our present thoughts build our life of tomorrow: *our life is the creation of our **mind***". (Page 1)[99].

In ***my view***, it would be more accurate to say (or to ***begin*** by saying):

(1) "What we are today comes from *our thoughts (and **feelings**) about our experiences*…"

So, we are not talking about *disembodied thoughts*, devoid of a stimulus in an ***external reality***.

And we are not talking about beings that can *think independently of their basic emotional wiring!*

People are emotionally wired up by their earliest relationships, and they live in the real world of good and bad experiences!

They have body-minds, and *their thoughts are strongly affected by diet, exercise, relationship support or its lack, external stressors*, and so on.

(2) "...and our present thoughts..." (*Plus our* **feelings** *and* **actions**, *including* **eating, sleeping, relaxing, exercising,** *etc.*) "...build our life of tomorrow...".

So our *thoughts* (about our *experiences*) ***do not act alone***; they are not the *sole determinant* of our lives.

Let us then move on to the third element of the Buddha's statement:

(3) "...our life is the creation of our *mind*". E-CENT theory would suggest that that should be change to this: Our life is the creation of our body-brain-mind-environment complexity. This includes the real world; *plus* our relationships; plus our experiences; plus our diet, sleep pattern, exercise; and our stressors – including economic and political circumstances, family life – and our coping resources - and on and on).

So the Buddha can easily *mislead the unwary*; as the unwary were misled by Albert Ellis and Aaron Beck – who both *downplayed* the role of the environment in human experience; with Ellis denying the role of early childhood in shaping the later life of the social-individual. Those theorists also overlooked the importance of our eating of unhealthy diets; and our failure to exercise our bodies; and our modern neglect of the importance of sleep; all of which impacts our emotional states.

To serve our clients well, counsellors and psychotherapists need to be *critical thinkers* (meaning *critical perfinkers!*); to be awake; to be well informed (meaning widely read, and subject to multiple influences); and to think (or perfink) for ourselves.

Buddhist ideology downplays the impact of the environment upon human organisms, in a way which is corrected by modern social psychology.

Social psychology is an attempt to understand and explain the various ways in which "we, as individuals are influenced by the actual, imagined or implied presence of others". Allport, (1985)[100].

If we are to develop a theory of human emotions, we must not follow the Buddhist dumping of this impact of the social environment on the thinking, feeling and behaviour of our clients, lest we end up **blaming the client** for their disturbance, as was done by Freud, Klein, Ellis and Beck. (Indeed, it was Dr John Bowlby who most strongly emphasized the importance of early childhood relational experiences: the impact, for better or worse, of our early social relationships upon our attachment style, and our chances of having a happy marriage in adult life. Because this went against both Freud's and Klein's perspective - [both of which blamed the child for their own emotional disturbances {which were assumed to result from phantasy!}] -

Dr John Bowlby was ostracized by the British psychoanalytic community for decades – because they insisted upon *blaming the clients' 'phantasies'* for their upset emotions.)[101]

~~~

However, the mindfulness aspect of Buddhism, especially Zen meditation, is very helpful for all of us, counsellors and clients alike, because it stops us ruminating on past problems, or anxiously anticipating future difficulties. Here is an illustration of how to understand 'mindfulness', or awareness of the present moment:

"The greatest support we can have is mindfulness, which means being totally present in each moment. If the mind remains centred, it cannot make up stories about the injustice of the world or one's friends, or about one's desires or sorrows. All these stories could fill many volumes, but when we are mindful such verbalizations stop. Being mindful means being fully absorbed with the momentary happening, whatever it is – standing or sitting or lying down, feeling pleasure or pain – and we maintain a non-judgemental awareness, a 'just knowing'." Ayya Khema[102].

However, here's one serious caveat: It is *not* a good idea to try to use mindfulness to suppress or deny our feelings about our distressing experiences. That will not work. We have to **file** our distressing experiences in the past, or they will **insert** themselves into our future! And the only way we know to file our distressing experiences in the past is to *experience their emotional content fully*; to *digest* those emotional experiences; to *complete* them; and thus to burn them up; and *file* them in inactive files in our long-term memory. This should also be combined with a re-framing process – like the Six Windows model – so that we get to *re-frame old traumatic experiences*; to see them differently; and to drain them of their original meaning.

~~~

7.2(b). Regarding Stoic theory:

The most famous saying of the Stoic philosophers in the world of cognitive counselling systems today is this *extremist* belief:

"People are *not* upset by the things which happen to them, but rather by their *attitude* towards those things".

This *extremist* belief is central to Rational Therapy (REBT), and, though recent attempts have been made to shift to a conception of emotional upsets as being caused by the interaction of negative activating events and our beliefs about them, the basic instinct of REBT is to blame the client for holding 'irrational beliefs'. (Byrne, 2017).

Beck's Cognitive Therapy (CT) and CBT in general hold a more ambivalent attitude than REBT, with some emphasis given to the idea that "the event does not make you feel anything" - (Willson and Branch, 2006; page 12) - and the idea that it is only "sometimes" that the client "may assign extreme meanings to events", causing them to feel disturbed. (Willson and Branch, page 13). See also, Byrne 2017).

These extreme beliefs, of REBT, and certain aspects of harsh CBT, are also very similar to the opening statement of the *Dhammapada*, in that it both **blames the client** for their interpretation of their experience, and ascribes to them *the capacity to be indifferent* to their environmental insults, hurts and defeats. (This inference is clear from verses 2 and 3 of the Dhammapada, page 1). But only a lump of wood, or a stone, or some other inanimate object, can be truly indifferent to particularly intense environmental stimuli.

A *wise person* may well choose to ignore some environmental insults, hurts and defeats; to downplay them; or to *reframe them*, so they seem less painful. But not all of our clients can claim to be *wise* upon first encountering us. (And many of them will fail to achieve significant levels of wisdom; and almost none will rise to the level of Stoic functioning, just as most Stoics fail to rise to the level of the theoretical '**indifference to externals**' which Stoic theory demands of its adherents).

In time, we might teach some of our clients to be somewhat wiser - using some *moderate* Stoic principles – but we **should not** attempt to teach them the more extreme principles, such as that shown above; partly because we would have to **blame them** for their distress, to begin with; and then we would have to move on to *advocating super-human goals for mere humans.*

But there are some *moderate principles* of stoicism that we should try to practice and preach.

The most helpful principle of Stoicism, which is also found in Buddhism, is this, from Epictetus's *Enchiridion*:

> "Freedom and happiness consist of understanding one principle: There are certain things we can control and certain things we cannot control. It is only after learning to distinguish between what we can and cannot control – and acting upon that knowledge – that inner harmony and outer effectiveness become possible".[103]

If some of the things that negatively affect me, in my current social environment, are within my control, then it makes sense to try to correct and control them: to change them. And if something proves to be beyond my control - (or *most likely* beyond my control – including my ability to move to a new environment!) - then it makes sense not to rail against that, but *to learn to* **accept** *it* (which will take time and effort, and courage and fortitude).

But that is *not* (ultimately) what is taught by the major Stoic philosophers, when they deploy their more extreme principles.

For example, in his *Meditations*, Marcus Aurelius defines 'harm' as being the ability of some outside agency to damage his 'individual ethical stance'. And he then declares an absolute principle that: **Nobody has the ability to damage my individual** *ethical stance*. Hence, *logically*, nobody has the ability to **harm** him. Hence, his final conclusion: *Nobody can disturb me!*

(See the *Introduction* to the *Meditations*, by D.A. Ross)[104].

The problem with that conclusion is that only a rare sage could live a life based on the idea – the *fantasy* – that *a hatchet through my skull does not constitute harm, since it leaves my individual ethical stance intact.*

Or, that somebody murdering my baby and raping my wife cannot disturb me, *because it leaves my individual ethical stance intact.*

These are *unreachable* goals, and *inhuman* beliefs, which could never be *universalized* as an approach to life. And therefore, counsellors and psychotherapists should not (morally) imply that these are goals which are achievable by average counselling clients; and that the client is somehow remiss for not acting like a lump of wood!

~~~

So, while we can learn some things about *moderating our desires* and *distinguishing* between what is a *realistic* goal (to be pursued) and an *unachievable* goal (to be abandoned) – we must not spread *the lie that our clients are not disturbed by their social experiences! They are!* (See Figure 4.1, above, and the subsequent text, for a description of the *six or more factors* which - jointly - cause human disturbance - one of which is the External Activating Event [A1], which is to say, *what happens to the individual* who then goes on to experience a consequent emotion!)

7.3: Another point of departure – Evolutionary psychology

While Buddhism and Stoicism mainly apply *the **negative** theory of emotion* – which assumes that *all* emotions are problematical - evolutionary psychology promotes the idea that our emotions arose, and were selected by nature, because *they **served** to keep our ancestors alive*. This is a *positive* theory of emotion.

Evolutionary psychology is an attempt to build a science of psychology, based on inferences - (many from anthropological studies; and many which appear to be little more than applied logic, or philosophical thought experiments) - about the ways in which our ancestors adapted to their environments, and how and why some psychological adaptations were most likely selected by nature for their survival value. For examples:

Without your innate tendency towards anger, there would be nothing to stop selfish individuals taking advantage of you, even to the extent of threatening your survival (by stealing all the available food, for example).

Without anxiety, you might sit and watch with curiosity while a lion approached you and then ate you.

Without distress (or sadness) you might be unable to attract social support when you are weakened by illness, or when you are otherwise disadvantaged and in need of extra support.

Without feelings of lust and romantic love, you might fail to attract a mate; fail to reproduce yourself; and the quality of your life might seem so poor (relative to social norms) that you could easily abandon the attempt to stay alive.

So feelings - even apparently destructive or painful emotions - can be seen to serve useful survival functions, *except when they are taken **too** far, and then they cause more harm than good.*

And, paradoxically, as pointed out by Siegel (2015), emotions are both **regulated** and **regulatory**. They are regulated (or controlled) by both internal and external factors; and we also tend to internalize those external, social factors over time. (This external factor often takes the form of verbal or non-verbal feedback from significant others [mother, father, others] about their experience of our emotional expression [or expression of affects]).

Some of our emotive-cognitive experiences (including that feedback from significant others) help us to regulate other of our emotive-cognitive urges.

Another way to say this is as follows: We have our innate affects, or emotions, *socialized* by mother/father; and this shapes *our **subsequent capacity** to perfink* (or perceive-feel-think). Then, when some new event impinges upon our consciousness, we use our historical capacity to perfink to regulate our current perfinking response to this new experience. (Of course, this is *an exaggerated statement of 'agency'*. In fact, it is not "*us*" that does anything! It is not so much that "we use" our historical capacity to perfink; but rather that "we are used by" our historical capacity to perfink. It is rather more that *our historical **capacity** to perfink* – which is electro-chemical, body-brain-mind, culturally shaped memories - *automatically regulates our subsequent perfinking* about new and novel incoming stimuli).

While cognitive therapists elevate 'thinking' to the driving seat of human behaviour; and affect regulation theorists elevate 'feeling' to this role; we in emotive-cognitive (E-CENT) theory, attribute overall control of the body-brain-mind to *perfinking* – which is *integrated, interwoven, perceiving-feeling-thinking*; which is so hopelessly intertwined that *it is not possible to **separate** out the strands* from each other.

The *modelling* (or *demonstration*) of emotional self-regulation by our parents – as they engage in *their own **perfinking** performances* - is another of the major internalized sources of self-regulation that we have (which begins outside of us, but ends up encoded in our neurological, higher cognitive emotions, probably largely in the right orbitofrontal cortex [OFC]).

An example of the excessive use of negative emotions would be the driver who is so angry about being frustrated by other drivers that he (or she) gets out of their car and assaults somebody – killing or maiming them; resulting in great harm to both parties.

Or the person who is so anxious they cannot go out of their own home, and thus they miss out on all kinds of social pleasures (and the possibility of earning a living!)

Or somebody who is so distressed (sad/ depressed) that they cannot relate to others, and they lose their life partner as a result.

Some of these overly-emotional responses may come from our family of origin; and some may come from changes in our lives today, including in our relationships, our stress levels, our diets, or the balance/ harmony of our lives; or even from pharmaceutical drugs we take to 'cure' ourselves[105].

~~~

On balance, in E-CENT counselling, we see emotion as being more positive than negative, and more helpful than unhelpful – though it is obvious that our emotions can complicate our lives and cause us suffering when we do not manage them well.

~~~

But we still have not defined emotion, nor said anything about the origin of emotions in the historical processes of evolution of species.

7.4 The origin of human emotions

Charles Darwin was the first major theorist to publish a serious study of the ways in which life on earth most likely evolved, and the principles that seem to control the evolutionary process – primarily *natural selection* of those *randomly arising features* of *organisms* which best fit an available ecological niche or habitat. Or, to state it in another way: Those organisms which were well adapted to survive in their local environment were the ones which survived to pass on their genes; and those who were poorly adapted did not survive.

Darwin noted, in his book on emotions in humans and other animals[106], that all mammals displayed similar emotional arousal patterns. This he saw as evidence for a common ancestor. But he considered that those emotions were a *residue* of more primitive times, while recent research suggests that **emotions are fundamental to all brain-mind functioning**, being **primary processes** which *modulate* cognitions (like attention, perception, thinking and memory processes); *generate* evaluations; *drive* goals; and *dictate* behaviours. (Panksepp, 1998).

Much later, Paul Ekman, an American anthropologist, set out to prove that Darwin was **wrong** about the *universality* of all basic primate and mammal emotions; and that, in fact, many cultures are wired up emotionally to be very *different* from each other – the major example being westerners versus the oriental mind. This is the famous (or *infamous*!) concept of 'cultural relativity'. However, despite the rigour of his studies, Ekman only succeeded in *proving Darwin to be right*. There is **no** *cultural relativity in respect of the* **basic** *human emotions* of anger, fear, distress, surprise, disgust and joy[107]. There are some cultural differences in *how* those emotions are *expressed* – for example the American and southern European tendency to be very open about feelings and emotions, on the one hand; and the Japanese tendency to be concealing of their feelings and emotions – but *the basic emotions – which are being revealed or concealed - are* **common** *to all cultures.*

~~~

Professor Jonathan Turner[108] has written an extensive study of the origins of human emotions. He draws attention to the *social* nature of humans and the relatively *solitary* practices of other kinds of apes; and argues that the development of our increased *sociality*[109] was brought about to facilitate living in the more exposed environment of the savannah, where **banding together** provided the best chance of survival. This need encouraged strong emotional ties, "allowing our ancestors to build higher levels of social solidarity". So *the social nature of human emotions* (or, rather, our higher cognitive emotions) can be explained in this way – as a constructive adaptation to a new foraging environment. But we still share our *basic emotions* with all mammals (as argued by Darwin and confirmed by Ekman, as mentioned above).

Jaak Panksepp is one of the foremost researchers in the field of affective neuroscience. In his book on the archaeology of mind, he "reveals for the first time the deep neural sources of our values and basic emotional feelings". These patterns in the human brain "are remarkably similar across all mammalian species"[110].

And we know from some brain studies that **some** emotional disorders result from damage to those emotional centres of the brain. However, **most** emotional disorders probably arise out of disruption of the *higher cognitive* and *social* emotions, (like guilt and pride), which will be introduced and discussed later.

7.5 The proximal cause of emotional disturbance

According to Dr Gordon Coates, all emotions can be understood as a result of our *wanting* something to happen (hope), and/ or *wanting* something else *not to happen* (fear)[111]. (This is very similar to the Buddha's view that all our emotional distress, or human disturbance, results from our desires. And it also reminds us of Freud's conclusion that humans are innately programmed to seek pleasure and to avoid unpleasure [or pain]).

But these conclusions by Coates could be a lightly concealed circular argument. What they seem to suggest is this: I experience **hope** because I **want** something to happen; and/ or I **want** something to happen and **therefore** I feel hopeful. Not only is this argument circular, but it also does not account for **wanting** as the 'prime mover'.

Why do I *want* **anything**? And *why* do I *want* **the specific things** *that I seem to want*?

If **wanting** is the *prime mover* of our actions/ thoughts, resulting in a cascade of emotions, *what accounts for the state of wanting itself?*

We will return to this problem, but first let us complete Coates' model. This little model, called *the Wanter-fall chart*, has two branches which flow downwards:

Branch 1. When I **want** something to happen, I experience **hope**. When the desired outcome **occurs**, I experience **happiness** (plus something called 'propathy', which is the opposite of antipathy). But since I am now happy, and I **want** *that state to continue*, I now experience **fear**.

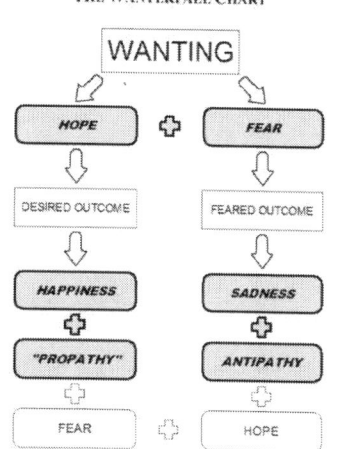

Branch 2. The second branch runs like this: I **want** to **avoid** a particular outcome, so I experience **fear**. When the feared outcome occurs, I experience **sadness** and antipathy.

This little model is too circular, and cannot account for the *origins* of emotion as such. And neither can it account for the *determinants* of human wants.

Figure 7.1: The Wanterfall Chart

7.6 The evolutionary view

The perspectives of *evolutionary psychology* and *affective neuroscience* are better sources of explanation of human emotions. According to Panksepp and Biven (2012) our evolutionary adaptations (as mammals) laid down certain subcortical structures in the limbic areas of the brain. These neurological structures underpin seven emotional systems as follows:

1. **Seeking:** This emotional system is about how the brain generates a euphoric and expectant response. (I am wired up by nature to seek: human faces; comfort; food; and as I grow, to seek novelty, stimulation. (I 'want' what I am *programmed* by nature to 'want'!) So when I am 'wanting' many experiences, I am expressing an innate, biochemical urge laid down by natural selection. Of course, my list of wants can be, and is, expanded by my cultural conditioning and experience).

2. **Fear**: This system is about how the brain responds to the threat of physical danger and death. (I am wired up by nature [natural selection] to fear threats and dangers, because my ancestors who survived long enough to reproduce were kept alive by their fear of predators; and they passed that fear down the line, biochemically. This is my innate 'flight response'. I 'want' to survive, because I am programmed by nature of 'want' to survive! [Again, of course, I can learn to fear things that are not real threats or dangers]).

3. **Rage**: This system is about sources of irritation and fury in the brain. (I am wired up by natural selection to respond ragefully to serious frustrations, and to those threats and dangers in response to which I can overcome my natural fearfulness, presumably because this tendency in my ancestors helped to keep them alive long enough to reproduce. This is my innate 'fight response').

4. **Lust**: This system is about how sexual desire and attachments are elaborated in the brain. (I am wired up by natural selection to feel love and sexual desire. Without this lust and desire for sexual congress, and close physical comfort, my ancestors might not have bothered to reproduce, and I would not exist. Because they survived, they passed on their loving-lusting tendencies to me).

5. **Care**: This system is about sources of maternal nurturance. (Mothers do not 'decide' to care for their young. Among our ancestral tribes, any non-caring mothers - [who lacked a strong, innate caring urge], would have been unlikely to keep their offspring alive long enough to reproduce, so non-caring attitudes tended to die out. Those mothers who kept their offspring alive long enough to reproduce were most likely those with neurologically wired tendencies to care sufficiently: to be 'good enough' mothers).

6. **Grief**: This system drives feelings of intense loss when I lose a significant 'attachment figure', whether they are sexual or non-sexual attachments. (I attach myself to significant others [especially mother {or my main carer}], by innate urging. This maximizes my chances of survival, so I can live to reproduce, and pass on to my offspring this same urge to attach to me and their other carers. But the downside of my strong attachment is that when my attachment figures die, or become unavailable to me, I experience an intense sense of loss [grief]). This is also the foundation of sadness and depression.

7. **Play**: This urge explains how the brain generates joyous, rough-and-tumble interactions. (I have innate urges to play, driven by a sense of joy in my own playfulness, and the responses of my playmates. This may have survived through evolutionary time because my playfulness makes me attractive to my carers, and so they want to protect me to keep me alive and near them. Less playful and joyful children might have been abandoned in tough times, and so their less-playful genes died out).

~~~

The general point arising out of Panksepp's research on the brains of animals, and other studies, is that all mammals have these seven basic emotional systems hardwired into the limbic system (or mammalian brain). These seven systems probably should not be seen as the end of the matter, since Panksepp himself included *panic* in his original list, and omitted *grief*.

The take-home message seems to be this: Every human being is carrying a set of basic emotional, motivational and automatic control systems (or the developmental capacity to create them) in the subcortical areas of their brains, at birth. Their neocortex, on the other hand, is available to be wired up by social encounters. Their social encounters, initially, are managed from their basic emotions, which, through social interactions become woven together with social experiences, into 'higher cognitive emotions'. This most likely takes place in the right orbitofrontal cortex, where the limbic system and the neocortex overlap. (Hill, 2015).

Contrary to Albert Ellis's view, *emotion*, on the one hand, and *conscious thought*, on the other, begin as two **separate**, brain-based systems, which interact and moderate each other, so that reason (when it emerges over developmental time in the child) **depends upon** basic emotions [in the limbic system], (plus socially influenced emotions [based in the orbitofrontal cortex]), which are required to evaluate (value) the significance of thoughts, options, actions, etc. (Siegel, 2015; Damasio, 1994).

Logic **cannot** tell us what to value, what to like, or what to love (Damasio, 1994)[112]. Those evaluations are made by our emotional systems (including our basic emotions and our higher cognitive emotions, including our moral emotions of guilt, shame and elevation [Haidt, 2006]).

7.7 Understanding emotive-cognitive interactionism

Before we move on to look at the *socialization of emotion*, as discussed in interpersonal neurobiology (Siegel, 2015)[113], let us review the E-CENT model of mind as developed in one of our main papers in 2009[114].

In this paper I reviewed the main theory of REBT regarding the connection between thinking and emotions.

Albert Ellis began (in the mid-1950's) with the thesis that thinking, feeling and action were all *interconnected*, and in many respects *essentially the same thing*.[115]

In Figure 2 of Byrne (2009a), which is reproduced in Figure 7.2 below, I presented the classic ABC model of REBT, with the embellishment that, at point B, in the middle of the model, I showed:

B1 = Emotive processing (quick, primary)

B2 = Cognitive processing (slow, secondary)

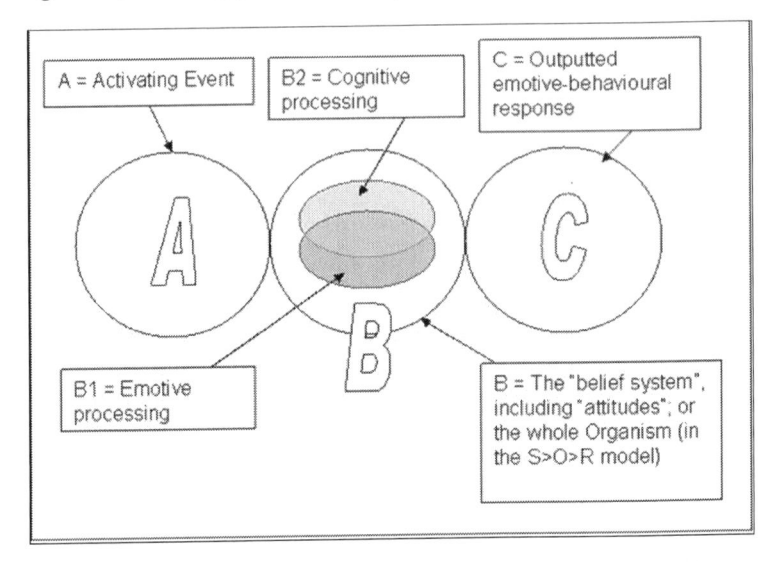

[Diagram: Venn-style diagram with three overlapping circles labeled A, B, C. Labels point to: A = Activating Event; B2 = Cognitive processing; C = Outputted emotive-behavioural response; B1 = Emotive processing; B = The "belief system", including "attitudes"; or the whole Organism (in the S>O>R model)]

Figure 2: The overlapping of thinking and feeling in Ellis (1958)

Figure 7.2: The interaction of thinking and feeling in the complex ABC model

And B1 and B2 are shown to be partially overlapping, to reflect Albert Ellis's claim that thinking and feeling are interactional and partly-overlapping in nature.

However, now, in the light of Panksepp and Biven (2012) and other modern sources on neurobiology, I want to amend that to say this:

The individual human has innate emotional control systems in their limbic system, which are relatively standardized.

If we take the example of a seven year old boy, he also has, by this stage of his development, acquired some limited cognitive processing capabilities based (or managed from) his frontal lobes.

And what we used to call the overlapping aspects of B1 (emotion) and B2 (thinking) we now see as being the ways in which his limbic system and his frontal lobes *interact*.

And, from the time of his birth, those interactions will have been strongly influenced by his social relationships, especially with mother (and later father and others).

What follows is an illustration of how Panksepp (1998) lists the elements of, and lines of communication between, a stimulus and a human response.

See Figure 7.3 below:

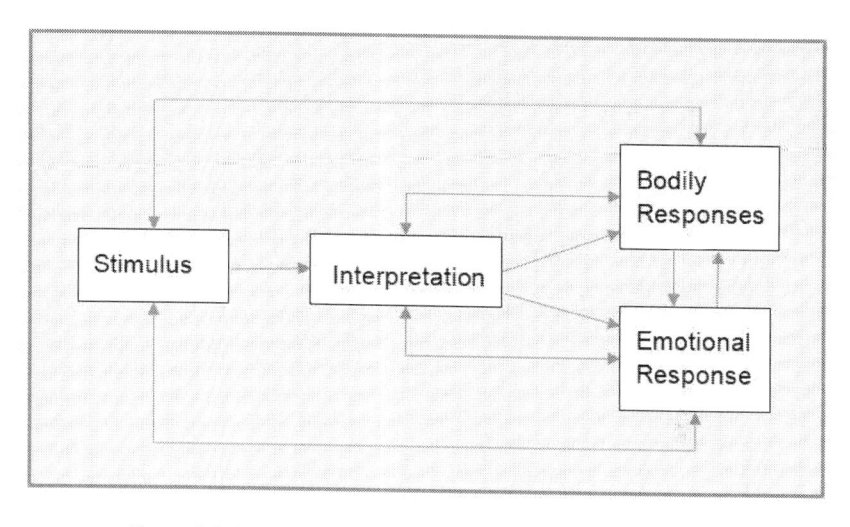

Or how to integrate nutritional insights, exercise and sleep coaching into talk therapy

Figure 7.3: From a presentation by Jaak Panksepp (Slide 12)[116]

This one of several ways to conceptualize the relationship between an organism and its environmental stimuli. And it is probably the most complete, and convincing model I've seen.

At the very least, we would claim that the incoming stimulus is interpreted, on the basis of the organism's innate wiring, and its memorized experiences. That interpretation triggers both a bodily response and an emotional (feeling, or affect) response. (Indeed, it would be more accurate to say: The interpretation is *both* (a) triggered by past physical-emotional experiences, and (b) triggers new, similar physical-emotional responses in the present moment).

The bodily response and the emotional response communicate with each other and send signals back to the interpretation, which will tend to modify it.

The bodily response and emotional response may also change the stimulus, (for example: if the stimulus is a comprehending being that reads body language and facial expressions).

The E-CENT perspective (in Figure 7.4 on the next page) accords with – or overlaps and lines up with - this model by Jaak Panksepp, in Figure 7.3 above.

That is to say, as we see it: A stimulus (A1) is interpreted (at A2) and that interpretation sets off a pattern-matched set of bodily and facial responses, as well as innate and socially shaped emotional responses.

Those responses feed back to the interpretation, to refine, modify or intensify it, and a feed-back signal goes to the bodily responses and the emotional responses to modulate them.

As the emotional state stabilizes, the higher cognitive functions (reflective thinking/ feeling/ appraising) begin to kick in, and may radically modify the original interpretation.

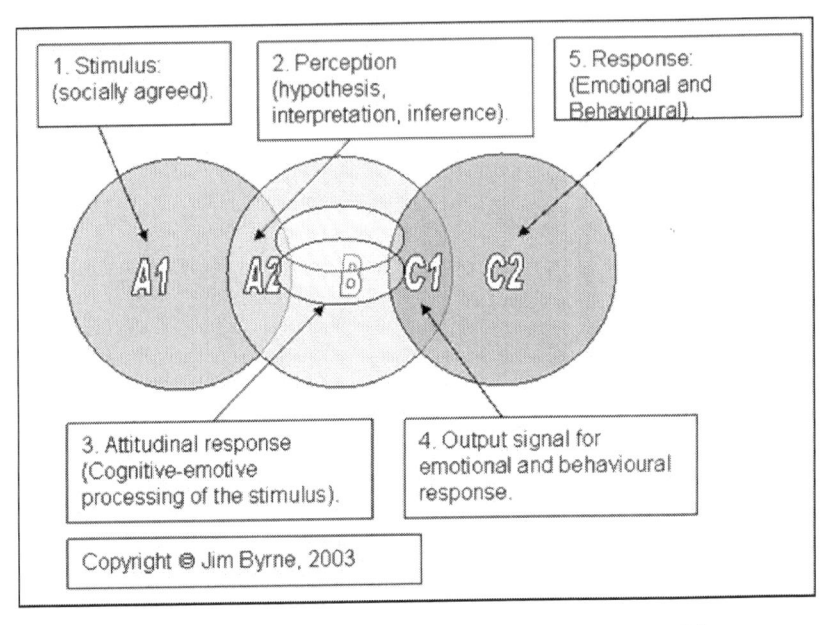

```
┌─────────────────────────────────────────────────────────────┐
│  ┌──────────────┐  ┌──────────────┐  ┌──────────────┐      │
│  │ 1. Stimulus: │  │ 2. Perception│  │ 5. Response: │      │
│  │ (socially    │  │ (hypothesis, │  │ (Emotional and│     │
│  │  agreed).    │  │ interpretation,│ │ Behavioural) │      │
│  └──────────────┘  │  inference). │  └──────────────┘      │
│                    └──────────────┘                         │
│                                                             │
│          A1      A2    B    C1    C2                        │
│                                                             │
│  ┌─────────────────────┐  ┌─────────────────────┐          │
│  │ 3. Attitudinal      │  │ 4. Output signal for│          │
│  │ response            │  │ emotional and       │          │
│  │ (Cognitive-emotive  │  │ behavioural         │          │
│  │ processing of the   │  │ response.           │          │
│  │ stimulus).          │  └─────────────────────┘          │
│  └─────────────────────┘                                    │
│  ┌─────────────────────┐                                    │
│  │ Copyright © Jim Byrne, 2003 │                            │
│  └─────────────────────┘                                    │
└─────────────────────────────────────────────────────────────┘
```

Figure 7.4: Further elaboration of the complex ABC model

This model is predicated upon (or based upon) well known and reliably inferred interactions between the various elements of the neocortex and the limbic system. And this is a change from Figure 7.2 above.

The ABC model in Figure 7.4 was influenced by both Ellis (1958, 1962) and also Damasio (1994).

Ellis described thinking and feeling as overlapping, and Damasio (1994) seemed to suggest that there was an area of the frontal lobes where reasoning and emotion interacted and moderated each other.

Now, it seems from Panksepp's anatomical studies, that rather than a 'place' where that happens, there are, instead, *a number of interactional connections between the emotional and reasoning centres of the brain*, which are themselves *discrete* and *separate* entities.

See Figure 7.5 on the next page.

This is one way to rethink the structures of cognitive-emotive functioning.

But there may still be a place where this happens, as suggested by Siegel (2015), which is the orbitofrontal cortex (or OFC).

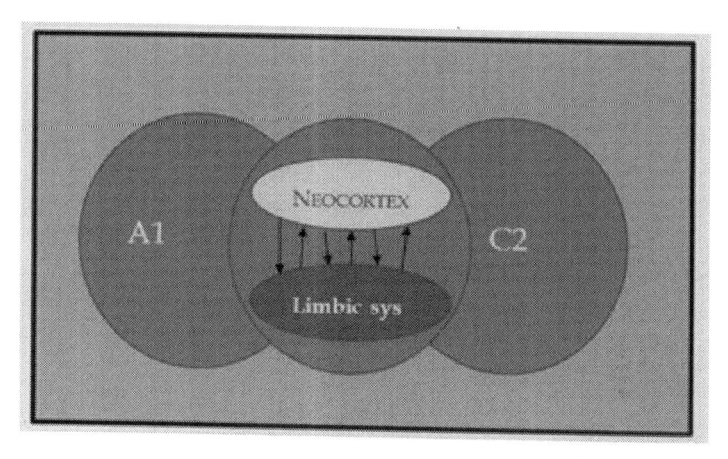

Figure 7.5: A new (hypothetical) model of the complex ABCs

In this new view, a stimulus in the external environment (A1) triggers an interpretation/inference/pattern-match, in the limbic system (initially), which – if the stimulus is sufficiently strong (for example, frightening) causes a signal to be sent (via the limbic system) to C1 (the 'output-manager' or 'action-controller') to take immediate defensive or self-protective action, as argued by LeDoux (1998)[117]. On the other hand, if the stimulus is sufficiently non-urgent, then a slower route towards forming a response is taken, via the neocortex and the individual's history of similar situations (again as clarified by LeDoux, 1998).

From the point of view of a counsellor sitting with a client in their counselling room, the take away message is this:

For most practical purposes, the client is more like a stimulus-response organism than not. They have *emotive-cognitive processing* going on at point B in the ABC model, but that is either handled by their automatic limbic instincts, or by their habitual patterns of response, laid down by their social history, which is most likely managed from the orbitofrontal cortex.

And we may be able to sustain the original idea of the overlapping areas of thinking and emotion, if we accept the description of the orbitofrontal cortex in the writings of Jaak Panksepp (see Panksepp and Biven, 2012). Panksepp describes the orbitofrontal cortex as a prefrontal cortex region in the frontal lobes of the brain which is involved in the cognitive processing of decision making. *But it is also considered to be a **part of the limbic system**.* If it belongs to both the limbic system and the frontal lobes, then is seems like the kind of entity described in the 'overlapping' of brain functions and brain areas.

~~~

Daniel Siegel (2015) suggests a tripartite model of the human 'individual', in which the brain of a child, interacting with its mother, gives rise to 'mind'. This is very similar to the basic E-CENT model which will be reviewed below, but which is essentially about the ways in which the mind of the baby and mother interpenetrate and give rise to the 'ego' or personality of the child.

Daniel Hill's (2015) description suggests a broader, four-part model of human functioning which looks like Figure 7.6 below. This new model by Hill suggests that, far from language, or thoughts, or beliefs being the intervening factor between a person's experience of challenges in their environment and their emotional/behavioural response, the emotional limbic system seems like a better candidate for this role, given its centrality to the organism-environment whole.

This is it:

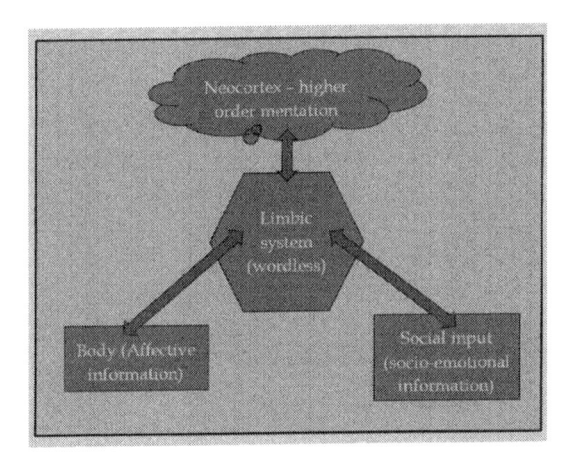

Figure 7.6: Daniel Hill's (2015) four-part model

The wordless limbic system was our original (emotional) control centre, and it continues to be in ultimate control, and it continues to be wordless.

But the overlapping area with the neocortex, the orbitofrontal cortex (OFC), should be seen to store *social learning*, much of which was derived from *language-based instruction*. And if my personality (or 'ego') has a physical (electro-chemical and hormonal base) then it most likely is my orbitofrontal cortex (OFC). (See Damasio on Elliott, in Damasio, 1998).

7.8 Language and mentation

With regard to Daniel Hill's (2015) emphasis upon the *wordlessness* of the limbic system, I should emphasize that the orbitofrontal cortex, which is most likely the seat of the personality and character – the ego – must be assumed to be wired up by *an integration of socialized experience* (including language, actions and paralinguistics) with the innate emotional control systems. (Mahrabian, 1981)[118].

This would mean that, although therapists' nonverbal, emotional communications are very important, so also are their statements, pronouncements and actions in the world.

The client *interprets* what the counsellor or therapist does and says. And those interpretations are largely automatic and non-conscious. Some small elements may enter consciousness.

If the client spots a contradiction between the counsellor's words and the counsellor's actions, s/he will most likely trust the actions and discount the words.

The client interprets what the counsellor says and does, on the basis of their past experiences. They may discount words which they found, earlier in life, to be hollow, or insincere. If they are not accustomed to kind words, or praising words, they may discount them. They may discount anything that they have previously decided to be untrue; or untrue about themselves.

Just as the client *perfinks* – or perceives, feels and thinks – all in one grasp of the mind; so the counsellor must be seen to *communicate* – or to speak, act and metalinguistically emote – all in one act of the self.

And the counsellor does not *know (precisely)* what s/he is communicating to the client, because:

> (a) S/he is a habit-based, socialized, organic being (which is what *all humans* are!). S/he is a largely non-conscious, automatic, stimulus-response organism, just like the client – except a good therapist has been trained to respond as a helpful person. And:

> (b) The client interprets the counsellor's words and actions in the light of the client's own experiences, and not in the light of a glossary of the counsellor's meanings!

However, a good, holistic counsellor often knows the kind of being she is, and therefore gets adequate sleep and hydration and exercise and nutrition (and perhaps meditation) before coming to a counselling session.

Furthermore, a good counsellor should have a better 'map of the good life' to share with the client, who most often has a *dysfunctional map* of life.

And both of those life maps include non-verbal experiences, emotional-cognitive responses, and linguistically-derived elements.

Finally, that brings us neatly to the *social model* of the individual, which I also developed in 2009.

7.9 The social individual

After reviewing the complex ABC model, I went on to lay down the basic E-CENT model of the mother-baby dyad, in Figure 5 of Byrne (2009b)[119], as shown in Figure 7.7 below.

This model helped us to explore the ways in which the mother of a new-born baby has to colonize the baby; take it over; and run its life, for the sake of its survival. The first couple of years of each of our lives is spent in close proximity to mother (or a substitute carer), who is more or less sensitive to our needs; more or less responsive, attuned, and timely in responding; more or less gentle and caring; and so on.

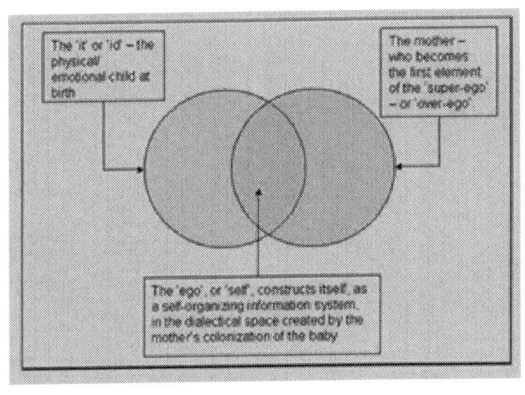

Figure 7.7: The most basic model of E-CENT counselling theory

The personality of the mother dictates the kind of care we get; and the kind of care that we got is internalized as the foundations of our first **Internal Working Model** of relationship. If she can provide us with a 'secure base', then we will grow up with a secure sense of attachment to subsequent love objects, including the individual(s) we marry[120].

It may be that the OK-Corral from Transactional Analysis (TA) captures the core decision of significance which is at the centre of the *Internal Working Model*. This is how the OK-corral model looks:

Figure 7.8: The OK Corral from TA

Thus my basic decision about my relationship with mother might be this: "I'm okay, and so is she!" But it could equally be that "I'm not okay, but she is!" And so on. That early decision, about who I am and how I feel valued or devalued, marks me for life!

This model can be translated (theoretically; propositionally) into a *Working Model equivalent*, in the form of **adult attachment styles**, like this:

		Thoughts-feelings about self	
		Positive	Negative
Thoughts-feelings about partner	Positive	**Secure:** (comfortable with intimacy and autonomy)	**Preoccupied:** (Anxious-ambivalent about relationship: Clingy)
	Negative	**Dismissing:** (Avoidant attachment, cool and remote)	**Disorganized:** (Confused, dissociating, blanking out: Approach-avoidance)

Figure 7.9: Adult attachment styles and appraisals of self and others

This is not a perfect fit with attachment theory, but it has some useful features, and some caveats. For example, the **preoccupied** mind-set of the anxious-ambivalent individual is based on a negative view of the self (or at least a view of the self as *not self-sufficient*, and of *desperately* needing the other person to stick around). And this causes their tendency to cling. On the other hand, they may not see their partner as 'positive' as such (and they may even cling angrily!) but they view their partner as a *'positive asset'* to which they must hold on!

We can also infer, in the average case, that if the mother's (and father's [or main carer's]) way of relating to the baby results in a positive self-appraisal (which is emotive-cognitive), and in a positive appraisal of the care provided by the main carer, then the baby (and later adult) will form a **secure** attachment style, in which they are comfortable with intimacy and autonomy.

On the other hand, in the absence of good-enough parenting, the individual is likely to develop an avoidant, or anxious-ambivalent, or disorganized attachment style.

Of course, there is more to attachment styles than is suggested here.

In particular, each individual builds up a non-linguistic, non-conscious picture of *"How 'they' related to me; who that 'makes me'; and how I had to relate to 'them'; and how I must relate to any new (significant) person in front of (adult) me today."*

We do not have to think about any of this. It's all automatic and non-conscious; a set of pre-patterned ways of relating, based on foundational experiences.

~~~

It takes five or six months for us to distinguish ourselves from our mothers, and we rely upon her, not just for food and comfort and taking care of our colic, and changing our soiled clothing, and so on; but also, and perhaps much more importantly, for her ability *to sooth our **uncontrollable** emotions*.

Young babies cannot soothe themselves, and need external assistance with this challenge. As we grow up, we take back some of those controls, but we never completely outgrow the need for external assistance with 'affect regulation'. (Lewis, Amini, and Lannon, (2001))[121]. We need our mothers to love us if our socialized brains are to grow and provide us with an adequate measure of social and emotional intelligence (Gerhardt, 2010)[122].

As mother interacts with her baby, the baby internalizes representations of the experience of those encounters – at least those which seem emotionally significant. (Siegel, 2015)[123]. And out of those encounters, the baby constructs its *ego*, or *personality* (as illustrated in Figure 7.7 above).

As I wrote at that time:

"Thus the mother wires up the brain of her baby, initially by handling and managing its body; and later by introducing the baby to her language, her linguistic culture, her rules, and her language-based world." (Byrne, 2009b).

But today I would also want to add this: It is not all about language and culture. It is also about the mother's behaviours, and the child's interpretation of those behaviours; which show up as both *narrativized* and ***non-narrativized experiences***!

Of course, the baby brings something to the party – his or her innate wiring in the brain stem and the limbic system; and its enteric brain (in its guts). All of which is instinctive and emotional. There are no 'innate beliefs', since 'beliefs' are linguistic constructions.

So, it is more useful to see the ABC/SOR/EFR models differently. The major mediating variable between

(1) new Activating Stimuli – coming into the senses of the child – and

(2) outgoing emotional and behavioural responses,

can now be seen to be

(3) **Experiences**, and **not** Beliefs!

That is to say, we are wired up for today by our **Previous Experiences**, from the past; *some of which have been **narrativized*** (or can be articulated in language today); and *some of which were **never narrativized***, and cannot be accessed today - because they are totally non-conscious, and beyond retrieval. But they nevertheless play a role in ***guiding** our reactions* to new events today!

~~~

Or how to integrate nutritional insights, exercise and sleep coaching into talk therapy

I have argued above that there are seven innate emotional control systems, and there is an evaluation capacity – 'good' – 'bad' – which guides the baby's reactions to incoming stimuli. A felt experience seems either negative or positive to the newborn baby and young infant; and this triggers one of the emotional control systems: (e.g. anger or fear, or joy, etc.)

The baby, as it develops, shows signs of having pro- and anti-social tendencies, but these are shaped overwhelmingly by the mother's level of skill. A skilful mother can soothe a truculent baby; while an unskilful mother can aggravate and irritate a calm baby and render it truculent.

As the baby grows and encounters mother and father and perhaps a sibling or two, and perhaps *granny*, and *babysitters*, and then perhaps *nursery teachers*, and so on, s/he increasingly internalizes their ways of being: their Parental tendencies; their Adult tendencies; their Child-like tendencies.

And the child can also link those states to its own child-like tendencies, and, from age two years onwards, increasingly to act like a Little Professor, asking questions and exploring its environment.

But s/he (the child) mainly learns from instruction and modelling, and trial and error, and eventually can organize all those Parent, Adult and Child experiences – with good and bad aspects – into coherent wholes, below the level of conscious awareness, until his or her personality (C) emerges (through the interaction of A and B) like this:

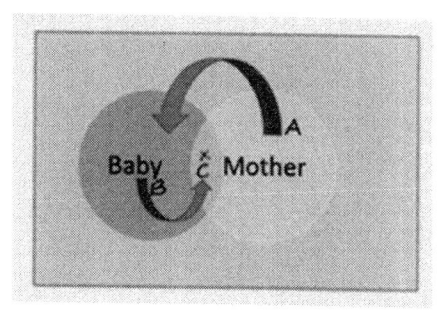

The child internalizes representations of its encounters with mother, and in the overlapping space of encounter, a cluster of ego state possibilities arise, which are later triggered by external stimuli. (See Figure 7.10 below). And in the overlapping space of their emotional encounters, the child constructs its own sense of self.

The child knows how to act like the child it is today, and the child it was in an earlier period (regressing to that state when stress levels are high).

The child knows how mother and father act and speak.

So children know not just *how to be scientific* and *inquiring*, and *how to be playful*, but also *how to order mother* to do things, and *how to comfort mother* when she is apparently unwell. (In other words, children have a number of *different* embryonic ego-states, or ways of being, which they copied from their social environment; and which we commonly call **Parent Adult** and **Child** ego states). See Figure 7.10, below:

143.

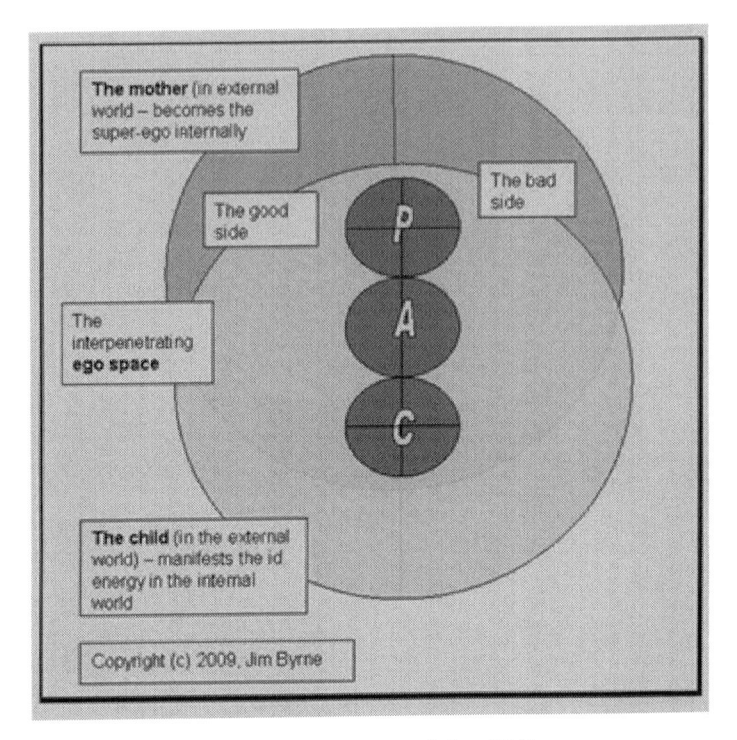

Figure 7.10: The structure of the child's ego

Each of those 'ego state' possibilities – Child, Parent, Adult - has a **good** side and a **bad** side. The good side is constructive and pro-social; and the bad side is destructive and anti-social. (These two states are also known as *Eros* and *Thanatos* [in Freud's language] – or the *Good Wolf* and the *Bad Wolf* [in the language of the native American Cherokee people]).

Figure 7.10 above shows a summary of those developments.

The emergent ego of every child contains the embryonic components of Good and Bad Nurturing Parent; Good and Bad Controlling Parent; Good and Bad Adult; Good and Bad Adapted/Rebellious Child; and Good and Bad Free (or Natural) Child.

~~~

In Byrne (2009b), I explored the nature of a physical/social human by exploring my own nature. This was my conclusion:

Perhaps I am just this physical organism (body/brain/mind)

Including its feeling/affective foundation (in the limbic system)

And its language based – or language-aided - cognitive/emotive superstructure (in the neocortex, and the orbitofrontal cortex)

With all of its cumulative, interpretative experiences

Including internalized representations of good and bad aspects of significant others

And all of my good and bad adaptations towards them

And my good and bad reactions and rebellions against them

Which gave rise to my Internal Working Models, of how they (my significant others) related to me (positively or negatively), and how I related to them (positively or negatively)

All of which is stored in long term memory

*In the form of electro-chemical equivalents of stories, scripts, frames, schemas and other narrativized **and non-narrativized** elements*

Below the level of conscious awareness

*And **permanently** beyond direct conscious inspection.*

Perhaps that is what I most fundamentally am. And thus, although I am *distinct* from others, I carry many others inside my head, and I am indeed made up of many 'social/ relational/ interactional bits and pieces'. So I am both individual and social. But I am very far from being a 'separate entity'.

Because my sense of 'self' develops in lockstep with my sense of 'society', and with my biological development, none of these three 'levels' of 'me/I/us' can exist (for any significant period of time) without the other.

~~~

From the point of view of an E-CENT counsellor, working with a client, it is important to note that the individual is hard-wired by nature to be *an emotional being*. This emotional being (as a baby) is thrown into a family with its own cultural shape, which impacts the baby so powerfully that it leaves its mark on the baby like a die stamps a pattern on a copper or silver coin. The coin is malleable, and can be melted down and re-stamped, but not easily. (It takes a lot of heat to melt it!) And the child, once grown up, retains some neurological and psychological malleability, but also lots of rigidity or habit-based inflexibilities.

Counselling and therapy can begin to work on restructuring the emotional/ neurological shape of the socialized individual (by 'melting it'), but the outcome depends upon how good the client is at taking on the necessary hard work (of melting into the possibilities offered – many of which will involve feeling previously unfelt pains!).

The counsellor can be available as a secure base for the client - and a safe harbour to come back to again and again - and thus hope to re-parent the client (which also means: *to re-educate the emotions and thinking* of the client). But none of this is easy, and it's certainly not automatic.

When a client sits before me, I do not see a discrete, separate, stand-alone individual. I see the outworking of a complex family history. I sense the many Internal Working Models from which this social-individual relates to the world. I am aware that this is *an emotional being*, with some capacity to *think* (or *perfink*!) and learn; but also most likely s/he is a "community of sub-personalities"[124] with some strongly *frozen schemas!* Those 'frozen schemas' are fixed *frames*, or ways of perceiving-feeling-thinking about the world as interpreted. And, because those frames are non-conscious, the client cannot offer them up for examination in counselling. They have to be 'stumbled upon' by serendipity!

~~~

Let us now look at how we can tackle some typical emotional disturbances - like anger, anxiety and depression - in counselling or self-help contexts.

7.10 Managing human emotions

Like Panksepp (1998)[125] and Schore (2015)[126], Daniel Siegel in his (2015) book on the developing mind, emphasizes that what we call 'appraisal' is an *emotive* rather than a *thinking* process. The emotional centres of the brain can appraise an incoming stimulus as either 'good' or 'bad' from the beginning of life, long before we have any form of language labels. (This has been tested empirically, with either a sweet or a sour drink for the baby's first drink after birth, combined with observation of their facial responses!)[127] And from this innate appraisal process, and using our emotional control systems (described by Panksepp, 1998), we elaborate some basic emotional reactions, of anger, sadness, fear, surprise and/or joy[128].

In E-CENT theory we see that slightly differently.

In the beginning, the baby uses its innate, basic emotions to evaluate the goodness or badness of a situation.

But over time, and especially in the first two or three years of life, the new child is taught by its carers to modulate its affects - through rewards, penalties, modelling, soothing, and so on, and it may be that that integration of socialized-emotions, or higher cognitive-emotions, are stored in the Orbitofrontal Cortex (OFC).

Thereafter, appraisal becomes *a learned emotive-cognitive process*. And it should be thought of as a function of *perfinking*, rather than either *thinking* (which is the CBT preference) or *emoting* (which is the Affect Regulation Theory preference).

Thus it is clear that E-CENT does not follow either of the extremes – the *cognitivists* or the *emotivists* – but rather that we have *'perfinked'* our own way to a *novel, balanced* solution, which takes account of the innate (emotive) affects, and the later (linguistic-cultural) shaping, both of which are woven together into the *perfinking body-brain-mind*.

~~~

Siegel's (2015) argument is that the baby's 'primary feelings' - (which can be expressed by us as 'this is good'; 'this is bad'; or 'this feels good'; 'this feels bad') - are elaborated over time into (categorical) emotions (of anger, sadness, joy, fear, etc.).

Furthermore, babies need external regulation (soothing), and it's the quality, quantity and timeliness of that soothing that shapes the baby's dominant mood and habitual emotional profile. (Siegel, 2015, page 183).

As we grow and develop, interact with our care-givers, learn to read their nonverbal emotional states, and increasingly acquire language, we also evolve/ acquire higher cognitive emotions (like guilt, shame, pride, love, embarrassment, elevation, envy, and jealousy, etc.): and the flow of basic emotions, and socially-shaped emotions, is what *creates **meaning** in our lives*, and allows us to appraise our situations in life. According to Siegel (2015): Emotions do not follow from thinking. Thinking follows from socialized-emotion. Attention and perception are also modulated by emotion. Emotions are basic to who we are and who we become. And the central features of emotion are *(non-conscious) appraisal* and *(non-conscious) arousal*. (Siegel, 2015. Pages 184-185).

Our ability to manage our emotions, to "regulate our affects", is a function of our history of attachment with our primary carers and subsequent significant others. (Bowlby, 1988/2005; Schore, 2015; Siegel, 2015; Wallin, 2007[129]).

In E-CENT theory, we see that slightly differently. Firstly, innate feelings precede, and are the foundation for, subsequent socialized perfinking (perceiving-feeling-thinking). What we call 'thinking' never was a separate function of the brain-mind. *It is one of our delusions* (Gray, 2003) that we are thinking being; that we think; that we have thoughts; that we can reason, separately and apart from feelings and automatic perceptions!

To an E-CENT counsellor, a client has two major aspects:

First, s/he is:

(1) A *physical/cultural organism*, with all of his/her cumulative, interpretive (*perfinked*) experiences, stored in long-term memory, below the level of conscious awareness, and permanently beyond conscious inspection: (Byrne 2009b). But the client is ***also:***

(2) A *subjective*, felt-being, and feeling-being, a *virtual self* which feels like a **concrete** reality in the world. (Erwin, 1997)[130].

I do not *think* it ethical – or *perfink it* to be ethical - that we relate to the client exclusively on the basis of aspect (1) above. We must always recognize aspect (2) as *the dominant **reality** for the client*; while aspect (1) is the dominant reality for science.

But although E-CENT counsellors use science to find our way through the swamp of social and individual psychology, *we are **not** primarily scientists*.

*We are primarily **healers** and **feeling – perfinking** - beings.* We not only show our clients cognitive empathy (like all other systems of counselling and therapy) but also emotive empathy. We feel for the client; and with the client: (as do 'affect regulation' therapists – Hill, 2015).

And our obvious pain upon learning of the client's suffering is part of what heals them! (Because they 'feel felt'!)

We care deeply about our clients, because there is "only one being", and we all participate in that being. The universe is one big living being!

And then – if it is possible to anticipate what we normally do' - we try to get the client to tell us what is going on (confession) and we investigate that situation (explication), and then we set about educating the client, like a good parent – a good *re-parenting* 'secure base'.

In between the *explication* and the *education*, is the process of 'agreeing a story' of 'what is going on', or 'what is going wrong', which makes sense to us and to the client, *so we can **agree** a **potential** way forward.*

7.11 Managing anger, anxiety and depression

So let us look, briefly, at those three common emotional problems mentioned above.

7.11(a). Anger:

The E-CENT theory of anger says that anger is one of our basic emotions. It's innate. It was selected by nature for its survival value. We would not survive for long without an innate sense of *angering* in response to abuse or neglect. We also would not survive for long if we did not quickly learn how to *moderate* our anger as young children. My anger is a two-edged sword. It can help to protect me, and it can attract hostile reactions from others.

My **basic** emotion of anger is elaborated into a *higher cognitive emotion* through modelling by my mother and father and significant others in the first few years of my life. My ability to become *emotionally intelligent* in relation to my innate anger urges depends on the emotional intelligence of my parents. My first angry outbursts are with them. How successfully I and they handle those angry episodes will shape how I manage my anger in the school playground. And my socialized anger management strategies continue to evolve through my successful and my unsuccessful experiences of engaging in conflict with others: siblings, school peers, and so on.

I may become an *exploder*, who erupts in the faces of others. I may become an *imploder*, who keeps his anger inside. Or I may hide my anger from myself (repress it) and then project it into my environment where it may frighten me.

So anger is a socialized emotion, and if you grew up with angry people, you are likely to be prone to angering yourself when provoked; or you might feel fearful of your own anger, or the anger of others.

~~~

Healthy anger is present-time defence of your legitimate rights in the face of inappropriate behaviour by another person. Healthy or *reasonable* anger is the fuel that drives our **assertive** behaviours. It pushes us to engage in *constructive conflict*, when that is *necessary*!

To ask for what you want, which is legitimately yours to request, requires a certain level of 'fire in your belly'. If you lack that fire (that *reasonable* level of anger), then you will tend to 'wimp-out'; to act passively and let other people control you, or intimidate you, or deny you your reasonable share of the social stage. One of the problems that we encounter in therapy is this: Some parents, anxious to socialize their children to be 'nice' and 'civilized', go too far in 'switching off their fierceness' – instead of teaching them to manage their fierceness appropriately. And one of the things we do for passive clients is to help them to switch on their 'fierceness switch' – but to only use their fierceness assertively, up to the boundary of their personal space – and never to invade the personal space of another – or to use their fierceness aggressively!

Unhealthy or ***unreasonable*** anger is an over-reaction to a frustrating or insulting stimulus from another person or external force. Unhealthy or unreasonable anger leads to **aggressive** actions and destructive conflict. It is an excessive use of fierceness, and an under-use of communication and negotiation strategies.

We teach the following eight insights to our anger management clients:

1. You were born with *an **innate capacity** to develop angry*, anxious and depressed responses to your social environment - in response to frustrations, threats and losses.

2. You then encountered your mother, who already had a 'style of relating', based on her attachment experience of her own mother and father. She would inevitably have shaped your emotional expression by:

(a) Modelling an approach to relationship and emotions; and:

(b) Rewarding and penalizing you for your daily emotion expressions, including your angry outbursts in the first couple of years of your life.

3. Your father's approach to relationship, including emotion expression, especially his way of expressing (or suppressing) anger, would have been the next major influence on the development of your emotion expression, including your way of being angry - implosive or explosive; appropriate or inappropriate.

4. If both of your parents had a secure attachment to their own parents, they would have had a warm but assertive approach to relating to you. From them you would

have learned to be secure in your relationship with them, and, by extension, in virtually all subsequent people-encounters. You would have learned to express healthy or appropriate anger in an *assertive* way - to ask for what you want, and to say no to what you do not want. And to strive to be treated with respect as an equal human being. You would not have any significant problems with anger.

5. However, if one or both of your parents had an insecure attachment to their own parents, they would have had an insecure attachment to you, and been either explosively or implosively angry with you when you frustrated them or broke their *personal* rules, or their *culturally shaped moral rules*. From them, you would have learned to engage in unhealthy or inappropriate anger expression of an explosive or implosive type, or a mixture of the two, varying from situation to situation. (Or you might have learned to be *passive* in those situations in which you felt frightened or fearful of reprisals, but *aggressive* in those situations where you felt no constraint of fearfulness!)

6. If you want to change your relationship style today, you need to experience secure relationship with another person - possibly a romantic partner; a very good friend; or a good therapist who understands how to build a secure relationship with you. You need to learn the difference between **appropriate** and **inappropriate** anger. And also that **explosive** anger - (like shouting and using aggressive body language) - costs you, in terms of damage to relationships and careers, for examples; and that **implosive** anger – (like sulking and stewing in your own angry juices, or withdrawing aggressively) - damages your ongoing happiness, your relationships at home and at work, and ultimately your physical and mental health.

7. You can improve your relationship and attachment style by studying and applying new ideas from emotional literacy and self-assertion. And I (and/or other counsellors) can teach those ideas and skills to you.

8. But you are also a body-mind, and so your approach to managing your diet, physical exercise, sleep pattern, self-talk (or inner dialogue), and relaxation/meditation, are also important. And it is easier to develop a secure attachment style if your romantic partner is already secure.

9. See Chapter 4 – sections 4.3 to 4.7 - for specific dietary guidance and advice.

~~~

When an E-CENT counsellor works with an angry client, they may work on deep, emotional and attachment issues from early childhood; or on present-time assertiveness skills; or advice on important dietary changes; or recommendations regarding regular physical exercise, or improvements to sleep patterns; or teaching the client how to reframe their anger-inducing experiences; or changing some elements of their philosophy of life (as they show up in their inner dialogues about anger-inducing situations) – and even to change some aspect of their social or physical environment with which they have been putting up or tolerating unnecessarily!

~~~

Managing anger with diet and nutrition

In Taylor-Byrne and Byrne (2017), we explored - among other things - the key ways in which *diet can influence anger*. Some of the key findings were as follows:

Firstly, (unlike in the case of depression) there is at least one study which supports the idea that there is a link between low serotonin levels and the expression of anger, annoyance and irritation (specifically, low serotonin was linked to a reduced ability to self-manage rising levels of anger). We also presented evidence which showed that 5HTP, a natural nutritional supplement (from a West African medicinal plant called *Griffonia simpicifolia*), can be effective in restoring serotonin, an important neurotransmitter within the brain, thus reducing the expression of angry and hostile behaviour, as evidenced by Julie Ross's (2002) case study example.

The levels of copper and manganese in the client's body can have an effect on levels of anger; so vitamin and mineral supplementation seems to be important to address.

The link between violent behaviour - by young offenders (in prison) - and the condition known as 'reactive hypoglycaemia' (where blood sugar levels fall too low after eating high carbohydrate meals) - has been established by scientific research. There is thus an obvious connection between fluctuating blood sugar levels and anger management problems, and this can guide us in recommending particular (low sugar, slow-burning) foods to our angry clients.

A number of studies have established a definite link between a reduction in the consumption of sugar and refined foods, (on the one hand), and anger and anti-social behaviour, (on the other). In a similar vein, reductions in diets containing trans-fats, mainly involving hydrogenated fats in processed foods, led to a reduction in impatience, irritability and aggression in research participants.

Conversely, the link between pro-social behaviour and a healthy diet has also been evidenced by research. Dietary changes which increase the nutritional content of people's diets (especially introducing omega-3 fatty acids, as found for example in oily fish; plus vitamin and mineral supplements) result in improvements in pro-social behaviour, and better emotion and mood control. Anger levels declined in prisoners whose diet had been supplemented with fish oils, vitamins and minerals: and it has been shown that omega-3 fats have a rapid and significant impact on aggression in children and adults.

For further information, please see sections 4.3 to 4.7 above; and also Taylor-Byrne and Byrne (2017), for specific dietary guidance and advice.

~~~

How anger can be reduced by exercise:

According to the British National Health Service website, anger is effectively reduced in intensity by exercising, including walking, swimming and yoga. Research studies have supported this view, and here are some examples which have provided valuable evidence on the role of exercise in anger reduction:

Research conducted by Joseph Tkacz, *et al.*, (2008), found that aerobic exercise regimes reduced anger expression among obese children. It was the first study which had been conducted to assess the value of having structured aerobic exercise sessions for overweight children, and the findings pointed to the value of exercise sessions after school.

Also, there was a study which investigated levels of anger amongst undergraduates at the University of Georgia. It looked at whether physical education (exercise) could moderate anger: (Reynolds, 2010); and it was reported in the *New York Times* magazine.

The 16 students selected were regularly oversensitive to provocations, and their anger was easily triggered.

They were subjected to different research conditions (*provocations*), designed to arouse their anger.

Firstly, those provocations were experienced without the benefits of exercise;

Secondly, they were experienced after the benefits of exercise.

The research results revealed that, the provocations had a stronger angering effect – producing a higher level of anger - ***before*** the exercise than they did after the participants had engaged in physical exercise.

After they had exercised, they were able to show composure and self-assurance in the face of emotional provocation. The physical exercise program did reduce their levels of anger, prompting the lead researcher, Nathaniel Thoms, a stress physiologist, to say:

"Exercise, even a single bout of it, can have a robust prophylactic (therapeutic) effect against the build-up of anger…it's like taking an aspirin to combat heart disease. You reduce your risk".

This result is echoed by the advice of the Mayo Clinic Staff, who have written that the higher the levels of stress a person is experiencing, the more likely they are to have high levels of anger, and that these effects can be diminished by vigorous and pleasurable exercise.

For further information, please see section 4.10 above; plus Taylor-Byrne and Byrne (2017), for more specific information on research into different forms of exercise.

~~~

7.11(b). Anxiety:

The E-CENT theory of anxiety says that we are born with an innate sense of fear: (Darwin, 1872/1965; and Panksepp, 1998). Babies begin to display a pronounced sense of fear from about the age of six or seven months. This sense of fear is of something that is present – like loud noise; a furry animal; something that looks like a snake; etc. In time, we learn to feel anxious, which is to say, fearful about things that are *not* present, but which we 'think-feel' (consciously and/or non-consciously) might represents threats and dangers just a little while in the future.

People feel different intensities of anxiety, depending upon the seriousness of the threat or danger that they are anticipating, and how that degree of seriousness interacts with their felt sense of 'coping capability'. That is to say:

1. *The less serious the inferred threat is assumed to be* - and the more coping capability we sense that we have - then the *lower* our intensity of anxiety is likely to be.

(Our coping capability seems to be a combination of physical solidity or confidence; emotional stability and optimism; and security of attachment. And these capabilities are fed by healthy diet, regular physical exercise, relaxation/ meditation, social connection, adequate sleep, and so on)

2. *On the other hand, the more serious the inferred threat is assumed to be* - and the less coping capability we sense that we have - then the *higher* our intensity of anxiety is likely to be.

~~~

REBT theorists distinguish between anxiety (which is intense) and concern (which is much less intense); and some others theorists distinguish between anxiety (which is helpful) and panic (which is unhelpful): Kashdan and Biswas-Diener (2015)[131].

In E-CENT counselling we do not go along with those kinds of distinctions. We see our clients as having a range of anxious-feeling potential, from very low to very high; and we normally work with clients whose anxiety level is high or very high, and our aim is to help them to reduce it until it is low, or very low. But they will never get rid of it; nor should they try to do so, as we **need** each of our basic emotions. *What needs to be reformed is* **how those basic emotions became socialized!** If we come from *emotionally less intelligent families*, then we will need to **re-learn** how to *emote*, as we become adults, so that we behave ***appropriately*** with those people with whom we work, rest and play.

We also work with clients whose anxiety gets out of control, and becomes panic – which we conceptualize as *anxiety about anxiety about anxiety* – spiralling out of control.

And we teach panicky clients the following guidelines:

(1) Accept your panic as your own creation (embrace it rather than trying to push it away. You **cannot** push your **own** *agitated lungs and guts away*!)

(2) Recognize that panic passes in a matter of a couple of minutes, so 'play a waiting game'. And:

(3) Take yourself outside and lean against a wall; focus on your breathing, and make your outbreath longer than your inbreath. You can guess at that, or you can count your outbreath to the count of eleven, and your inbreath to the count of seven. Or, if that's too complex, *breathe* **out** *for a much* **longer** *period that you breathe in*. Try to empty your lungs completely, before allowing the inbreath to return.

Here is some advice for managing anxiety in general:

Practical strategies for managing anxiety

1. Make sure you get enough sleep.

2. Arise in a timely manner to get on top of the challenges of the day.

3(a) Eat a hearty breakfast of either complex carbohydrates, or protein, but it is perhaps best not to mix them (according to Dr Hay; although Patrick Holford advises mixing them!)

3(b) Avoid caffeine drinks and sugary drinks. (One mug of real coffee each day is a good upper-limit guideline. But if you are particularly sensitive to caffeine, avoid it completely!) Avoid junk foods because they are high in sugar and bad fats (trans-fats).

4. Make sure you have a mid-morning snack – e.g. a piece of fruit, or some nuts and seeds (assuming you are not allergic to fructose and seeds.)

5. Do not skip lunch or evening meals. Eat a healthy, balanced diet. (The Mediterranean diet is widely recommended. As is the Nordic diet; and, to a lesser extent, the Paleo diet. But we recommend that you develop a personalized diet, by trial and error; perhaps with the support of a nutritionist).

6. Meditate after breakfast, and then do about thirty minutes of physical exercise at the start of each day. (If it helps, you could start off doing five or ten minutes of each, and then gradually increase the time over the first couple of years, until you reach thirty minutes of each [meditation and exercise], every day – or at least five or six days per week). These two processes tend to calm your central nervous system, making it less reactive.

7. Whenever you feel tense, take a mental break, and take five deep, slow, relaxing breaths. If that does not relax you, then stand up and walk around, counting to twenty silently in your mind. (Sitting around for too long can increase your anxiety level. Sedentary lifestyle is bad for both physical health and emotional wellbeing. So, take frequent breaks and walk around)[132].

8. Set a few (3-6) *realistic* goals for the day, and try to achieve them. Do not aim for perfection. Only try to control what seems likely to be controllable, and leave the rest. Accept the things you cannot change.

9. Watch comedy shows on TV or DVDs, when you get home, instead of *bad News*, or stressful *Current Affairs*. Have a hobby. Read something enjoyable before bedtime.

10. Work at developing good, supportive relationships, at home and at work, and in your community.

11. Keep a journal, and write about your anxiety symptoms. What are the triggers? What about those triggers is controllable? What could you do to problem-solve in that area of your life? Set goals to change those changeable aspects of your life that cause you anxiety. And accept the rest!

12. Identify a good counsellor or psychotherapist to whom you can talk about your anxiety problems, with a view to changing what can be changed, and learning to accept what is beyond your control.

13. Additional dietary advice might include the following:

- You might need to supplement your vitamin intake from food with a good multi-vitamin and mineral tablet; plus B-Complex; plus omega-3 fatty acid capsules (or strong cod liver oil; or Krill oil capsules); and perhaps *kava kava*.

- Drink lots of water, (six to eight glasses of filtered or glass-bottled water per day), and limit alcohol consumption to one unit every other day, or less.

- Drink herbal tea instead of caffeinated drinks, especially if you have difficulty reducing your anxiety by other means.

~~~

Anxiety management: The impact of diet and nutrition

It has been proven empirically that dietary changes can reduce the experience of anxiety: as demonstrated in Taylor-Byrne and Byrne, 2017.

Firstly, 2011 was the first year in which there was a double-blind trial establishing that there was a link between omega-3 fatty acids and a reduction in anxiety. This connection has been confirmed by many hundreds of anecdotal accounts by clients (to their professional practitioners) in which those clients have attested to the benefits in anxiety reduction, which they personally gained from omega-3 fatty acids.

~~~

Secondly, both magnesium and GABA (gamma-amino-butyric acid) are very valuable for the body-brain-mind in terms of reducing tension, anxiety and hyperarousal. The recommended foods are as follows: dark green leafy vegetables, (like spinach and kale); nuts (walnuts and almonds); and seeds; fruit (e.g. bananas); and oats; and extracts of Reishi (described as the power mushroom).

~~~

Thirdly, the management of our blood sugar levels can stop the following vicious circle happening:

(1) A person (ill informed) eats white bread, or white pasta, white rice, chocolates and drinks fizzy drinks;

(2) As a direct consequence of this ill-advised activity, this person experiences a rapid rise in blood sugar.

(3) Soon afterwards, this is followed by a big drop in blood sugar levels, as the person's body releases insulin to cope with the sudden influx of sugar. And then,

(4) **Because** of the sudden drop in blood sugar, the hormone, adrenalin, is released into the bloodstream. This results in experiencing a racing heart and rapid breathing, and negative *perfinking* (or perceiving-feeling-thinking) processes, which create the symptoms of anxiety.

(The vicious circle, of course, is this: When some people feel anxious, they reach for 'comfort foods', which boost their blood sugar levels – and the whole cycle begins all over again!)

The recommended solution is to alter the combination of foods that you eat, so the release of energy, from the digestion of the food, is slowed down. Also it is recommended that people avoid refined carbohydrates, and simple sugars. Eating vegetables, oily fish and reducing meat consumption; plus eating nuts and seeds; would mean that the blood-sugar roller-coaster effect would be avoided. (This is called 'eating slow-burning fuels').

~~~

Fourthly, there is growing evidence that the state of our guts, including our gut bacteria, is very important in managing the experience of anxiety. This view is expressed by Dr David Perlmutter (2015). He cites many research studies which establish several facts:

(1) When we eat foods containing gluten, this affects the junctions between cells in the intestines, called the 'tight junctions'. This makes them leaky, and this enables toxins that come from within the bacteria in the intestines to enter the bloodstream. As a consequence they bring about a massive inflammatory response in the body-brain.

(2) Perlmutter (2015) also considers that there are physical vulnerabilities which can precipitate high levels of inflammation in the body, such as antibiotic use, manner of birth, and the balance of bacteria in the gut.

(3) Dietary changes therefore are necessary to heal the gut, such as:

>(a) Giving up gluten-containing foods (like: wheat; rye; [non-organic] oats; and barley – and any foods containing those grains); and:

>(b) Consuming oral probiotic supplements, and vitamin supplements. (Specific probiotics [e.g. *lactobacillus* and *bifidobacterium*] reduce anxiety and return the intestines to full health and proper functioning.)

(4) But he also considers lifestyle changes such as sufficient sleep and aerobic exercise as necessary to complete the process.

~~~

There is also research supporting the conclusion that the consumption of caffeine, sugar, artificial sweeteners and alcohol actually *create* anxiety in the human body. Two relevant examples to mention are the consumption of caffeine and sugar. High levels of caffeine in coffee bring about a sudden increase in tension and anxiety, and sugar causes a drop in our blood sugar as the body tries to cope, and this results in feelings of anxiety and weakness in the body.

For further information, please see Taylor-Byrne and Byrne (2017), for specific dietary guidance and advice. (But also remember to 'find out for yourself'; perhaps by consulting a nutritional therapist or alternative or lifestyle medical practitioner).

~~~

Anxiety management: How anxiety can be reduced by exercise:

If we do not exercise, we are asking for trouble, for our body-minds. This is because, as human animals, we have evolved to handle threats and dangers *by taking physical action*. If we don't take physical action when presented by a threat, we will experience anxiety and a build-up of stress hormones in our body-mind.

We need to process the stressors in our daily lives and remove the stress hormones from our body-mind by taking physical action. Exercise is a form of managed stress exerted on the body-brain-mind, which actually reduces stress hormones and the feeling of anxiety.

Joshua Broman-Fulks proved this in 2004 with students suffering from anxiety. Two weeks of exercise reduced their anxiety levels, and made the students less sensitive to anxiety.

If our bodies are tense, the brain-mind registers this and starts to go on red alert. But if we exercise, this action reduces the tension in our muscles – and if our bodies are relaxed the brain-mind does not worry. So exercise stops the anxiety 'feedback loop', whereby we become anxious about being anxious, which then activates the brain into starting the 'fight or flight' response.

Exercise works by making chemical alterations in our bodies. As our muscles move, fat molecules are broken down to provide energy for this extra demand on the body. This then releases fatty acids into the bloodstream, and tryptophan and serotonin - (which some theorists call *the 'feel-good' hormone*) - increase, and (it is thought by some), serotonin calms us down and also increases our feelings of safety.

For further information please see sections 4.9, 4.12, and 4.13, above; plus Taylor-Byrne and Byrne (2017), for information about exercise benefits.

~~~

7.11(c). Depression:

The E-CENT theory of depression says we have to distinguish between ***transient grief*** and ***stuck depression***.

Our primary stance on depression and grief is this:

Grief is 'depression' which is *appropriate* to some significant loss or failure in the recent past. While ***depression*** is stuck-'grief' which is *inappropriate* to loss or failure in the more distant past.

But we also have a secondary stance:

Inappropriate depression can also come from *exaggerating* the degree of badness of a current or recent loss or failure; or refusing to accept its inevitability; or trying (in your mind) to reverse an irreversible loss or failure.

Our (primary stance) distinction (between grief and depression) is equivalent to saying that there is ***appropriate depression*** (called 'grief', which *gradually* heals itself) and ***inappropriate depression*** (called 'depression', which *gets stuck* and needs some kind of psychological intervention).

Grief and depression are intense forms of sadness about real or symbolic losses (or failures), combined with a sense of hopelessness and helplessness.

Grief is a helpful emotion which has enhanced human survival; while there is also a kind of ***inappropriate-depression*** which indicates a grief process that is stuck, and which is not being processed over time; or an ***exaggerated sense*** of recent loss.

When clients present with grief about a recent (significant) loss or failure, E-CENT counsellors offer sympathy and understanding, and sensitive attunement to their emotional state. Over time, we encourage the client to cry, to grieve, and to heal. There is only so much crying that a person can do about a loss (or failure), if they are gradually *completing their experience* of that loss (or failure).

Stuck-depression is an <u>unhelpful</u> emotion: When client-grief goes on for more than about eighteen months, we consider that the process is stuck and needs to be moved forwards. Two common scenarios are encountered by us:

Scenario 1: Sometimes that stuckness is caused by *trauma* – arising out of the fact that the client was already overly stressed when they experienced the loss or failure in question. So we assist this client by suggesting that we help them to work through our desensitization process (outlined in Appendix C of Byrne, 2016).

Or we guide them through a process of getting in touch with their depressed feelings; naming them; describing them in words; and reflecting upon their growing understanding of *what it means* (to them) to have these feelings (about their loss [or failure]).

Scenario 2: On the other hand, sometimes the process of grieving gets stuck because of temperament/character problems within the client. This normally takes the form of *excessively strong* **demands** *that the loss or failure* **must be reversed**, somehow – even if somebody has died, or the lost thing no longer exists.

And it does not even have to extend to *strong* **demands**. It can simply be *an unrealistic desire* which is so important to the client that they cannot let it go, even when it clearly cannot be achieved! ("One hairsbreadth difference between what you want and what you've got, and heaven and earth are set apart!")

In this latter kind of stuck-depression, (which we have labelled as **Scenario 2** above), we might use the *Six Windows Model* to teach the client to *reframe* their depressing loss or failure: (See Chapter 6 above). And/or we might recommend that they write out a Gratitude List, every night, for thirty or sixty nights, containing five or six items for which they can be *grateful*. Thus, they can learn to focus upon *what they've* **got**, for which they can be grateful, instead of *what they have* **lost**, which they cannot (presently) retrieve!

And we would tend to give the following dietary advice: Avoid sugary foods, but do have complex carbohydrates, from vegetables, fruit and (some experts say) whole grains. (However, the Paleo Diet theorists claim that *all grains* cause inflammation in the body-brain, beginning in the guts: and anything that causes physical inflammation will make our emotional well-being worse, not better!) Gluten-free oats might be a good compromise. And brown rice seems to be a safe grain.

Lots of nutrient-rich salads can help; plus good fats, like olive oil, and coconut oil (if you can tolerate fats!) Salmon, sardines, trout and other oily fish are good for brain health. (All of these foods provide a good supply of omega 3 fatty acids).

Avoid factory-farmed chicken, as it contains lots of antibiotics, which tend to kill off your friendly gut bacteria, and there is a link between healthy gut bacteria and emotional well-being. (Borchard, 2015)[133].

Also, avoid trans-fats (which are super-heated, hydrogenated fats).

And make sure you get lots of vitamin D, mainly from daily exposure to sunlight, but supplement with tablet form if necessary: (Mercola, 2013) And a good, full spectrum multivitamin and mineral, plus B-Complex, are also recommended by many theorists. (E.g. Ross, 2003).

For more information on diet, nutrition, and healthy gut bacteria, please see sections 4.5-4.7, in Chapter 4 above; plus Taylor-Byrne and Byrne (2017).

~~~

Depression: How diet and nutrition can reduce and eliminate it
In Chapter 4 above, we present a lot of research evidence for the link between diet and depression. For examples:

Both Dr Kelly Brogan (2016) and Dr David Perlmutter (2015) are convinced that depression doesn't come from chemical imbalances in the brain. They consider that the health condition of the gut, if addressed, can eliminate the experience of depression. The main culprit in the creation of mental disorder (or emotional distress) is inflammation in the body; and specific dietary strategies can eliminate this.

Reducing (or, preferably, eliminating) sugar consumption - and getting rid of processed or refined foods - is considered to be very important. So dietary changes which improve nutrition are essential, as well as meditation and exercise. These are daily strategies for the reduction of depression.

Apparently, according to Dr Perlmutter (2015), the health and balance of our gut microbes are very important, as they regulate cortisol and adrenalin (which are the major hormones of the stress response). Interestingly, our guts contain about 70-80% of our immune system (and about 80% of our serotonin – which some theorists see as intimately linked to controlling depression; but some disagree).

The ways in which depression can be reduced, according to Dr Perlmutter (2015), include following these dietary recommendations:

Switch to gluten-free foods;

eat healthy fats (and get rid of and avoid trans-fats);

take *prebiotics* (like psyllium husk, and fibrous vegetables), and *probiotics* (like Acidophilus);

eat fermented foods, like sauerkraut, kimchi, etc.;

and stick to low-carb foods.

Patrick Holford (2010) and Dr Sarah Brewer (2013) are of the opinion that fish oils (which contain lots of omega-3 fatty acids) are very important to help prevent depression. Holford recommends supplementation with natural herbs, minerals and chemicals which balance our neurotransmitters. He further considers that there are also psychological factors present in depression, which are related to a person's life and whether they are living it in a way which is true to themselves. These latter issues benefit from talk therapy.

Finally, Robert Redfern (2016) cites evidence that the nutrient B9, which is folate, is one of the main nutrients in a healthy diet that can reduce the risk of depression. The research which he quotes, which was conducted at the University of Eastern Finland, showed that eating a healthy diet, free from processed foods, reduced depressive symptoms and created an overall lower risk of severe depression.

For further information, please see Taylor-Byrne and Byrne (2017), for specific dietary guidance and advice.

~~~

Depression: How it can be reduced by exercise

The value of exercise for reducing depression is very well-proven, and this has been confirmed by Blumenthal *et al.* (1999). They carried out what became known as a landmark study, which contrasted the value of exercise with the drug Sertraline, (which is also called Zoloft).

There were three different patient groups for the research procedure:

a group of patients on Zoloft;

an exercise group,

and a group on a combination of exercise and Zoloft.

The exercise group had supervised exercise three times a week.

All three groups showed a marked reduction in their levels of depression, after the research experiment, and approximately half of each of the groups went into remission.

The results showed that *exercise was as beneficial as medication*, and led Dr John Ratey and Eric Hagerman (2009) to recommend exercise for depression. Their conclusion was that exercise altered the brain chemistry of the exercisers, in positive ways, which would help patients with depression.

Ratey and Hagerman (2009) declared that:

"The results should be taught in medical schools and driven home with health insurance companies and posted on the bulletin boards of every nursing home in the country, where nearly a fifth of the residents have depression."

(Ratey and Hagerman, 2009: Page 122).

They also mention the follow-up survey Blumenthal and his colleagues (2010) did six months later. *The researchers found that exercise performed more effectively than medicine in the long term*: About 30% of the exercise group were still depressed, as opposed to 52% of those on medication, and 55% in the combined treatment group.

This means that *70% of those on exercise alone got better*, compared with just 48% on Zoloft alone.

Blumenthal and his researchers found that the most revealing indicator of whether someone would have increased feelings of well-being, was the extent to which they exercised.

> *"Specifically, every 50 minutes of weekly exercise correlated to a 50% drop in the odds of being depressed."*

(Ratey and Hagerman, 2009, Page 124).

These research results refer to major depression – not just mild depression.

Both the British National Health Service and the Mayo Clinic recommend physical exercises as effective in treating depression.

A valuable reminder is also given by Dr Alan Cohen (a GP with a special interest in mental health). He considers that in order to have the *motivation* to perform exercise regularly, we need to *enjoy* it, and he recommends 150 minutes of moderate-intensity exercise every week.

For further information about exercise for depression, please see section 4.11 of Chapter 4 above; plus Taylor-Byrne and Byrne (2017).

~~~

Chapter 8: Counselling individuals using the E-CENT approach

8.1: Quick introduction

There is no standard or invariable structure that can be applied to all E-CENT counselling and therapy sessions. There are several core models that we use to guide our counselling process – and they will be reviewed below - but they tend to occur in various, unpredictable patterns, depending upon the client's narrative, and various *automatic* counsellor-judgements.

There are at least twenty standard principles that guide the thinking of the therapist, but not all of these is activated by any particular client, or client-problem: (See Chapter 3). And the order in which they become relevant cannot be anticipated or pre-specified.

Furthermore, the E-CENT counsellor is guided from non-conscious levels of mind, rather than consciously working out how to respond.

So, given these facts, how can I quickly provide you with an *overview* of a 'fairly typical' individual E-CENT counselling session, as a map of the territory to be explored? The most important things to bear in mind are these:

1. Right-brain to right-brain, non-verbal, emotive communication is probably the most potent thing that goes on in emotive-cognitive therapy: (Hill, 2015; Siegel, 2016; Rass, 2018; Forgas, 2001).

2. We are attachment therapists first; affect regulation therapists second; and only then cognitive-behavioural-informational.

3. We aim to build a warm relationship of *attentive awareness* and *acceptance* with the client. We aim to become a safe-harbour and a secure base.

4. We also practice sensitive attunement to the emotional state of the client.

Beyond that point, here is my 'quick tutorial' on how to apply E-CENT counselling in practice, drawn from my impressions of thousands of counselling sessions. If I have to try to summarize 'the process', here is my best approximation to what the counsellor is trying to do:

1. Build a relationship with the client, while trying to find out what they want and need.

2. Get an outline of the client's story – the 'confession stage' (in the Jungian tradition) - about the client's presenting problem.

3. Help them to explore their story, and to refine it, so it becomes more accurate – more complete; or more digested; more known. For example, help them to check if their story has been subjected to any (or many?) deletions, distortions or over-

generalizations. Help them to explore their story of origins and their story of relationships (to begin with).

4. Help them to see that their stories (including their emotions about events) could be *edited* ('re-framed')[134] so that they are less disturbing, less painful, and more tolerable than they originally seemed[135].

5. Teach the client that the quality of *the story that they inhabit* – or live inside of – is strongly and *unavoidably* affected by their diet[136], physical exercise regime, sleep pattern, relaxation processes, relationship support (adequate or inadequate), physical and socioeconomic environment, and social connections (good and/or bad)[137], etc.; as well as their inner-dialogue (or self-talk; mainly at non-conscious levels of mind).

6. Teach the client:

(a) To dedicate themselves to *reality* at all cost![138] (Even though it is hard for a human to know what is 'real', because we *automatically interpret* every event/object on the basis of our prior, cumulative, interpretive, cultural experience.)

(b) To accept the things they cannot change, and only try to change the things they can. (Even though it is actually very difficult to find out what might be controllable!)

(c) To live a moral life (on the basis that "You cannot live *The* Good Life unless you are willing to live *A* Good [Moral] Life!"). This involves growing their Good Wolf side (or virtuous side), and shrinking (starving) their Bad Wolf side (or the vicious, evil side of their character). See Appendix H of Byrne (2016).

(d) To keep their expectations in line with reality. (Even though it is difficult to identify what is actually 'real'!)

(e) To understand their emotions, and also how to manage them. (See Chapter 7, above, on human emotion).

(f) To grow their Adult ego state, and to shrink the *inappropriate elements* of their Controlling Parent, Critical Parent, and Adapted/Rebellious Child ego states[139].

(g) To restrain their tendencies towards passivity or aggression, and to mainly try to engage in *assertive* communication with others.

(h) To love some significant individual(s) in their lives; and to *offer love* to one of those significant individuals, as a way to get love: meaning, to establish a couple relationship.

(i) To take *responsibility* for their life. Nobody is coming on a white charger (or in shining armour) to rescue them. If it's to be, it's up to them!

(j) To commit themselves to personal and professional development; and, if they are up for it, some form of spiritual development; or community involvement; or political activity.

8.2: Validity of our models and processes

Most of the models and processes which went into forming the theoretical foundations of E-CENT counselling come from one or more of the ten systems of therapy which were evaluated by Smith and Glass (1977), and found to be not only *effective*, but fairly *equally effective*![140] So I do not feel any need to waste resources funding a Randomized Control Trial to 'prove' the efficacy of E-CENT. (West and Byrne, 2009[141]). You *cannot* use research to *'prove'* anything anyway: according to Karl Popper's philosophy of science.

The main types of therapy 'validated' by Smith and Glass (1977, 1982)[142], and also by later studies[143], and used in E-CENT counselling, are:

Transactional Analysis;

some small residue of (moderate) Rational emotive therapy;

Psychodynamic approaches;

Gestalt therapy;

Client-centred counselling;

and Systematic desensitization.

The *main exceptions* to this rule – that E-CENT has been constructed from *validated systems* of counselling and therapy (validated by the Common Factors School of research – Smith and Glass [1980]; Wampold and Messer [2001]; and others) – include the use of:

1. Elements of **Attachment theory** (which is perhaps the most researched and *validated* approach to developmental psychology in use today). See Wallin (2007); and Bowlby (1988)[144].

2. Aspects of **the most popular approaches** to Moral philosophy (including The Golden Rule; Rule utilitarianism; Duty ethics; and Virtue ethics.)[145]

3. **Moderate aspects** of Buddhist philosophy, including elements of the Zen perspective on language; and some of the insights of the **Dhammapada**.[146] Plus moderate aspects of Stoic philosophy[147].

4. The Narrative approach to counselling and therapy, which has become increasingly popular, mainly as a result of the work of White and Epston; and Kenneth Gergen; plus Theodore Sarbin[148].

5. And the paradigm shift "...from the primacy of behaviour, cognition, and content to the primacy of emotion, relationship, and context..." promoted by Allan Schore and others, is a new, but highly rated scientific re-evaluation of the nature of the human brain-mind and how it is shaped by social-emotional experience. (Rass, 2018; Siegel, 2016; Hill, 2015; Forgas, 2001).

8.3: Imaginary 'typical' session structure

Most systems of counselling and therapy have a characteristic 'session structure' to which trainee counsellors are expected to conform, and this seems to carry on into full professional practice for many systems (including Rational Emotive Behaviour Therapy)[149].

The publishing industry has tended to accentuate this requirement: that a system of therapy *must* have a beginning, a middle and an end phase, which are distinct and clearly specifiable, with common tasks for each phase. (See in particular the Sage Publications' *'Counselling in Action'* series).

However, as stated above, E-CENT counselling does **not** have a predetermined or predictable session structure. On the other hand, it may be *necessary* to *imagine* a 'typical' (though not invariable) structure, in order to *teach* some of the standard models and processes that we commonly use.

For example, in this chapter, it might help to explore the models and processes of E-CENT counselling by using the standard Jungian therapy session structure. The Jungian approach has the following four stages: (1) Confession; (2) Elucidation; (3) Education; and (4) Transformation.

If we are to use this approach, then we must begin with the confession stage:

~~~

8.3(a): Confession

Stage One

The Confession Stage

The main model that I want to emphasize in **the 'confession' stage** is our own version of *the RCFP model*, (or the *Rapport→Contract→Focus→Process* model), which is described below.

By using the concept of 'confession' we evoke memories of the Catholic confession box. However, it is important to note that E-CENT has a *secular approach to spirituality*; and a link to moderate Buddhism and moderate Stoicism, rather than any brand of Christianity.

Confessions we do hear, but we do **not** begin our counselling and therapy work by asking the client to confess, or even to open up. We actually begin with a very gentle process, based on our *Rapport→Contract→Focus→Process* (RCFP) model.

This model determines and structures how we meet and greet our clients, and how we work slowly towards a therapy focus; and thereafter we (spontaneously, intuitively) select additional models to guide the processing (P) of the client's communications.

~~~

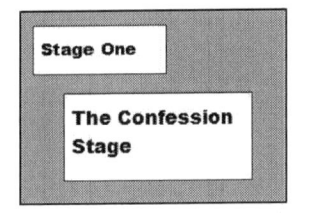

The RCFP model:

R = Rapport. Build rapport[150] (or attentive attunement) with the client as a basis for a strong therapeutic alliance. (This is increasingly seen as our role of providing a 'secure base', and a 'safe harbour', as defined in Attachment theory. [See Wallin, 2007, and Bowlby, 1988]). It also includes the core conditions of genuineness, empathy and non-possessive love (agape)/caring[151].

C = Contract. Find out what the client wants to work on, as a contractual undertaking. But bear in mind that this might be the first of more than one 'presenting problem', before the client feels secure enough to reveal the 'real' problem. (Sometimes this does seem as if the client has decided to 'confess', or 'own up' – or to arrive at some new stage of conscious awareness of some previously hidden aspect of their problem).

F = Focus. Focus in on an area of work that will assist in the pursuit of the client's goals, as implied by the contract (C).

P = Process. Process the client's communications and concerns about this 'area of work' through one (at a time) of the various models available; some of which are discussed below.

(This RCFP model was inspired by a similar model developed by Dr Ed Jacobs, in his system of Impact Therapy)[152].

Some of the unsolicited client testimonials, which I often receive, testify to the importance of our emphasis on building rapport.

Here are two recent examples (in which the clients' identities and locations have been concealed):

> ♣ "Hello Jim, I am so grateful to you for all the skilful help you've given me over the two years that I've been seeing you. You have given me a new kind of life; new ways of relating; and an improved view of myself as a person in the world. Thank you so much."
>
> P.A.G., Crag Vale, Calderdale. (20+ sessions of face to face counselling for a range of attachment, relationship and self-esteem issues).

~~~

> ♣ "Dear Jim, I want to express my gratitude for the help you gave me over the past few weeks. I was in a bad way, lost, and not understood elsewhere – but you understood me, believed in me, and helped me to work out a better understanding of my condition. You were right to focus on my diet and lack of physical fitness, rather than the psychiatric emphasis on my 'brain chemicals'! I am now back on my feet, and back in my university

studying. (In fact, I did a resit exam last week, and got a 'grade A' pass.) Thank you for your excellent diagnostic and humanitarian skills."

> H.H.G., Bradford. (Six sessions of face to face counselling for unusual physical sensations and panic about personal identity difficulties).

~~~

Questioning strategies:

From the beginning of the counsellor's relationship with each client, and especially as rapport is achieved, there is a need for *effective, systematic* questioning. Effective, systematic questioning has a number of features:

In the opening encounters with a new client, I normally offer *an invitation to speak*, rather than a tightly focused question. I am trying to *establish a relationship*, tentatively, carefully. I want to hear the client's story, in their own words, and in their usual way of conversing.

I then explain that I want to arrive at a *contract* which will involve me in working on the client's key issues. Of course, I also know that they may begin with a 'presenting problem' which is not their main concern. I may have to wait some time before they feel safe enough to present the real issue.

~~~

In the **confession stage**, we are still mainly dealing with the client's presenting problem, which may not go deep enough in terms of understanding what is really causing the client's main difficulties in life.

When thwarted goals seems to be a significant part of the problem, I might use the WDEP model. From Dr William Glasser's 'Reality therapy', this model asks:

> W = What do you ***Want***?
>
> D = What are you ***Doing*** to get what you want?
>
> E = How well is this going (the ***Evaluation*** stage)? And:
>
> P = Let's re-***Plan***, or produce an explicit ***Plan*** linked to what you Want.

Out of this questioning process normally come some fragments of story, which may or may not fit well together, and with which we work to make sense of the client's overall life narrative.

If there is a tension between what the client **wants** and what they are **doing**, we are immediately into the **elucidation** stage; helping the client to change either what they want, or what they are doing, so they both line up.

If there is no tension between what the client wants and what they are doing, I often switch to the Egan Model

The Egan model: This is a more detailed exploration of the client's goals and resources for making progress. In its simplest form it includes asking the client the following three questions:

> 1. Where are you now (in your inner and outer life)? Or what is the problem with which you are stuck?
>
> 2. Where are you trying to get to? Or what would need to change for the problem to be resolved?
>
> 3. What (new or revised) action could you take to get from 1 to 2? Or how could you begin to build a bridge towards your goal?

This process often gives us a 'focus area' to begin to work upon. It also often reveals blind spots that they client has, which we can clarify; and we can often help them to identify resources for solving their problem, about which they were unaware.

~~~

However, we should note that, in E-CENT counselling, we are not just interested in the so-called 'thinking' side of the client; or the so-called 'feeling' side of the client. We are also interested in these questions:

> *How well do you sleep? How many hours per night do you sleep?*
>
> *Do you get up in time to have a slow and gentle start to the day, or do you begin late, with tight time deadlines, which push up your stress level?*
>
> *What do you have for breakfast, and is it the healthiest option possible? (It is never a good idea to skip breakfast!)*
>
> *How well do you manage your time and your stress, in your daily working life?*
>
> *How good are your relationships with your significant others? At home and in work?*
>
> *How much physical exercise do you do, and how many days per week do you do it?*
>
> *How much water do you drink during the day?*
>
> *What do you eat for lunch?*
>
> *What snacks do you have mid-morning and mid-afternoon?*
>
> *How much alcohol do you drink?*
>
> *Do you consume any of these toxic foods: sugar; alcohol; caffeine; gluten; trans-fats (or hydrogenated fat, in junk foods); and highly-processed foods (with added sugar, salt, trans-fats, colours, flavours, and other denatured components)?*

Tell me about your childhood? Was it broadly happy? Or not? Are you secure or insecure in your relationships?

What is the problem that brought you here today? And how does it relate to the questions I have asked above?

~~~

During **the confession stage**, some clients have admitted to serious wrong-doing, such as being unfaithful to their partner, or stealing family assets. At this point I switch from confession to education, and begin to teach the importance of pursuing a virtuous life, and avoiding vice, because of the inevitable outcome of 'bad karma'[153]. We tend to reap what we sow, and we cannot have a happy life if we live in an unprincipled manner. (Of course, I also teach the importance of morality for the sake of being a moral agent – a good person; which is a social requirement). And I teach that immorality also tends to undermine our sense of self-esteem.

Furthermore, I also teach the Golden Rule[154] - which requires us to treat other individuals at least as well as we would want them to treat us, if our roles were reversed - and I often recommend reading of the ***Dhammapada*** (which outlines basic Buddhist teachings)[155].

~~~

8.3(b): Elucidation

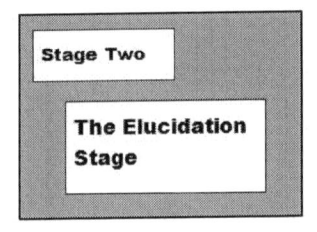

Stage Two
The Elucidation Stage

There are a number of models that I use for the purpose of **elucidating** the client's concerns, dilemmas, goals, etc.

Chief among them is our own holistic version of the *Stimulus→Organism→Response* (or Holistic-SOR) model.

The original SOR model (created by the neo-behaviourists) suggested that, when an animal (or human) notices a stimulus (S), it outputs a response (R), because of the way the organism (O) processes the stimulus.

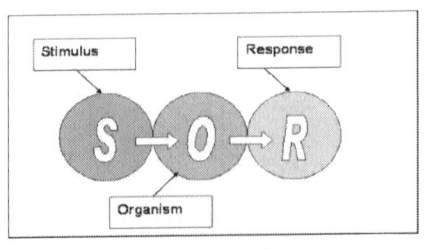

Figure 8.1: The classic S>O>R model:

That original SOR model of neo-behaviourism was dumped by Dr Albert Ellis, the creator of Rational Emotive Behaviour Therapy (REBT), and replaced by the simple ABC model, in which the client is assumed to be always and only upset because of their 'irrational beliefs'. (And Freud's 'ABCs' were no better, in that he implied that when something happens [let's call it an 'A', or activating event], the client responds with their own phantasy [let's call it a 'B', or belief], which upsets them [at point C – consequence]: though Freud did not use that 'ABC' lettering system)

Aaron Tim Beck (despite being a medical doctor, and theoretically aware of the importance of the human body) also adopted this simple ABC model. (Beck 1976).

So one of the main contributions of E-CENT counselling has been *'adding back the body'* to the client; and accepting that the client's *body-mind-environment-whole* is implicated in all of their emotional and behavioural states.

In the process we developed a more holistic version of the *Stimulus →Organism → Response* model. (See Figure 8.2 below)

In the simple, classical SOR model, an incoming stimulus (S) – (which is a sensed experience) – impacts upon the nervous system of the organism (O) – (or person, in our case) – causing a reactive response (R) to be outputted (or generated), to cope with the stimulus (or incoming experience).

In the early stages of our explorations, after looking at Freud and Ellis – on the ABC model and the Experience-Phantasy-Neurosis model – we turned our attention to the *Parent-Adult-Child* (PAC) model of TA, plus this simple, classic SOR model.

But then we began to ask ourselves what factors are most likely to affect the capacity for a human organism to be able to handle difficult incoming stimuli, or activating events. We came up with an extensive list, which includes:

> **Diet:** (meaning balanced, healthy, or otherwise). (Does the individual/ organism have enough blood-glucose to be able to process the incoming stimulus, physically and mentally?)
>
> **Exercise:** (meaning regular physical exercise designed to reduce stress, versus a sedentary lifestyle)[156]
>
> **Self-talk, scripts, frames and schemas:** (Including conscious and/or non-conscious stories and narratives/ thinking-feeling states/ self-signalling/ attitudinizing / framing, etc. Plus other culturally shaped beliefs and attitudes, expectations, prophesies, etc. Plus non-narrativized experiences stored in the form of schemas and frames, etc.)
>
> **Relaxation:** (or release from muscle tension and anxiety, versus tension and anxiety);
>
> **Family history:** (including attachment styles [secure or insecure]; childhood trauma; and personality adaptations, etc.);
>
> **Emotional needs:** (including deficits and/or satisfactions);
>
> **Character** and **temperament:** (as in Myers-Briggs or Keirsey-Bates)[157];

Environmental stressors: (including home environment, work situation, economic circumstances, and so on);

Sleep pattern; and the balance between work, rest and play.

~~~

By keeping our focus on the fact that the client is a complex, socialized body-brain-mind; steeped in storied- (or narrativized-) experiences (plus non-storied experiences) of concrete experiences in a concrete world; and living in a complex relationship to an external social environment - which is often hostile and unsupportive, resulting in stress-induced over-arousal of the entire body-brain-mind - we never fall into the trap of *foolishly* asking the client: "*What do you think you are **telling yourself** in order to cause your own problem?*"

And we do not *foolishly* tell the client that the thoughts which (in reality, very often) *follow on* from their emotional experiences are **causing** those emotional experiences!

~~~

We focus on the client's story and the client's physical existence, both with roughly equal, but variable, emphasis. Sometimes the story needs most attention, and sometimes the state of the body-brain-mind, in terms of diet, exercise, etc., is more important.

Traditional medical doctors were guilty of separating the body from the mind, and trying to treat the body as a 'faulty machine' – which was in line with Newtonian mechanics of the nineteenth century, which lasted well into the twentieth century and beyond.

Sigmund Freud, as a trained neurologist and MD, came out of that tradition and began the process of moving towards some kind of appreciation of *the mind*.

However, many generations of counsellors and psychotherapists have gone too far in this direction, and *forgot all about the body.*

Some modern medical doctors are beginning to realize their original error.

Here's how Dr Ron Anderson, Chairman of the Board of the Texas Department of Health, describes his aim for all the doctors he influences:

> "*I try to have people understand wholeness if I can, because if you don't understand the mind/body connection, you start off on the wrong premise.*
>
> *You also have to understand the person within their family and community because this is where people live*".[158]

Using the Holistic SOR model

Figure 8.2 below shows how we present the holistic SOR model for our clients.

The Holistic Stimulus-Organism-Response Model (H-SOR)		
Column 1	Column 2	Column 3
S = *Stimulus*	O = *Organism*	R = *Response*
When something significant happens, which is apprehended by the organism's (or person's) nervous system, the organism is activated or aroused (positively or negatively)	The organism responds, well or badly. The incoming stimulus may activate or interact with: (1) Innate needs and tendencies; (2) Family history and attachment style; (3) Recent personal history; (4) Emotive-cognitive schemas (as guides to action); (5) Narratives, stories, frames and other storied elements (which may be hyper-activating, hypo-activating, or affect regulating); (6) Character and temperament; (7) Need satisfaction; goals and values; (8) Diet and supplementation, medication, exercise regime, sleep and relaxation histories; (9) Ongoing environmental stressors, state of current relationship(s), and satisfaction with life stages, etc., etc.	The organism outputs a response, in the form of visible behaviour and inferable emotional reactions, like anger, anxiety, depression, embarrassment, etc.

Figure 8.2: The E-CENT holistic SOR model

As indicated in Figure 8.2, E-CENT theory takes a holistic view of the client as a social-body-mind, with a habit-based character and temperament, living in a particular social and physical environment, with stressors and supports.

The client has a personal history which is unique to them; plus some social shaping that extends to their family, and some to their community; some to their nation/ race/ gender, etc.

This illustration should be read as follows: Column 1 - 'S' = (or equals) a **stimulus**, which, when experienced by an O = **Organism** (in our case a human), may activate or interact with any of the factors listed in column 2; and this will produce an R = **Response**, as shown in column 3.

To be more precise: The holistic SOR model states that a client (a person) responds at point 'R', to a (negative or positive) stimulus at point 'S', on the basis of the current state of their social-body-mind.

How well rested are they?

How high or low is their blood-sugar level (which is related to diet)?

How well connected are they to significant others (which is a measure of social support)?

How much conflict do they have at home or at work?

What other pressures are bearing down upon them (e.g. from their socio-economic circumstances; physical health; home/ housing; work/ income; security/ insecurity; etc.)

And how emotionally intelligent are they? (Emotional intelligence is, of course, learned, and can be re-learned!)

Within the Holistic-SOR model (in Figure 8.2 above), in the middle column, what we are aiming to do is to construct a balance sheet (in our heads) of the *pressures* bearing down on the client (person), and the *coping resources* that they have for dealing with those pressures.

~~~

So this is a *historical-social-stress model*. It is not a purely 'cognitive distortion' model; nor a purely 'biological/ sexual urges' model; nor a purely 'prizing and listening' model.

~~~

The exploration process

Once we have established rapport, and worked on a contract and a specific focus, we move on to the detailed work of processing the client's communications about their concerns.

Process = The process of E-CENT counselling can have formal and informal aspects; including: discussion and questions; or the use of questionnaires to explore possibilities. And/or the use of a range of models and techniques and strategies, as described and explored throughout this chapter.

And the process tends to vary considerably from one client to another, as each client is unique. Although there is no one right way to begin, one fairly typical or common approach could be to:

> 1. Explain the **H-S-O-R model**, and then:
>
> 2. Explore the details of the client's Diet, Exercise, Sleep patterns, Self-talk, Relaxation/Meditation (as first priorities) – if appropriate.

3. Then, explore the client's relationships (current and historic), as the next priority – if appropriate. (Of course, for some clients, the order of items 2 and 3 would be reversed).

This **elucidation** sometimes involves the use of explicit questionnaires, but more commonly we stick to informal questioning about:

Diet and vitamin supplementation; Exercise routine and frequency; Sleep quality and duration; and Relaxation and/or meditation practice.

Also: What's going on at home, and/or in work? What has changed recently?

And, if called for, what went on in the family of origin.

And so on.

Other instruments

The emotional needs assessment questionnaire (adapted from the Human Givens approach): This allows the client to identify any unmet needs which may be affecting their equilibrium, and thus causing emotional disturbance. (See Appendix B of Byrne 2016).

A brief Depression inventory (from Dr David Burns' handbook[159]): This is sometimes used to check the intensity of a client's depression; and sometimes to check on progress over time.

A brief Anxiety inventory (from Dr David Burns' handbook): Like the depression inventory, this is sometimes used to check the intensity of a client's anxiety; and sometimes to check on progress in reducing anxiety over time.

Other models: We also use some other models, to help the client to understand their marriage, or to help them to understand stress, or the handling of panic, etc. For examples, we teach eighteen principles of happy relationships – some of which come from Professor John Gottman's books[160].

We teach twenty-one principles of stress management, from a broad range of sources[161].

And we use our own desensitization process to help clients to reduce their traumatic stress and panic symptoms. (See Appendix C of Byrne 2016).

~~~

Questioning strategies

Various questioning strategies have been adopted, adapted or evolved within E-CENT; and these are particularly important at the **elucidation stage**:

As we move into the Focus stage (of the RCFP model), we begin to ask a range of open and closed questions; and as we enter the Process stage, we begin using funnelling questions – going deeper and deeper into the client's problem.

If we get stuck, and no longer understand the shape of the client's presenting issue, we may have to use one of the following questioning techniques:

(a) **The 5W's & 1H model**: In this approach, the counsellor asks: Who…? What…? When…? Where…? Why…? And, finally, How…? (Or some relevant sub-set of those questions, in whatever order makes most sense).

(But be careful. Questions can trigger anxiety in the client!)

(b) **The Five Why's model**: This model is a form of drilling down into the problem: *Why did it happen? Why did you respond the way you did? Why did you not try X instead? Why…?* (And I will explain later how we modify these questions to substitute 'For what reason…?' - instead of the word 'Why?' And we do that to avoid making the client anxious).

(c) **Other approaches**: Of course, the WDEP model (which we mentioned above) is also primarily a questioning model. And we also use the simple Egan Model of the Skilled Helper:

> 1. *Where are you now?*
>
> 2. *Where are you trying to get to?*
>
> 3. *How could you build a bridge from 1 to 2?*
>
> 4. *Reflection and insight:* (The counsellors watches out for blindspots and unutilized resources or sources of strength, and discusses them with the client).

Dangers of questioning!

This is a good point to mention our reservation about *excessive* questioning, or the *intensive* or *insensitive* use of questioning, especially when the client is particularly stressed.

The main problem here is that the client may become anxious and even feel that they are being 'interrogated' or 'treated as the villain of the piece'.

If the client has an avoidant attachment style, they are highly likely to become stressed if questioned about their feelings: (Hill, 2015, pages 208-209).

And many clients become upset if they are questioned about their actions or behaviours. CBT/REBT therapists are completely unaware of the disturbances they may cause by misguided questioning strategies.

In particular, we need to be aware of the insights of Joines and Stewart (2002), on *personality adaptations*. These authors clarify that each of our clients will have a particular adaptation to their parents.

This theory asserts that:

(1) Some people respond to life by thinking; some by feeling; and some by acting unthinkingly.

(2) Some people have their behaviour "walled off", unavailable for inspection or consideration; while some will have their thinking walled off; and some their feelings. And:

(3) The challenge for therapy is to identify the element of their mental processing – thinking, feeling or behaviour – which the client leads with; and which needs to be integrated with that element.

The most helpful aspect of this book is that it allows us to see and understand that some clients will lead with their thinking, and thus be happy to engage in encounters where we ask questions which cause them to think.

Some clients will have their thinking "walled off", so that they lead with behaviour or feelings, and cannot think without digging holes for themselves. So we would be doing such clients a disservice by questioning them about their thinking.

And, some clients will have their behaviour "walled off", and they will be ultra-sensitive about having their behaviour challenged or questioned, so we should not use questioning of behaviour with them.

So, in practice, we do not use the *Five Why's*, as such, but rather the gentler, *'For what reason?' times 5*. "For what **reason** did you go there?" "For what **reason** did you respond the way you did"? Etc.

(We might use this approach with the first four personality adaptations:

[1] the *Enthusiastic-Overreactors*, who lead with their feelings, and need to integrate their thinking with their feelings;

[2] the *Responsible-Workaholics*, who lead with their thinking and need to have their feelings integrated with their thinking;

[3] the *Brilliant-Skeptics*, who lead with their thinking, and need to integrate their feelings with their thinking; and:

[4] the Creative-Daydreamers, who lead with behaviour, and need to integrate their thinking with their behaviour.

See Joines and Stewart, 2002. Pages 42-47).

However, we do not use *questioning, which causes thinking to start up*, with those clients who have their thinking "walled off". (These are the *Playful-Resisters* and the *Charming-Manipulators*. See Joines and Stewart, 2002, pages 47-49).

In the 'bad old days', when children were asked *'Why?'* at home or in school, this was often a signal that they were *'in trouble'* and that they should *'button their lip'* to avoid being punished.

When we ask (of the clients who do not have their thinking walled off): "For what reason...?" we are clearly focusing on *causality (or causation)* and/or *motivation*, and not *blame!*

("I would be *interested* to know the *reason* that... [you did X]", is an even better formulation.)

However, overall, in E-CENT counselling (with clients whose thinking is not walled off), we try to stick to **the five functions of questioning** that are outlined in G.I. Nierenberg's (1987)[162] book on negotiation skills.

Those five functions of questions, are as follows:

Q1. To cause the client to focus upon a particular point (event, or object);

Q2. To cause their thinking to start up;

Q3. To ask them for some information;

Q4. To pass some information to them (rhetorically); and:

Q5. To cause their thinking to come to a conclusion.

Nierenberg also argues that you can arrange those five questions in a grid, like this:

	Q1.	Q2.	Q3.	Q4.	Q5.
Q1.			Q1+3		
Q2.					
Q3.					
Q4					
Q5.					

Figure 8.3 Gerard Nierenberg's question grid

Using this grid, you can see that a question can be in two parts. For example, in Figure 8.3, I have illustrated a combination of Q1 + Q3. *Q1 Should/could/can aim to cause the clients attention to focus on a specific event/experience, and Q3 should/could/can ask them for some information about that specific event/experience.*

Here is an illustrative example:

> "(Q1) With regard to (event X), (2) *for what reason* did you experience it as (an insult, [for example])?"

The great beauty of this system is that it gets rid of the "Socratic smart-arse" aspect of questioning the client, which is prevalent in rational therapy (REBT).

The problems with classic *Socratic Questioning* (as used in REBT/CBT) include:

1. That the client may interpret the therapist as 'picking a fight' with them; making them wrong; or putting them down;

2. That the client may become anxious when asked particular kinds of right/ wrong questions (perhaps because of re-stimulation of one or more of the many humiliating experiences of being a child in classrooms in school and being subjected to interrogations, the aim of which was to find *a reason to punish* the client when they were a child).

3. That the client may - (as suggested by the research studies of Asch, Milgram and Zimbardo)[163] - simply go along with the therapist's inferences, as a form of obedience or conformity to authority.

4. That the client may have their **thinking** *"walled off"*, is described in our discussion of Personality Adaptations, a la Joines and Stewart 2002, above. Asking them questions will not help, since they cannot think well or clearly enough to benefit from this approach.

5. That the client may have their behaviour "walled off". The first three Personality Adaptations looked at above – the *Enthusiastic-Over-reactor*, the *Responsible-Workaholic* and the *Brilliant-Skeptic* - have their behaviour "walled off", such that, *any questions* about *their behaviour* will tend to make them feel bad (not-OK), such as shamed or humiliated!

6. That the therapist never gets to know the client, because s/he (the therapist) is always tilting at the windmills of 'innate irrational beliefs' – or 'negative automatic thoughts' – and not paying attention to *the actual story* the client is telling them. Or the actual wiring of the client's personality – such as walled off thinking – is never noticed, and thus the possibilities of *effective therapy* are seriously compromised!

And so on.

The point is *not* to avoid questions completely (as some Rogerian, person-centred counsellors do), but to use questions skilfully, sparingly, and appropriately. And to be particularly aware of the client's personality adaptations, and to try to avoid using questions with those people who **cannot** *benefit from them!*

~~~

> **Stage Three**
>
> **The Education Stage**

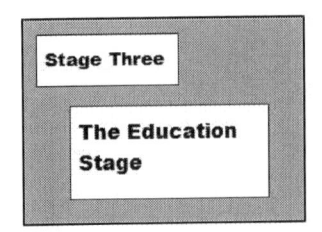

8.3(c): *Education*

Education of the client is a key aspect of our work. We teach the client that they are socialized-body-minds, interacting with social and physical environments, and not just *'floating heads'*.

We teach them (or try to *help them to learn* – to be more accurate) that *everything* they put into their body – and some of the things they *fail* to put into their body - will have some (positive or negative) effect on their mind.

And we try to clarify that, everything they do with their mind or mental processes – like 'thinking' (which is really *perfinking*!), feeling, ruminating, worrying, planning dire outcomes, *et cetera* - will have some effect on their body – which will in turn rebound on their mind (because the so-called *body and mind* are really a *unified, integrated, body-mind*).

We try to get them to see that it is most sensible to work at taking care of their body-brain-mind as a holistic activity. And also to work at managing their relationship to their social and physical environment.

But we also try to educate our clients like a good enough mother of a young child tries to educate: by *modelling* certain attitudes and behaviours; by providing gentle and kind *developmental feedback*; and by showing *care and concern* for the *feelings* of the client.

General teaching points, including diet and exercise

We teach our clients that they are storytelling animals, which live in a sea of stories – but *not disembodied* stories. Rather, they live in a sea of stories *about experiences* – their own story, their family's stories, their community's scripts and legends, and their nation's narrative; as well as the stories of their religion/ race/ creed/ gender/ sexual-orientation. But we also help them to see that they must pay attention to their own *physical* existence; their own *social* existence, including their key relationships.

Our stories live in our bodies; and the stories we can generate about our present and our future depend upon the state of health of our bodies.

We teach some basic principles of diet and physical exercise; sleep hygiene; meditation and relaxation; and we recommend that clients follow up on this introductory *educational input* with more extensive study of these fields of self-care, perhaps with the *support* of a *nutritionist* or *dietician*; a sports coach; a meditation teacher or relaxation class or audio program; or with a *holistic healthcare practitioner*.

We teach assertive communication strategies, in order to improve relationships and social connection, which are essential to good physical/emotional health. We also teach *dedication to reality at all cost*; and the importance of *accepting the things we cannot change*.

~~~

We sometimes make general or explicit recommendations to our clients regarding the kinds of changes to make to their diet[164] and/or physical exercise[165] practices. (And we sometimes refer them to see a nutritional therapist, or a sports coach at a local gym).

We also recommend particular relaxation programs (normally audio CD, or DVD based programs by Glenn Harrold or Paul McKenna); and teach them simple approaches to meditation[166].

And we have explored, and teach, particular (non-drug-based) approaches to sleep promotion; and where to get more holistic professional help for sleep problems.

If we begin to suspect that character or temperament may be part of the client's problem, we suggest a self-analysis using the Keirsey-Bates approach[167]. And we discuss their results with them.

When insecure attachment style seems to be a part of the client's problem, we might recommend that they assess their own attachment style at a particular website.[168] We use those (attachment style) results to adjust our approach to the client, and to expand our understanding of their life story. And we follow Wallin's (2007) approach to being a secure base for the client. Being a good-enough re-parenting figure.

To help clients change their self-talk (or how they frame their problems) we use the Six Windows Model.

~~~

The Six Windows Model(s): We have already outlined this model in Chapter 6 above. We created the Six Windows Model mainly from some of the more moderate insights of Buddhism and Stoicism. Initially there was only one model of the Six Windows, though we recognized that there were likely to be at least 66 different ways of looking at any problem, and possibly even 666. (See Figure 6.1(b) above).

(We are now working on two additional 'Six Windows' Models, one for dealing with *couple relationship* problems, and the other for dealing with *anger management* problems.)

Our aim in developing the Six Windows model was this: We wanted to develop a way of introducing the client to six different ways *to re-frame their problem*, which would hopefully break up their automatic, (non-conscious), mono-focal (or single focus) way of viewing their problem.

This theoretically involves them in integrating new ideas 'in their left brain' with old emotions 'in their right brain'. (Hill, 2015).

In other words, we wanted to help them to *re-story their approach* to the presenting problem; to create *a new narrative* about it. This has worked well in practice. An example was shown in Chapter 6, above.

~~~

Applying the Six Windows Model

This is how we apply the model:

1. We ask the client to rate a particular presenting problem, on a scale of 1 to 10, where 10 is as bad as it could possibly be. (These are called 'subjective units of disturbance' – or SUDs, for short).

2. We then ask them to view their 'presenting problem' through Window No. 1, and to decide if the problem shows up as less bad (reduced SUDs) when viewed in this way. (**Typical question for Window No. 1**: "Since life is difficult for all human beings, at least some of the time, and often much of the time, does this help you to see your situation as any less negative or challenging?")

3. We repeat step 2 with each of the six different window frames, each of which has a particular perspective (or framing statement) written around it. (The *typical question* obviously varies from window to window, and reflects the slogan written around each particular window).

4. The process is simple: The client is asked to consider how – taking each of these six *perspectives* into account – their problem shows up differently, each time, for them. They are not obliged to reach a definitive answer (or specific SUDs rating) at the end of each window. We are happy to wait to the end of the process, to see what the overall effect might be.

5. The ultimate question is this: "Does your *'presenting problem'* seem any better when viewed through any or all of the new (window) perspectives?" (Other questions could be: "And, on a scale of 1 to 10, how bad does your problem now seem? Has your 'subjective units of disturbance' [SUDs] rating declined as a result of considering these six new perspectives?")

~~~

The first three windows (or framings; or perspectives) are as follows:

Window 1: Life is *difficult* for all human beings at least some of the time, and often much of the time, (so why must it not be difficult for me right now?)

Window 2: Life can be *significantly less difficult*, provided I pick and choose modestly, realistically, and reasonably. (We cannot give up picking and choosing outcomes completely; but we can moderate our choices and expectations!)

Window 3: Life is ***both difficult and non-difficult***, (so if all I can see through this window is my difficulty, then I need to be aware that I am *overlooking* [or *excluding*] non-difficult things for which I could be grateful!)

~~~

Testimonial about the Windows Model: Here is an example of the kind of feedback we receive from our clients about the usefulness of the Six Windows Model:

> "Thank you, Jim. I use your Six Windows Model every time I'm emotionally disturbed; ... and the specific applications you developed for dealing with depression, anger, and stress are very helpful. ... I normally rely upon my ... religious beliefs to get me through my life ... but the Six Windows philosophy made the difference recently."
>
> P.J.L., Argentina. (Three sessions of email counselling for a variety of emotional problems).

Once the client is familiar with the Six Windows Model, it **might** sometimes be helpful (in face to face counselling) to prompt them to use it, by applying the EFR model, which follows next:

Using the EFR model

In 2010, the EFR model was at the core of E-CENT, alongside *the Six Windows Model*. But this has now changed, and this model has been somewhat downgraded.

The EFR model is structured like this:

> **E = Event**. What happened in the client's life, about which they are disturbed.
>
> **F = Framing**. How did the client frame this experience? (They normally *will not know* this, as it is mainly non-conscious. And the way they frame it varies from situation to situation, depending upon the current state of their body-mind. But they can often *infer* what their attitude towards the Activating Event, or Life challenge, **seems** most likely to have been, especially after they have been using the Six Windows model for a while).
>
> **R = Response**. How did the client respond to their Framing (F) of the Event (E)? What emotion did they feel? How did they act? Is this response something they want to change?

Today, in 2018, we have almost completely given up on the simple ABC model. We have also downgraded the EFR model (to a lower priority; or a later stage in counselling) – and, as mentioned above, instead we now mainly emphasize our own holistic version of the SOR model: which involves exploring *the total state of the client's body-mind*, and not just their verbal-framings, or beliefs or attitudes.

Whenever we do use the EFR model, the next element after the 'R' is this:

Narrative inquiry

NI = Narrative inquiry: This step normally involves questions to the client (assuming their *personality adaptation* does not make questioning them *counterproductive* or *iatrogenic*). For examples:

> *What seems likely to be going on 'in the basement' of your (the client's) mind to produce the kind of feelings and behaviours that are a problematic Response for you?*
>
> *What do you think the story could be that produced this 'R' response to this particular 'E' (or activating Event or Experience)?*
>
> *What is the narrative that is implied by this reaction? How helpful, logical or reasonable is this implicit narrative (or frame)?*

We need to find out (if possible):

> (1) What could the client change in their *implicit* narrative, which would make it more positive?
>
> (2) How could they *reframe* this experience to produce a better outcome for themselves?

Very often, all of this remains hidden; and it is only by using the Six Windows Model to help the client to **rethink** and **reframe** their situation that we can produce any real, lasting change for and with the client.

Teaching the client about human disturbance

In Chapter 7, we outlined our approach to understanding the core of human emotional and behavioural disturbances.

Stress is often part of the client's problem – meaning too much pressure in their life, relative to their coping resources. So we help them to work on reducing those stressors which they **can** reduce, and building up those coping resources which they **can** increase.[169]

One area of **education** involves helping the client to learn how to 'reframe' their identified problems.

As we have already seen, we have a strategy to get the client to rethink how they *frame* the problem, beginning with some conscious re-framing, which will become non-conscious with practice. And that strategy involves teaching them the Six Windows Model, which we have already reviewed, above.

We also teach the client just how automatic and instantaneous their emotional reactions tend to be.

One of the ways we do this is by teaching them the APET model, from the *Human Givens* approach (Griffin and Tyrrell, 2004, 2008).

Or how to integrate nutritional insights, exercise and sleep coaching into talk therapy

The APET model:

Because the ABC model (of REBT) tends to emphasize 'beliefs' – assuming that the disturbed emotions experienced by the client (at point C in the ABC model) are *caused* by *linguistic beliefs* (at point B) we had to reject this model. Furthermore, REBT theory talks about clients 'choosing' to upset themselves, whereas in E-CENT theory we see the client as *a largely **non-conscious** and **automatic** organism*, responding emotionally to environmental cues. Therefore, it may often be more realistic to use the APET model, from the Human Givens school of thought, as a corrective. This model illustrates just how *automatic* human disturbances tend to be. The key elements of the APET model are as follows:

A = An Activating event (as before): Something frustrating, challenging, frightening or saddening in some way, happens to the client.

P = Pattern matching. Our 'organism as a whole' recognizes this activating event, and 'matches it' to an appropriate response. Our brain-mind recognizes any particular event or object because it can be *assimilated* to (or fitted into) an existing 'schema' (or recognizable pattern, or frame) in long-term memory. (Pattern matching can also be thought of as habit-based *perceiving-feeling-thinking* [or *perfinking*] in which the incoming stimulus is apprehended,/identified and responded to all in one automatic grasp of the body-brain-mind).

E = Emotion. Our organism as a whole then 'outputs' a standard, habitual, emotional response to this stimulus (from 'A' above), in a fraction of a second, which is much too fast for any thoughts to occur.

T = Thoughts. Thinking follows on from consciously registering the fact that the emotional response has **already occurred.**

Whereas the ABC model tends to focus attention on the B (or *belief system* of the client), and what the client can do to change their beliefs/ attitudes about the A (or Activating stimulus), the APET model often focuses attention on the possibilities of **changing the A**, or activating stimulus. Or coming up with a new E (or emotional response) which is more self-helping than the old emotional response.

This can be done by asking: *What would be **a solution** to the problem posed by the Activating event (A)? What could you do – or do differently - to achieve that solution?*

However, because the 'A' often cannot be changed – e.g. in the case of redundancy from employment, for example - the APET model also can draw attention to the need **to change the client's inappropriate patterns of *automatic* responses** to particular stimuli. This can be done by the therapist telling relevant 'educational stories', using metaphors, or using appropriate humorous images.

More importantly, we can get the client to use the Six Windows Model to come up with new ways of framing their noxious stimuli (or unpleasant activating events). According to E-CENT theory, this tends to (eventually, after several repetitions) produce *non-conscious insights*, and *revised evaluations*, which tend to modify the client's (or users) *current pattern-matching options* which are stimulated by a particular Activating stimulus (A). (Or, to put it differently: the client learns to *perfink* more self-supportingly about particular, noxious activating events!)

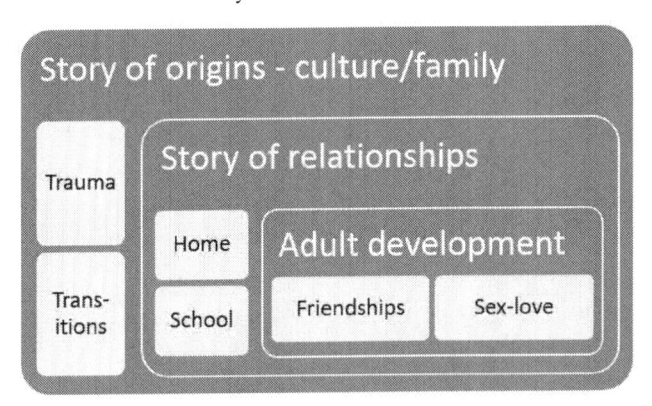

~~~

Fragments of disconnected story

We might also want to use the Jigsaw-story model at point P in the RCFP model. (**Point P** involves *processing* the client's communications about their Contract/Focus issue).

The Jigsaw-story model is a kind of *notional mental-matrix* in which we accumulate bits and pieces of the client's story or stories, over time.

Figure 8.4: The Jigsaw-story model

Part of the challenge here is to try to make the various bits and pieces cohere. You might ask yourself: *What is the overall storyline? How well do the transitions work? How healthy are the foundational stories: of **origins** and **relationships**. Are there any gaps, blind spots, or contradictions?*

(This is similar to *case formulation* in cognitive therapy, except that the CBT therapist seems to mainly focus on the client's thoughts and behaviours, which are assumed to drive their feelings. In E-CENT, we focus on the client's *stories* about their *lived experiences*. We assume that the external environment has a very powerful effect upon the client's body brain mind. We assume that they client is doing the best they can with what they have to make sense of their lived experience. And our aim is to help them to 'straighten out' their stories, so they are consistent, reasonably accurate, hopeful and self-helping).

In E-CENT counselling, the Jigsaw-story model is utilized at various points, when the counsellor spots a discrepancy between stories; or senses that a new revelation may make a lot of sense of an earlier mystery.

This is part of the detective-investigator role of the counsellor. And we often need to use *systematic questioning,* (when appropriate) as described earlier in this chapter, to resolve a jumbled jigsaw arrangement of stories.

The Parent-Adult-Child model

When the problem involves interpersonal conflict, we often turn to the Parent-Adult-Child (PAC) model of Transactional Analysis (TA).

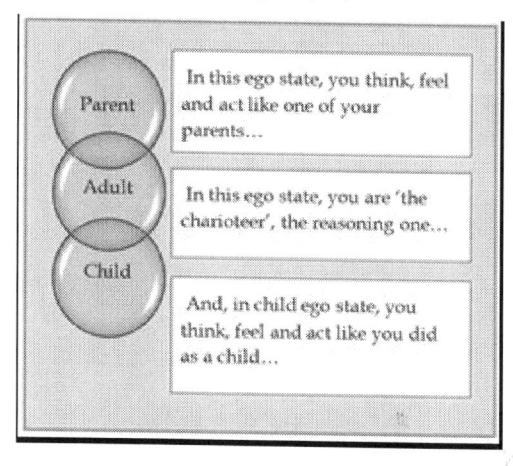

Figure 8.5: The PAC Model of TA

This model is used to teach clients how they move around between *ego states* (or ways of being – or distinct *styles* of thinking-feeling-acting); how those ego states can be managed; and how to grow **the Adult ego state**, and keep the *Adult ego state* in **the Executive position** in the personality.

The **Adult ego state** is the highest expression of our integration of thinking-feeling-acting which is guided by what Freud called *the Reality Principle*. Thus, our *perfinking capacity* is a measure of the balance between the Parent, Adult and Child states of being (or ego states).

The **Adult ego state** can be characterized as a compromise between:

1. The *Controlling* and *Nurturing* aspects of the *Parent ego state,* on the one hand; and:

2. The *Rebellious* and *Conforming* aspects of the *Child ego state,* on the other.[170]

We internalize *models* of *Controlling* and *Nurturing* ego states – or 'states of the ego', 'ways of being', or 'sub-personalities' - from our parents and parent substitutes. And our *Rebellious* and *Conforming* child ego states are *memories* of how we actually responded to our parents and/or parent substitutes during our childhood.

When a client shows up as being 'too high' on **Bad** *Adapted Child* – that is to say, they are too *conformist*; too *adapted* to their inner our outer **Bad Controlling Parent** forces – we set out to teach them to become 'higher' on **Good** *Rebellious Child*. *Good Rebellious Child* ego state is all about striving for socially-responsible ***Autonomy*** from **Bad** *(inner our outer) Parental Control*.

On the other hand, when a client shows as being 'too high' on **Bad** *Rebellious Child* – that is to say, too *resistant* to **Good** *(inner or outer) Parental Control* – we set out to teach them to become *more socially responsible*; *more morally reasonable*; more *adapted to reasonable social rules*.

And a good deal of our work involves trying to persuade clients to ***reduce*** their *Controlling Parent* ego state, in their relationships with others; and to ***grow*** their *Adult* ego state, which is guided by the *reality principle* – or *reliable data* about how the world *works*!

~~~

The OK Corral (from TA):

This model helps the client to understand that the healthy life-position to operate from is this: *"I'm OK and so are you (all)"* – assuming we are both (or all) committed to acting as moral and socially-responsible individuals. (See previous footnote).

		Your Decision About Others	
		OK	Not-OK
Your Decision About Yourself	OK	1. I'm OK - You're OK	2. I'm OK - You're Not-OK
	Not-OK	3. I'm Not-OK - You're OK	4. I'm Not-OK - You're Not-OK

Figure 8.6: The OK Corral

It also helps the client to understand if they are operating from ***negative attitudes*** towards themselves or others. In TA, these could be classified as conscious or non-conscious *not-OK life-positions* (about self or others).

A '*not-OK' life position* could include, any of the following attitudes:

(1) **"I'm not OK** because I cannot get a partner; (or I cannot get a job; or I cannot make a success of my career; or I cannot get along with others"; etc.) Or:

(2) **"You're not OK** because you're too rich (or too poor); (or because you frustrate me; or threaten my self-concept; or because you challenge me in ways that make me feel uncomfortable"; etc.) Or:

(3) **"The world is not OK**, because it does not give me what I want, when I want it; (or because it is too difficult; too boring; too painful; too uncertain or scary"; etc.)

We are committed to **teaching** our clients to reverse their *not-OK life positions*, by teaching them that *they are OK, exactly the way they are*, so long as they are striving to be good, moral citizens of their communities. (Byrne, 2010b)

We encourage them to forgive the imperfections of the people in their lives, so long as those individuals are not acting in an illegal or significantly immoral way towards our client.

When other people are treating our client badly, we teach our client to try to change what is not working for them - or to escape from the oppressive situation - and *then* to try *to accept what they cannot change.*

But we do **not** encourage them to *stay in intolerable situations* in order to grow their capacity to tolerate *anything* that life throws at them (which is a weakness of Albert Ellis's system, and other forms of extreme Stoicism).

We help the client to see that *they are OK* (so long as they are **committed** to *acting in a moral fashion*).

When the client is excessively passive in the face of pressures from other people, or from life forces, we teach them to fight back – to the degree that this seems reasonable and safe! We teach them to adopt this non-verbal attitude: "Don't F--- With Me!"; and we teach that lesson using a Gestalt-like Boundary Exercise of our own invention.

We also teach them that, no matter how *inefficient* or *ineffective* they might happen to be; or how *poor* their general judgements often prove to be – this just proves that they are *imperfect humans.* They can still *accept themselves* with all these *imperfections*, so long as they can honestly say they are *trying to live a good, moral life*[171].

And we teach them to keep their expectations of life in line with reality; to only try to change those things that seem likely to be changeable by them; and to take responsibility for steering the boat of their life through the choppy seas of frustration and challenge.

~~~

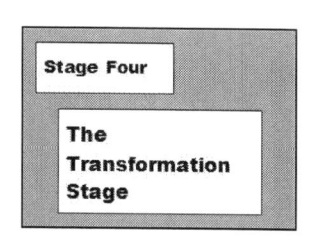

Stage Four

The Transformation Stage

8.3(d): Transformation

Transformation of the client's fundamental way of being in the world is slow work. Most clients do not stick around long enough for this phase to become very much of a reality. They mostly leave when they have had sufficient education to be able to resolve their *burning issues and questions,* and to resolve their *most painful* problems. And that's okay with us!

However, a small minority of clients, with major developmental needs, do stay on for quite long periods of time – between one and five years, to work on deepening their therapeutic change processes.

Six main therapy-deepening processes

The long-term work that is required for ***personal transformation*** involves at least:

(1) deepening the therapeutic relationship;

(2) facing up to painful insights and memories;

(3) more honest and exhaustive confession of personal insights of the client's own contribution to their disturbance;

(4) repeated use of the jigsaw-story model;

(5) some writing therapy work by the client, to clarify their stories further; and

(6) some, if not all, of the following processes:

Use of the Gestalt Chair-work model:

We use this model to help clients to explore incomplete relationships (e.g. with mother or father, etc.), by allowing the client to have *previously* **unexplored** *conversations* with the absent other.

This could be designed to help the client to heal psychological splits, or to become more fully self-expressed. (Source: Scott Kellogg[172])

The client sits in one chair, and imagines another person sitting in the opposite chair. They then have a previously uncompleted conversation with this significant other. Sometimes more than two chairs are used, if the client is badly fragmented in terms of ego states or sub-personalities.

And the E-CENT counsellor may often encourage the client to have dialogues between their Parent and Child ego states, to resolve old family conflicts.

~~~

Gradual desensitization:

We have evolved a four-stage gradual desensitization hierarchy, for problems of panic and trauma, with three processes at each stage in the hierarchy of ascending degrees of intensity.

It takes one session to complete each level in the hierarchy.

The three processes that we use are: (1) Full-body relaxation suggestions[173]; (2) Rational Emotive Imagery[174]; and: (3) Havening[175]. (See Appendix C of Byrne, 2016).

Or how to integrate nutritional insights, exercise and sleep coaching into talk therapy

~~~

Cutting the Ties that Bind:

This is a process which was developed by Phyllis Krystal[176], and adapted by us for use in a *secular form,* (though we sometimes use a spiritual form, for those people who *like* that approach). It is a kind of (often badly belated) ***puberty rite*** – or rite of passage into fully functioning adulthood. In the exercise, the client spends fourteen days visualizing a process of *cutting the invisible ties* between themselves and one significant other person (most often mother or father), who has had (and often is still having) a negative influence upon them (even – sometimes – if the parent has already died!)

After that 14-day visualization process is complete, the client attends the counsellor's office. The E-CENT counsellor then facilitates a process of:

(1) Complete physical relaxation;

(2) A ritual (visualization of) cutting the ties to the person in question;

(3) Mutual forgiveness (of client and significant other) for past transgressions; and:

(4) A release from past influences of the 'divorced' (or 'cut away') person (who is often a parent figure).

Clients report great relief as a result of this exercise, which often changes significant aspects of their interpersonal way of relating in the world today.

~~~

Meditation:

Regular daily meditation, for ten or more minutes, is a great way to relax the whole body-brain-mind; and to practice *detachment* from material grasping or unrealistic desiring. We teach - (to those clients who show an interest) - a form of secular, Zen meditation, as described on our web page[177].

~~~

Attachment system work:

This work is most often based on the attachment styles questionnaire. This questionnaire helps the client to learn whether they have a secure or insecure attachment style (to their original carers, and/or to their current partner). It also distinguishes between two types of insecure attachment, and I teach how differences in insecure attachment style play havoc with some relational patterns. This is where the *first* partner is 'anxious-ambivalent', and clings to the *other* partner. But if the *other* partner is 'avoidant', they will feel trapped by the clinging process, and withdraw, which makes the *first* (clinging) partner feel dreadfully abandoned.

The E-CENT re-attachment process involves the counsellor in providing a 'secure base' and 'safe harbour' for the client, so they can learn to feel securely attached to the counsellor; and this 'earned security' can then be transferred into their relationship with their partner, and also into the wider world.[178]

~~~

Exploring personality:

1. The Keirsey Temperament Sorter:

This can help some individuals more than others, especially those who have had a lot of negative programming from parents which has badly affected their self-concept. Knowing their temperament style can help the individual to understand their *potential* to grow into a very different person from their *parental scripting*. It can also help individuals in relationships to become much more tolerant of individual differences within that relationship; and it helps individuals to understand their career options.[179]

2. Personality Adaptations

We may also, as indicated earlier, use ideas from *Personality Adaptations* by Joines and Stewart (2002). This latter book can be particularly helpful in deciding whether to focus upon the client's thinking, feelings or behaviours, as dictated by their personality adaptation.

~~~

Additional processes:

We sometimes encourage our clients to take up physical exercises programs; to manage their diet and nutrition better; to take more care over their sleep patterns; to keep a reflective journal, and bring it to counselling sessions as subject matter for discussion; to write emails for analysis between counselling sessions; and many other processes.

8.4 Summing up

In this chapter we have mainly tried to describe (in briefest outline) the nature of an individual counselling session, so that we could illustrate the range of E-CENT theories, models and processes which are available for use.

In order to facilitate that outline, we used the standard Jungian session structure, of: Confession; Elucidation; Education and Transformation. This does not mean that we are Jungian, or that we have this structure explicitly in mind when seeing our clients. And it may be that there has *never* been a single E-CENT counselling session that has *corresponded closely* to the structure outline above!

In the process of developing this chapter, we clarified the status and role of some of the most important models used in E-CENT counselling; including:

1. **The holistic SOR model**, which helps us to focus upon the fact that the client is a socialized-body-brain-mind in an environment (especially their social environment), and that there are many factors that go into shaping the client's emotional and behavioural experiences apart from their beliefs and thoughts. (This model is supported by effective, systematic questioning strategies [where appropriate] – which are quite unlike so-called 'Socratic Questioning' – as well as the teaching of mind-body health promotion strategies).

2. **The Six Windows Model**, which allows us to educate the client regarding various alternative ways of viewing their current problems – which allows them to reframe their experience and to generate reduced levels of emotional arousal, and better forms of behavioural response. (And this is supported by various other models; including: the EFR (Event > Framing > Response) model; the Human Givens (APET) model. Plus the Parent-Adult-Child (PAC) model - and also the OK corral model - both of which are borrowed from Transactional Analysis [TA]).

3. **The Jigsaw-story model**, which helps us to keep track of the stories told to us by our clients, so we can spot tensions, contradictions, gaps, and so on; which we can use to help the client to revise and update their stories, and to get a better life from living within a more accurate set of narratives of their life.

4. And a broad range of **other models** which can be used to support the work done in paragraphs 1-3 above.

And all of this work is done in the context of aiming to provide the client with a secure base; to re-parent them; to help them to grow their Adult ego state; and to improve their ability to *regulate* their own *affects, or emotions,* within a more reasonable range than they could when they first arrived to see us.

~~~

Lifestyle Counselling and Coaching for the Whole Person:

Chapter 9: How to incorporate lifestyle and health coaching into talk therapy

By Jim Byrne

9.1 Introduction

One of the most exciting developments in the world of coaching, counselling and psychotherapy at the moment is the emergence of *lifestyle coaching* and *health coaching*. Those two disciplines, which overlap significantly, seem to appeal to growing numbers of counsellors, psychologists and psychotherapists, as an emerging aspect of their own areas of professional interest and practice. For those counsellors and therapists who want to teach the content of this book to their clients, many will find that it is simply a matter of reading this book, and then passing their learning along.

However, others may feel that they want *more support* than that.

One reason for feeling the need for such support is that, while lifestyle coaching and health coaching are compatible with talk therapy, and, indeed, *should, logically*, be part of what psychological therapists offer to their clients, there is a problem with the *mode of delivery*. This is so because most systems of counselling and therapy (apart from the cognitive/rational approach) rely upon the healing power of relationship, and therefore many counsellors and therapists lack experience of 'direct teaching', or 'facilitation of learning', or coaching.

The heart of coaching is the ability to (1) teach something; (2) observe the effect of that teaching/learning process; and (3) to provide corrective or developmental feedback. This we could call the 'coaching cycle'.

Because many counsellors who have no previous experience of coaching will want to make the transition towards lifestyle or health coaching, we have to look at some of the challenges that that will involve.

Therefore, we have to make provision for those individual readers of this book who may want to be *directed* towards the salient aspects of the challenge of *how to teach this material to their clients*.

For this reason, this chapter has been designed to help such individual counsellors and therapists to bone up on particular approaches to teaching and learning.

However, because it is not our intention to patronize anybody, we leave it to the individual reader to decide if they *need* this level of explicit guidance, or if they would prefer to figure it out for themselves through trial and error; or from previous teaching/learning experience. If you decide to study this chapter, then please read it in conjunction with the reading of Chapter 8, which provides insights into our typical approach to counselling; and also with Chapter 7, which explores our take on human emotions.

9.2 Guidance for those who feel they need it

In *Alice in Wonderland*, Lewis Carroll wrote of how the King advised Alice to "begin at the beginning", and continue to the end, and then stop.

This is a good, if simple, guide to action, in planning any journey.

So let us map out the journey we must now follow, and sort out both the beginning and the end. Four obvious elements of our journey have to be as follows:

1. Who to teach. This will include individual 'learning styles', as well as locations on the 'stages of change' model.

2. What to teach. This has to include the ordering of learning tasks, as well as the amount of change per unit of time.

3. When to teach it. This could include client readiness; priority of learning needs; and other elements.

4. How to teach it (and/or how to facilitate some learning). This is about the art of teaching; the promotion of learning; and the use of 'selling skills'.

So, without further ado, let us begin at item 1, and continue until we reach the end.

~~~

1. Who to teach

Counsellors from different traditions will have different approaches to teaching and learning.

Postman and Weingartner (1969)[180] were in favour of promoting student *enquiry* into problems. Their slogan was this: *"No question, no teacher"*. If the client does not have any questions (or curiosity) about the impact of diet, sleep or exercise upon their personal concerns, then it will be virtually impossible to 'teach them' anything in those fields (according to this theory).

Carl Rogers (1983)[181] was famous for saying that "I know I *cannot* teach anything to anyone. I can only create *an environment* in which they can *learn*". And for Rogers, the 'facilitative environment' was one in which the facilitator simply accepted and prized the learner, who was assumed (in line with the theory of Jean Piaget) to be *self-motivated*, and capable of learning everything by *exploration* **alone**.

I (Jim Byrne) have experimented with both of these approaches (in the previous two paragraphs), and find that it *sometimes helps* to be as non-directive as these theorists.

However, I have also found that, *sometimes*, it is important to move to a more *Gestalt-based* approach – or *social learning* approach – in line with Vygotsky and Bandura - which consists of:

    (a) *Building support* for the learner; and then

    (b) *Issuing a challenge* to them to cause them to think and learn; or

    (c) *Modelling* particular kinds of behaviour for them; or

    (d) *Providing them with guidance* in the form of instruction.

Building support for dietary change, for example, could include:

1. Teaching the *advantages* of healthy eating;

2. Teaching the *disadvantages* of junk food, and various toxic foods, like sugar and gluten, etc.

3. Identifying *one **small** change* that would produce the biggest improvement for the client.

4. And so on.

~~~

Then there is the *psychodynamic* approach to learning, which emphasizes the non-conscious motivations of the client; the childhood shaping of the client's personality; and the need to revisit the scene of our original learning – as in learning how to eat, and what to eat, from mother when we were very young[182]. (And current best practice in the UK, concerning issues of *eating disorders*, is that we need to combine the psychodynamic and the cognitive approaches).

Then again, Novak and Gowin (1984)[183], operating within the cognitive tradition, recommend the use of 'focus questions' about a relevant or important 'event or object'. (However, we are now moving into the area of '*how* to teach', which is item 4 in our list, and so let us return to this question later). For now, I want to look at teaching and learning in terms of strategies, styles and readiness:

(i) Teaching strategies:

(a) Sometimes we should ask ourselves: *Does this person have any questions about lifestyle or health issues?* If the answer is 'No', then perhaps we should let the matter lie. But if they **do** have some questions or concerns, then we move to item 2, 'What should I teach them?' (And we will answer that question when we get to item 2, below).

(b) Sometimes we should accept that we *cannot teach* anybody (including our current client) anything. We can only create an environment in which they can learn. The next question is: *How could we do that?* Again, this will be considered under item 4 below. And:

(c) Sometimes we should strive to *get our clients to* **think** about the things they eat, and don't eat (provided they don't have thinking 'walled off'). Or should we get them to think about the way they exercise their bodies, or fail to do so. And the way they understand and attend to their sleep needs.

But we still have not answered the question, 'Who should I teach?' We have simply looked at 'our side of the equation'. So let us try again, and look at the qualities or tendencies of the individual client:

(ii) Learning styles and learning readiness:

(a) *Learning styles:* Individual clients will be found to have somewhat differing 'learning styles'. Some of them will be *Activists/Pragmatists*, who learn best by exploring and doing – taking action and observing the results, for example. And some will be *Theorists/ Reflectors*, who learn well reading/ writing, and discussing/ debating. You can often find out a lot about your clients by asking them: "Do you find you learn easily and well by reading?" Very often, the answer will be some version of, "I hardly read at all!" In which case you know you are dealing with an Activist/Pragmatist, and you will have to devise *practical approaches* for such individuals, which involves a minimum of abstract theory and new concepts.

Then again, some clients will tell you they have learned a lot from books and articles. With those clients, you can have a strategy of having 'handouts' prepared in advance, which outline a good approach to managing diet and nutrition; a good approach to getting into regular physical exercise; and a helpful approach to managing sleep patterns; and so on. You can issue those handouts, as appropriate to individual clients, ask them to read the handout(s), and discuss the implications for the client at the next session.

(b) *Learning readiness:* However, not everybody can be easily helped via the simple approach outlined in paragraph (ii)(a) above. *Why not?* Because not everybody is at the same *stage* in terms of 'the stages of behaviour change'. (Prochaska et al, 1998)[184].

For example, if a client comes to you with a declared desire to change their diet, then they are (or seem to be) at the 'contemplation' stage of behaviour change. And if they are contemplators, they will be open to some form of guidance, instruction or advice.

On the other hand, if they are 'pre-contemplators' – that is to say, they are not contemplating any form of behaviour change – they will not be helped by advice, guidance or instruction. What they need at this stage is to be 'woken up'. Or 'sold' on the idea that some form of behaviour change is desirable, in their best interest.

So, 'contemplators' can be advised, in order to try to move them on to the next stage, which is to become 'determined'. It will take real *determination*, on the part of the client, to make any significant change in their diet, exercise, or sleep pattern. It matters less how determined *you* (the counsellor/coach) happens to be. Indeed, it matters not at all unless you can *help the* **client** *to become* **determined** on their own behalf.

Once a client becomes *determined* to change, you can help them to know how to change, which is discussed in item 4, below.

~~~

2. What to teach

The simple answer to the question of *what to teach* is this: teach your clients whatever part of this book is relevant to their health improvement, including their emotional health improvement. Teach them to value a good night's sleep; 'balanced diet'; and regular physical exercise.

However! You cannot teach everything at once! And you cannot expect progress on more than *one element* of change per client at any one time. So teach them *gradual change*, using the Kai Zen approach. (See Taylor-Byrne and Byrne, 2017 - [Section 1 of Part 6]).

So how do you decide 'what' to teach?

Firstly, you have to engage in some form of assessment of the client's situation and needs. This can be informal (and normally is within the humanistic and psychodynamic traditions), or formal (which is closer to the spirit of the cognitive behavioural tradition).

Let's say you have discovered that a client called Harry has problems with sleep sufficiency, junk food consumption, and sedentary lifestyle, leading to problems of alternating or mixed anxiety and depression.

If you asked Matthew Walker (2017) how to help Harry, then he would say you have to *prioritize* **sleep**. If the client's sleep is disrupted, then no amount of work on their diet or exercise patterns will make a significant or dramatic improvement. And we certainly agree with Walker.

(a) Coaching for sleep improvement

If you agree with Walker, then how should you proceed? If the client is a Theorist/Reflector, you could can get out your (previously prepared) handout on sleep, and talk him through the key points; ask him to take it away and read it three times, to get it into long-term memory; and suggest that you both review his thoughts about this handout at your next counselling session.

(But if he is an Activist/Pragmatist, you will have to keep the teaching approach *conversational*, and use yourself as a role model, by talking about how you manage your sleep pattern, and why this is a valuable and beneficial thing to do. What do you gain from it? Etc.)

At the next session, you should try to find out if the client is **contemplating** some change to their approach to sleep; or if they are stuck at *pre-contemplation*. Your teaching task – with a pre-contemplator – is to get them to understand the costs of not changing their sleep pattern, and the benefits of making some key changes.

With a 'contemplator', your challenge is to encourage them to become more **determined**, again by:

(a) Focusing on a cost-benefit analysis, and a description of how to do this using rewards (for success) and penalties (for slipping back). Or:

(b) By showing that there are *attractive substitutes* they can use for the old habits. (An example of this – from the realm of dietary change - would be where you persuade the client to get some stevia [which is a healthy sugar-substitute] and to try it out in lieu of sugar; and to see for themselves that the transition from sugar to stevia will be relatively effortless, and will involve no real loss of sweetness!)

(b) Coaching for nutritional and dietary improvement

We believe that, once the client's sleep pattern has been addressed, any problems with their diet should be looked at next. And, if Leslie Korn (2016) was here, she would certainly agree.

According to Korn (2016), the first task in helping a client with low mood, depression or mood fluctuations, is to eliminate refined carbohydrates and sugars; and to add protein to the diet. Unless the carbohydrate consumption is reduced, it seems unlikely that they mood problems can be resolved.

There are probably two major tasks that are required to make the change described in the previous paragraph:

(i) Food preparation: Many clients do not prepare food. They eat ready meals, and take-away food, and all kinds of junk food. So they have to be brought to focus upon how to shop for fresh wholefoods; how to store them; how to prepare both raw salads and cooked meals; and how to integrate those changes into their lives. (Korn, 2016; page 13).

(ii) Food and mood diary: Korn (2016) recommends the use of a food/mood diary with the following elements:

(1) *What did you eat?*

(2) *How did it feel?* And:

(3) *Did you do any physical exercise?*

(See table beginning on next page).

According to Korn (2016): "This diary is a valuable tool for revealing clients' self-care routines – or lack of them – and can greatly enhance awareness of what one eats and how it affects energy and mood". (Page 13).

When you review a client's Food/Mood diary, your capacity to spot problems will depend upon how thoroughly you have studied Chapter 4, above. And if you want to go deeper into the theory of nutritional and exercise science, then you could also study Taylor-Byrne and Byrne (2017), which is our book of diet and exercise, and the links to anger, anxiety and depression.

What did you eat?	How did you feel (in the subsequent hour or two)	Did you move about, do any exercise? Describe:
Day one: Breakfast		
Lunch		
Evening meal		

What did you eat?	How did you feel (in the subsequent hour or two)	Did you move about, do any exercise? Describe:
Day two: Breakfast		
Lunch		
Evening meal		

What did you eat?	How did you feel (in the subsequent hour or two)	Did you move about, do any exercise? Describe:
Day three: Breakfast		
Lunch		
Evening meal		

~~~

And when you decide to recommend to a client that they give up some item of food – such as sugar – make sure you do not try to 'take that away from them' without 'giving them' an acceptable substitute *first!* For example, Korn (2016) recommends that, before you ask a client to give up sugar, you should first introduce them to *stevia* – a low GI substitute. Get them using and liking stevia before you suggest the 'last day for sugar consumption'. The same principle applies to all other items of food and/or drink.

(c) Coaching for physical fitness

The most important principle in this area of lifestyle coaching is this: *You cannot teach any exercise system that you have not studied and applied in your own life*. You have to teach by example.

If you want to incorporate the promotion of Tai Chi or Yoga in your counselling practice, it follows that you have to incorporate them into your own life first. Then, when you find a client who is open to being introduced to *the system **you** use*, you will be able to *teach from **experience***, and be a good role model for them.

This brings us to the second most important principle which is this: Teach in small chunks. For example, in teaching Chi Kung, introduce the client to just one or two movements per week; break it down into simple elements; make sure they can do it while copying you; then without your modelling; then ask them to do it at home as homework; and check how they do it when they return the following week. Give any corrective or developmental feedback that seems relevant. And then add another one or two movements. Build up slowly.

The third most important principle is this: Use the Kai Zen approach. Teach the client that it is better to do **two minutes** of *enjoyable exercise per day*, to begin with, than to **bore** themselves or **frighten** themselves by taking on too much of a time commitment, or exertion commitment. Two minutes per day will quickly build up to fifteen, twenty or thirty, over a period of weeks and months. Too much too soon can be demotivating

The fourth most important point is this: Teach your clients to try to find an *exercise buddy*, to work with. Somebody who is normally available, and who will reinforce the habit.

Have a system of rewards and penalties in place. For example, if they do their daily physical exercise (about five days per week), then they get to read their favourite newspaper or magazine. But if they fail to do the agreed exercise program on any particular scheduled day, then they not only do not get to read their paper or magazine (or whatever the reward is), but they also have to drop £2 (or $5) down the nearest drain, as a penalty. Those rewards and penalties will help to keep them on track with their commitments.

(See Part 6 of Taylor-Byrne and Byrne, 2017, for more on how to change negative habits).

~~~

3. When to teach it

Because *relationship* is so important to counselling and therapy, we cannot put teaching about lifestyle *before* the task of establishing a warm relationship; which means becoming *a secure base* for the client.

And, because we know *nothing* about the client when they first arrive, we cannot put teaching about lifestyle before the task of finding out who the client is; what is not working in their lives; and what they would like to get from counselling and therapy.

Once we know a ***reasonable*** amount about the client's lifestyle and agenda; including the presenting problem that they have brought to the first and/or second session; we can begin to formulate a sense of who the client is, and what might be going wrong in their lives.

At that point, we should *begin* to teach the client our understanding of how the body, brain and mind are related to the current environment; and to the early childhood relationship; and how all of those elements interact; and are affected by current stressors; and how problems in any of those areas may be affecting their moods, emotions, behaviours and/or relationships.

Out of this conversation, opportunities will present themselves to explore whether or not there is a sleep problem; and whether it is serious enough to need urgent attention. Is it causing a mood problem? Or is the sleep problem a result of a pre-existing mood problem?

Or is alcohol involved?

Or does the client simply need to learn good sleep hygiene? Depending upon the answers to these questions, you can begin to teach what seems most appropriate.

If you suspect a link between mood and food as being more salient than attitudes or beliefs, or personal history, or personal philosophy of life, then that would be the time to explore the client's attitudes towards food; and to teach whatever seems to be missing from the client's understanding in this area of lifestyle knowledge.

Finally, if you become aware that the client is not doing any physical exercise, or very little, and that this seems to be an important link in the chain of causation of their emotional or behavioural problems, then this would be the time to teach the value and importance of avoiding sedentary lifestyle.

At a more general level, the time to teach might be when the client reveals that they are contemplating making some kind of lifestyle change in a particular area of concern.

And when a client declares that they are committed to making a particular change, and to getting into action soon, that would be the time to teach them how to break bad habits. (See Taylor-Byrne and Byrne, 2017; *Part 6: How to change for good*).

~~~

4. How to teach it

Let us assume you have satisfied the first four questions: *Who, what, and when to teach about lifestyle factors in mental health and emotional well-being?*

You then arrive at the final piece of the jigsaw puzzle of lifestyle coaching: *How to teach it*

As mentioned earlier, there are many schools of thought in both educational psychology and in counselling and psychotherapy. So we want to suggest a model which will not do violence to any particular school of thought. It occurs to us that, a good counsellor or therapist is somebody who cares deeply about their client, and that, no matter how non-directive they might be in terms of their approach to counselling and therapy, they would mostly be willing to 'sell' a better lifestyle to their client if that could be done ethically!

So let us consider a model which is often used by sales people. It's called the AIDA model, and it structured like this:

Attention: You have to gain the attention of the client before anything else can happen. You need to present something sufficiently dramatic, for example on the link between loss of sleep and reductions in emotional intelligence; or the linkages between gluten, leaky gut and brain inflammation. That kind of information would most likely grab the attention of any client who values the preservation of their brain-mind health, and their emotional intelligence – which includes their capacity to manage their own emotions, while understanding the emotions of others. Some will only be interested because emotional intelligence is said to be central to professional success; while others value the idea of being emotionally intelligent in their personal relationships.

Interest: Once you have caught their attention, you will need to get them interested in improving their sleep hygiene patterns (or whatever it is that you want to promote). One way to do that is to focus upon the *features* of a well-established set of rules for managing bedtime and bedroom details (such as those outlined in Chapter 5 of this present book).

Desire: Once they are clearly interested, you need to move them along to the next step; which is *to develop the **desire** to implement that list* – or some elements of that list – of lifestyle changes. The best way to do that is to focus on the *benefits* of making those changes. (See section 5.6 of this present book, above). If the client shows signs of being moved to take action, as a result of this review, then move to the next step:

Action: Help the client to draw up a *brief action list*, with **one** or **two** key points to be changed; which will then be reviewed at the next session. (Remember the Kai Zen approach: Small gradual steps are more durable than sudden, radical change! And they mount up surprisingly quickly, and durably).

Review the client's success at the next session, and give any corrective or developmental feedback which seems to be necessary.

~~~

That brings us to the end of this brief review of the E-CENT approach to incorporating lifestyle and health coaching into talk therapy

~~~

Jim Byrne, Hebden Bridge, March 2018

~~~

Chapter 10: Conclusion

10.1 Overview

Let us begin with a quick overview of the ground we covered in this book so far.

Chapter 1 began with two sections on the holistic nature of E-CENT counselling, and how we have placed feelings before thinking, and also emphasized the fact that our narratives are embodied. We then looked at the counselling and therapy theories out of which E-CENT was built, and how most of them are considered by the Common Factors School of research to be effective in about equal measure.

We moved on to describe how we – initially - accidentally created E-CENT theory while trying to defend Rational Emotive Behaviour Therapy (REBT). Subsequently, we moved on into incorporating elements of Attachment theory, Transactional analysis, and various outgrowths of affective neuroscience and interpersonal neurobiology; plus moral philosophy, and aspects of *moderate* Buddhism and *moderate* Stoicism.

We then looked at our approach to science and the use of case studies in defending systems of counselling and therapy, and decided against the use of case studies to 'prove' or 'verify' any aspect of our theory.

Next came a consideration of the roots of E-CENT in pre-existing forms of narrative therapy, and how we differ from those pre-existing schools of thought. There is then an elaboration of the E-CENT approach. And this is followed by a consideration of the E-CENT approach to Attachment theory.

Chapter 1 ends with a brief introduction to some of the core models used in E-CENT.

10.2 The core theory of E-CENT

E-CENT counselling theory sees humans as essentially emotional beings; or, rather, we seem to be socialized-physical-cultural-emotional-story-tellers. We tend to tell (emotionally significant) stories about our experiences, to ourselves and others, and we live in a world of (emotionally significant) narratives and scripts, (about *concrete* realities!), which include reasonable and unreasonable elements, as well as logical and illogical elements, and some defensible and some less defensible elements. However, because these stories have to be 'socially agreed', in the main, we cannot call this 'subjectivism'. It is actually *intersubjective*, and based on *social agreement*.

Furthermore, we are *not* involved in 'telling ourselves' things which upset us; since we are **perfinking** rather than **thinking** beings. We **perceive-feel-think** all in one grasp of the mind. So E-CENT theory clearly integrates the cognitive/thinking elements of CBT and the emotive/feeling elements of psychodynamic psychotherapy.

We humans tend to delete elements of our storied experiences; to distort some other elements; and to generalize from particular experiences. And we also have lots of early experiences which are non-narrativized, but which are still active or operational in the non-conscious basement of our emotional lives; guiding or influencing our moods, emotions and behaviours.

Humans often tend to push away (or repress) unpleasant experiences; to fail to process them; and to then become the (unconscious) victims of those repressed, and/or undigested experiences.

E-CENT theory also sees adult relationships as being the non-conscious acting out of childhood experiences (which occurred with parents and siblings), because some part of those earlier relationships have not been properly digested and completed. And/or because we modelled ourselves upon role models, and now tend to carry on our earliest patterns of habitual behaviour, as modified (slightly or greatly) by subsequent significant experiences.

10.3 Key Learning Points and Applications

This book was designed to be relevant to the learning needs of:

>(a) Counsellors, coaches, psychotherapists, psychologists, social workers, psychiatrists, psychiatric nurses, key workers, and others in similar lines of work;
>
>(b) Students of counselling, psychology, psychotherapy, psychiatry, and related disciplines and professions; and:
>
>(c) Self-help enthusiasts, or individuals who want to learn about the human brain-mind-emotions for their own personal development purposes.

Let us now suggest some key learning points for each of those reader-groups, which could be deduced from the reading of this book. And, for those readers who want to apply their learning from this book in their daily lives, so that they can learn about it in practice, we suggest the following activities:

(a) For therapists and counsellors:

The two main points that should interest counsellors and therapist are presented next, and linked to some activities designed to reinforce this learning:

Point 1: That human personality is conceptualized as an evolving *epiphenomenon* (or *outgrowth*) of a primarily *social body-mind*, which has innate potential to develop good and bad tendencies – in attachment to a social environment - and which accumulates *interpretative experiences* (in the form of narrativized and non-narrativized schemas and frames) which are stored primarily in *non-conscious forms*, and which manifest in **Parent**, **Adult** and **Child** forms of thinking/ feeling/ behaving (or perfinking). This effectively integrates the psychodynamic, the cognitive behavioural and the narrative traditions.

Because we are body-minds, the state of our bodies is crucial to our 'mental health', or *emotional wellbeing*; and the state of our mind is crucial to our physical health. Both must be taken care of. And counsellors and therapists need to pay as much attention to the diet and exercise practices, and sleep patterns, of their clients as they do to the client's stories and experiences.

Here are three suggested activities for active learners among our counsellor and therapist readers:

Activity 1: Experiment with physical exercise in your own life, and write a journal about how you feel when you are well exercised, and how you feel when you are not. Try – for example – seven days without any physical exercise, and write up how you feel, physically and mentally, every day. Then try – for example – another seven days with about thirty minutes of physical exercise each morning (which could be as simple as a brisk walk!), and write up how you feel, physically and mentally each day. Then compare the two periods to arrive at your own assessment of the effect of physical exercise on your body-mind. (This could then be turned into a handout for your clients).

Activity 2: Explore the ideal diet to reduce stress, and experiment with dietary changes in your own life. (Use the ideas in Chapter 4, and/or Part 1 of Taylor-Byrne and Byrne, 2017).

Again, you might try seven days on junk food, followed by seven days on a healthy diet.

Make journal entries about how you feel – in terms of mood and physical energy; and also monitor skin condition - on a good diet and a bad diet. (And again, these notes could be turned into a handout for your clients).

Activity 3: Keep a sleep diary. Try to track links between broken sleep or insufficient sleep, on the one hand, and low mood or anxiety or irritability, plus physical energy, concentration ability, and perfinking quality, on the other. Also, monitor good quality sleep, of sufficient duration, and try to track linkages to improved emotional intelligence; better moods; and clearer thinking (or perfinking).

~~~

Point 2: That humans (at the mental level) are essentially (emotional) story tellers, to ourselves and others, and storytellers who live in a world of narratives and scripts, which include reasonable and unreasonable elements, logical and illogical elements, and defensible and indefensible elements.

Humans often tend to push away (or repress) unpleasant experiences, to fail to process them, and then to become the (unconscious) victims of those repressed, undigested experiences.

E-CENT theory also sees adult relationships as being the acting out of childhood experiences with parents and siblings, as creatures of habit, and/or because some part of those earlier relationships have not been properly digested and completed.

Activity 4: In a journal, experiment with digesting stressful experiences from your own life in the form of stories. You could try:

First day at school;

Birth of a new sibling;

Childhood nightmares;

A childhood trauma;

Schoolyard stress;

Transition into and through puberty;

Early adult difficulties; or whatever stands out for you as being in need to clarification and digestion.

Write the experience up as autobiography. Then, to achieve some detachment, write it up as a short story about a fictional character. Try to re-author the experience, using any insights you can gain from considering the PAC model; or the OK-corral. Also, consider the middle column of the Holistic-SOR model. Or use the APET model and/or the WDEP model. If none of that helps, try taking an online attachment styles assessment quiz, to see if that helps you to understand your own role in the experience. You could also check out your own character and temperament, using the Keirsey Temperament Sorter, which might clarify why you were the way you were in relation to the experience and other people who were involved in the experience under consideration. And you could assess your own Personality Adaptation, to see what role that might have played.

~~~

Activity 5: In your personal journal, explore a stressful experience in your current life, using the Six Windows Model.

~~~

(b) For individuals interested in self-help and personal development:

If you are interested in developing yourself, and especially in managing your thinking, feeling and behaviours, then:

Point 1: The Six Windows model is likely to be of prime interest, because it is a powerful tool for reframing any problematical situation, so that it looks and feels better than before.

You can apply this model to several of your own current problems, and write up the results to get the learning into long-term memory.

Activity 1: In a journal, apply the Six Windows model to a current problem in your life.

Activity 2: On a notepad, help a friend to digest a current problem using the Six Windows Model. (Begin by writing it up as an E>F>R problem – *What did they experience* (E)? [Skip over the F (framing)]. Then, *What was their (emotional and behavioural) response* (R)? Then switch to Narrative Inquiry (NI), using the six windows).

~~~

Point 2: Learning to think 'globally' instead of in a 'mono-focal' (or tunnel vision) manner would be a useful goal. The brain-mind is an information processing 'machine' that jumps to conclusions, based on past experiences, using habit-based pattern-matching schemas.

Activity 3: Get a good friend to ask you how you are, and then answer the question using the six perspectives of the Six Windows model, instead of allowing your habitual way of responding to dominate your consciousness.

~~~

Point 3: Furthermore, if you (being human) are essentially a story-teller, what aspects of your life seem to be an outgrowth of a *defective narrative* that you wrote (with help from your family and community) when you were much younger than you are now?

Activity 5: In a journal, make a list of a few aspects of your life that seem to be *story-determined*. That is to say, try to identify areas of your life where you seem to be following an unhelpful 'script'.

Activity 6: Try writing about the issues arising in *Activity 5*, to see if you can re-author your life. Helpful questions might be:

Who am I? What was my childhood like?

Is my present life strongly influenced by my childhood? What might I have pushed away (repressed) when I was a child, that I now need to dig up and digest?

How could I 'reframe' a past experience (using one or more of the models in this book)? Do I need to get counselling help to do this work?

Write down your questions and answers, and then read back through them, and make any refinements or corrections that occur to you.

~~~

(c) For counselling and psychotherapy students:

If you are studying counselling and therapy systems, you might productively engage with the following five journal writing activities:

Activity 1: Write a page or two about how the Holistic SOR model might fit with the system of counselling and therapy you are learning on your course.

How much of the Holistic SOR view of the organism is omitted from your current approach to counselling and therapy?

Where do diet, exercise and sleep fit into the model of the human organism being taught on your counselling course?

~~~

Activity 2: Secondly, which of the other models used in E-CENT would be compatible with the system you are studying? Make a list.

~~~

Activity 3: Furthermore, if human personality is conceptualized as a primarily social body-mind, which has innate potential to develop good and bad (moral and immoral) tendencies, and which accumulates experiences which are stored primarily in non-conscious forms, and which manifests in Parent, Adult and Child forms of thinking/ feeling/ behaving – what does this say about how you should ***approach your role-play clients?*** Please write up your reflections in your journal. Think your way through a role-play session that you had recently, and ask yourself: *"Would I change anything about my approach to counselling a client, based on my learning from E-CENT?"*

(Role-playing counselling sessions – in trios [comprising a client, a counsellor and an observer] is a fairly standard part of counselling and therapy training).

~~~

Activity 4: Think about the following argument:

In this book, we have argued that humans are essentially (emotional) story tellers (about their concrete experiences), who tell stories to themselves and others. We have said they are storytellers who live in a concrete world of narratives and scripts – which include reasonable and unreasonable elements, logical and illogical elements, and defensible and indefensible elements. Considering this model of humans, please answer the following questions in your journal:

What does this say about how counselling sessions need to be conducted?

What problems does it present?

What obstacles does it place in the approach of the counsellor?

(Please write up your answers).

~~~

Activity 5: If it is true that humans often tend to push away (or repress) unpleasant experiences, to fail to process them, and to then become the (non-conscious) victims of those repressed, undigested experiences – *what must counsellors do to help them?*

~~~

Activity 6: And finally, consider doing the practical activities recommended in section (b) above, for people interested in self-help and personal development.

~~~

Some readers might want to go back over this book and identify their own key learning points.

~~~

The author would be pleased to learn of any attempts to apply these ideas in counselling and therapy settings; or to explore them in academic essays by counselling and therapy students; or of any experiments done using E-CENT for self-management.

Please send your correspondence to:

Dr Jim Byrne, ABC Coaching and Counselling Services, 27 Wood End, Keighley Road, Hebden Bridge, West Yorkshire, HX7 8HJ, UK

Or email: dr.byrne@ecent-institute.org

Copyright (c) Jim Byrne, March 2018

~~~

References

Ainsworth, M. (1967) *Infancy in Uganda: Infant Care and the Growth of Love*. Baltimore: Johns Hopkins University Press.

Ainsworth, M.D. (1969) Object relations, dependency, and attachment: a theoretical review of the infant-mother relationship. *Child Development, 40 (4):* Pages 969–1025.

Akbaraly, T.N., Brunner, E.J., Ferrie, J.E., Marmot, M.G., et al. (2009) 'Dietary pattern and depressive symptoms in middle age'. *British Journal of Psychiatry. 2009 Nov; 195(5):408-13.* doi: 10.1192/bjp.bp.108.058925. Available online at: https://www.ncbi.nlm.nih.gov/pubmed/19880930. Accessed: 22nd September 2017.

Amen, D.G. (2013) *Use Your Brain to Change your Age: Secrets to look, feel, and think younger every day*. London: Piatkus.

Anwar, Y. (2013) Tired and edgy? Sleep deprivation boosts anticipatory anxiety. Berkley News (University of California). Online: http://news.berkeley.edu/ 2013/06/25/anticipate-the-worst/. Accessed: 22nd January 2018.

Asp, K. (2015) Lack of Sleep and Depression: Causes and Treatment Options. The AAST blog: https://www.aastweb.org/blog /the-relationships-between-lack-of-sleep-and-depression. Accessed: 22nd January 2018.

APFHF (2008) The Links between Diet and Behaviour. The influence of nutrition on mental health. Report of an inquiry held by the Associate Parliamentary Food and Health Forum (APFHF). London: All Party Parliamentary Food and Health Forum.

Asch, S.E. (1956) A minority of one against a unanimous majority. *Psychological Monographs, 70 (416)*.

Aurelius, M. (1946/1992) *Meditations*. Trans. A.S.L. Farquharson. London: Everyman's Library.

Ballantyne, C. (2007) Fact or Fiction? Vitamin Supplements Improve Your Health. *Scientific American* (Online): http://www.scientificamerican.com/ article/ fact- or-fiction-vitamin-supplements-improve-health/May 17, 2007. Accessed 26th April 2016.

Bandler, R. and Grinder, J. (1975) *The Structure of Magic. Vol.1: A book about language and therapy*. Palo Alto, Calif.: Science and Behaviour Books Inc.

Bangalore, N.G., and Varambally, S. (2012) Yoga therapy for schizophrenia. *International Journal of Yoga* 2012; **5**(2):85-91.

Baran, J. (ed) (2003) *365 Nirvana: Here and now*. London: HarperCollins/Element.

Barber, L. K., Munz, D. C., Bagsby, P. G. and Powell, E. D. (2009) Sleep consistency and sufficiency: are both necessary for less psychological strain? *Stress and Health, Vol.26(3),* Pages 186-193.

Bargh, J.A. and Chartrand, T.L. (1999) The unbearable automaticity of being. *American Psychologist, 54(7):* Pages 462-479.

Bartlett, F.C. (1932) *Remembering*. Cambridge: Cambridge University Press.

Bastable, S.B. (2008) *Nurse as Educator*. Burlington, Mas: Jones & Bartlett Learning

Beauchamp, T.L. and Childress, J.F. (1994) *Principles of Biomedical Ethics*. Fourth edition. New York. Oxford University Press.

Beck, A.T. (1976/1989) *Cognitive Therapy and the Emotional Disorders.* London: Penguin Books.

Behere, R.V., Arasappa, R., Jagannathan, A., Varambally, S., Venkatasubramanian, G., Thirthalli, J., Subbakrishna, D.K., Nagendra, H.R., and Gangadhar, B.N. (2011) Effect of yoga therapy on facial emotion recognition deficits, symptoms and functioning in patients with schizophrenia. *Acta Psychiatrica Scandinavia, Vol 123 (2);* pp: 147 -153.

Benton, D. and G. Roberts (1988) Effects of vitamin and mineral supplementation on intelligence in schoolchildren. *The Lancet, Vol 1 (8578),* Pages 140-143.

Bjarnadottir, A. (2015) Why Refined Carbs Are Bad For You. Authority Nutrition - An Evidence-Based Approach (An online blog). Available online: https://authoritynutrition.com/why-refined-carbs-are-bad/. Accessed: 10th June 2016

Blanchflower, D.G., A.J. Oswald and S. Stewart-Brown. (2016) Is Psychological Well-being Linked to the Consumption of Fruit and Vegetables? Available online: http://www.andrewoswald.com/ docs/ October2FruitAndVeg2012BlanchOswaldStewartBrown.pdf

Bloom, P. (2013) *Just Babies: the origins of good and evil.* London: The Bodley Head.

Blumenthal, J.A., Smith, P.J., and Hoffman, B.M. (2012) Is exercise a viable treatment for depression? *American College of Sports Medicine Health & Fitness Journal.* July/August; Vol.16(4): Pages 14–21. Cited in: Ratey, J., and Hagerman, E. (2009) *Spark: The revolutionary new science of exercise and the brain.* London: Quercus.

Bond, T. (2000) *Standards and Ethics for Counselling in Action.* Second edition. London: Sage.

Borchard, T. (2015) 10 Ways to Cultivate Good Gut Bacteria and Reduce Depression. Everyday Health Blog. Available online: http://www.everydayhealth.com/columns/therese-borchard-sanity-break/ways-cultivate-good-gut-bacteria-reduce-depression/

Boseley, S. (2018) Half of all food bought in UK is ultra-processed. *The Guardian.* Saturday 3rd February 2018. Issue No. 53,323.

Bowell, T. and Kemp, G. (2005) *Critical Thinking: a concise guide.* Second edition. London: Routledge.

Bowlby J (1958) The nature of the child's tie to his mother. *International Journal of Psychoanalysis* 39 (5): 350–73.

Bowlby, J. (1988/2005) *A Secure Base: Clinical applications of attachment theory.* London: Routledge Classics.

Bowlby, J. (1969) *Attachment. Attachment and loss: Vol. 1. Loss.* New York: Basic Books.

Boyd, D.B. (2003) Insulin and Cancer. *Integrative Cancer Therapies.* Dec 2003. Vol.2(4): Pages 315-329.

Bravo, J.A., P. Forsythe, M.V. Chew, E. Escaravage, H.M. Savignac, T.G. Dinan, J. Bienenstock, and J.F. Cryan (2011) Ingestion of Lactobacillus strain regulates emotional behaviour and central GABA receptor expression in a mouse via the vagus nerve. Available online: http://www.ncbi.nlm.nih.gov/pubmed/21876150

Bretherton, I. (1992) The Origins of Attachment Theory: John Bowlby and Mary Ainsworth. *Developmental Psychology 28:* 759.

Brewer, S. (2013) *Nutrition: A beginners guide.* London: Oneworld Publications.

Broderick J., Knowles A., Chadwick J., and Vancampfort D. (2015) Yoga versus standard care for schizophrenia. Cochrane Database of Systematic Reviews 2015, Issue 10. Available online: http://www.cochrane.org/CD010554/SCHIZ_yoga-versus-standard-care-schizophrenia

Brogan, K. (2016) *A mind of your own: The truth about depression and how women can heal their bodies to reclaim their lives.* London: Thorsons.

Bruner, J. (1986) *Actual Minds, Possible Worlds*. Cambridge, MA: Harvard University Press.

Bryant, C.W. (2010) Does running fight depression? 14th July 2010. Blog post at HowStuffworks.com Available online: http://adventure.howstuffworks.com/outdoor-activities/ running/ health/ running-fight-depression.htm. Accessed 16th June 2016.

Bucci, W. (1993) The development of emotional meaning in free association: a multiple code theory; in A. Wilson and J.E. Gedo (eds) *Hierarchical Concepts in Psychoanalysis: Theory, research and clinical practice.* New York: Guilford Press.

Burns, D. (1999) *The Feeling Good Handbook*. London: Plume/Penguin Books.

Byrne, J. (2004/2011) Writing therapy: Applied to stress. Available online: http://web.archive.org/web/20160323004450/http://www.abc-counselling.com/id458.html

Byrne, J. (2017) *Unfit for Therapeutic Purposes: The case against Rational Emotive and Cognitive Behavioural Therapy (RE&CBT).* Hebden Bridge: The Institute for E-CENT.

Byrne, J. (2009a) Rethinking the psychological models underpinning Rational Emotive Behaviour Therapy (REBT). E-CENT Paper No.1(a). Hebden Bridge: The Institute for E-CENT. Available online: https://ecent-institute.org/e-cent-articles-and-papers/

Byrne, J. (2009b) The 'Individual' and his/her Social Relationships - The E-CENT Perspective. E-CENT Paper No.9. Hebden Bridge: The Institute for E-CENT. Available online: https://ecent-institute.org/e-cent-articles-and-papers/

Byrne, J. (2009c) The status of autobiographical narratives and stories: Regarding human non-conscious functioning. E-CENT Paper No.5. Hebden Bridge: The Institute for E-CENT. Available online at this web page: https://ecent-institute.org/e-cent-articles-and-papers/

Byrne, J. (2009d) A journey through models of mind. The story of my personal origins. CENT Paper No.4. Hebden Bridge: The Institute for E-CENT. Available online: https://ecent-institute.org/e-cent-articles-and-papers/.

Byrne, J. (2009e) How to analyze autobiographical narratives in Emotive-Cognitive Embodied-Narrative Therapy. E-CENT Paper No.6. Hebden Bridge: The Institute for E-CENT. https://ecent-institute.org/e-cent-articles-and-papers/

Byrne, J. (2009/2016) What is Emotive-Cognitive Embodied-Narrative Therapy (E-CENT)? E-CENT Paper No.2(a). Hebden Bridge: The Institute for E-CENT. Available online: https://ecent-institute.org/what-is-e-cent-counselling/

Byrne, J.W. (2010a) *Therapy after Ellis, Berne, Freud and the Buddha: the birth of Emotive-Cognitive Embodied-Narrative Therapy (E-CENT).* Hebden Bridge: The Institute for E-CENT.

Byrne, J. (2010b) Self-acceptance and other-acceptance in relation to competence and morality. E-CENT Paper No.2(c). Hebden Bridge: The Institute for E-CENT. Available online: https://ecent-institute.org/e-cent-articles-and-papers/

Byrne, J. (2011) Completing your experience of difficult events, perceptions and painful emotions. E-CENT Paper No.13. Hebden Bridge: The Institute for E-CENT. Online: https://ecent-institute.org/e-cent- articles-and-papers/

Byrne, J. (2011-2013) The Innate Good and Bad Aspects of all Human Beings (the Good and Bad Wolf states). E-CENT Paper No.25: Hebden Bridge: The Institute for E-CENT Publications. Available online: https://ecent-institute.org/e-cent-articles-and-papers/

Byrne, J. (2012) *Chill Out: How to control your stress level and have a happier life.* Hebden Bridge: CreateSpace.

Byrne, J. (2013) *A Wounded Psychotherapist: Albert Ellis's Childhood, and the strengths and limitations of REBT/CBT*. Hebden Bridge: The Institute for CENT Publications/CreateSpace.

Byrne, J. (2016) *Facing and Defeating your Emotional Dragons: How to process and eliminate undigested pain from your past.* Narrative Therapy Series (NTS) - eBook No.5. Hebden Bridge: The Institute for E-CENT Publications.

Byrne, J. (with R.E. Taylor-Byrne) (2016) *Holistic Counselling in Practice: An introduction to Emotive-Cognitive Embodied Narrative Therapy.* Hebden Bridge: The Institute for E-CENT Publications.

Byrne, J. (2017) *Unfit for Therapeutic Purposes: The case against RE&CBT.* Hebden Bridge: the Institute for E-CENT Publications.

Calm-Clinic (2018) How Sleep Debt Causes Serious Anxiety. Online blog: https://www.calmclinic.com/anxiety/causes/sleep-debt. Accessed: 25th January 2018.

Cameron, J. (1992) *The Artist's Way: a spiritual path to higher creativity.* London: Souvenir Books.

Campbell, T.C. and Campbell, T.M. (2006) *The China Study: The most comprehensive study of nutrition ever conducted and the startling implications for diet, weight loss and long-term health.* Dallas, TX: Benbella Books.

Cardwell, M. (2000) *The Complete A-Z Psychology Handbook.* Second edition. London: Hodder and Stoughton.

Chaitow, L. (2003) *Candida Albicans: The non-drug approach to the treatment of Candida infection.* London: Thorsons.

Christensen, L. (1991) The roles of caffeine and sugar in depression. *The Nutrition Report 1991*: Vol.9(5 Pt.1): Pages 691-698.

Coffman, M.A. (2016) The Disadvantages of Junk Food. A blog post at the 'Healthy Eating' website. Available online at this url: http://healthyeating.sfgate.com/disadvantages-junk-food-1501.html. Accessed: 30th April 2016.

Coles, M. (2018) People who sleep less than 8 hours a night more likely to suffer from depression, anxiety. Bing U News. New York: Binghamton University.

Colman, A. (2002) *Dictionary of Psychology.* Oxford: Oxford University Press.

Cordain, L. (2011) *The Paleo Diet Cookbook*. Hoboken, NJ: John Wiley and Sons.

Cummins, C. (2007) How to Start a Restorative Yoga Practice. *Yoga Journal*, Aug 28, 2007. Available online: http://www.yogajournal.com/article/beginners/restorative-yoga/. Accessed: 17th June 2016.

Cunningham, J. B. (2001) *The Stress Management Sourcebook. Second edition.* Los Angeles: Lowell House.

Damasio, A. R. (1994). *Descartes' Error: emotion, reason and the human brain.* London, Picador.

Darwin, C. (1872/1965) *The Expression of the Emotions in Man and Animals.* Chicago: University of Chicago Press.

Dawkins, R. (1989) *The Selfish Gene.* Second edition. Oxford: Oxford University Press.

Deans, E. (2018) Magnesium for Depression: A controlled study of magnesium shows clinically significant improvement. Psychology Today Blog: https://www.psychologytoday.com/blog/evolutionary-psychiatry/201801/magnesium-depression. Accessed: 2nd March 2018.

De Bono, E. (1995) *Teach Yourself to Think.* London: Viking/Penguin.

Deleniv, S. (2015) Is serotonin the happy brain chemical, and do depressed people just have too little of it? *The Neuropshere.* Online: https://theneurosphere.com/2015/11/14/is-serotonin-the-happy-brain-chemical-and-do-depressed-people-just-have-too-little-of-it/

Docherty, R.W. (1989) Post-disaster stress in the emergency rescue services. *Fire Engineers Journal,* August. Pages 8-9.

Doidge, N. (2008) *The Brain that Changes Itself: Stories of personal triumph from the frontiers of brain science.* London: Penguin.

Duraiswamy G., Thirthalli J., Nagendra H.R. and Gangadhar B.N. (2007) Yoga therapy as an add-on treatment in the management of patients with schizophrenia – a randomized controlled trial. *Acta Psychiatrica Scandinavia, 116 (3);* pp: 226-232

Egan, G. (2002) *The Skilled Helper: a problem-management and opportunity-development approach to helping.* Seventh edition. Pacific Grove, CA: Brooks/Cole.

Ekman, P. (1993) Facial expression and emotion. *American Psychologist 48 (4):* Pages 384-392.

Elliott, A.F. (2014) 'Can an Atkins-style diet really fight depression? Research suggests low-carb, high fat foods can drastically improve mental health'. Available online: http://www.dailymail.co.uk/femail/article-2590880/Can-Atkins-style-diet-really-fight-depression-Research-suggests-low-carb-high-fat-foods-drastically-improve-mental-health.html Downloaded: 2nd October 2017.

Ellis, A. (1958). Rational Psychotherapy. *Journal of General Psychology,* Vol.59, Pages 35-49.

Ellis, A. (1962) *Reason and Emotion in Psychotherapy.* New York: Lyle Stuart.

Enders, G. (2015) *Gut: The inside story of our body's most under-rated organ.* London: Scribe Publications.

Epictetus (1991) *The Enchiridion.* New York: Prometheus Books.

Ervine, W. (2009) *A Guide to the Good Life: The ancient art of Stoic joy.* Oxford: Oxford University Press.

Erwin, E. (1997) *Philosophy and Psychotherapy: Razing the troubles of the brain,* London, Sage.

Evans, D. (2003) *Emotion: a very short introduction.* Oxford. Oxford University Press.

Evers, E.A.T., Tillie, D.E., van der Veen, F.M., Lieben, C.K., Jolles, J., Deutz, N.E.P., Schmitt, J.A.J. (2005) Effects of a novel method of acute tryptophan depletion on plasma tryptophan and cognitive performance in healthy volunteers. *Journal of Psychopharmacology, Vol 178, No. 1.* Pages 1432-2072.

Eysenck, M.W. and Keane, M.T. (2000) *Cognitive Psychology: A student's Handbook.* Fourth edition. East Sussex: Psychology Press.

Fife, B. (2005) *Coconut Cures: Preventing and treating common health problems with coconut.* Colorado Springs, CO: Piccadilly Books Ltd.

Fonagy, P., Gergeley, G., Jurist, E.J., and Target, M.I. (2002) *Affect regulation, mentalization, and the development of the self.* New York: Other Press.

Forgas, J.P. (ed) (2001) *Feeling and Thinking: The role of affect in social cognition.* Cambridge: Cambridge University Press.

Freud, S. (1986) *Historical and Expository Works on Psychoanalysis. Vol.15.* London: Penguin Books.

Freud, S. (1995) Beyond the pleasure principle. In: Gay, P. (ed) *The Freud Reader.* London: Vintage Books.

Gergen, K. (1985) The social constructionist movement in modern psychology. *American Psychologist, 40:* 266-275.

Gergen, K. J. (1994). *Toward Transformation in Social Knowledge.* London: Sage Publications.

Gergen, K. (2004) When relationships generate realities: therapeutic communication reconsidered. Unpublished manuscripts. Available online: http://www.swarthmore.edu/Soc.Sci/kgergen1/printer-friendly.phtml?id-manu6. Downloaded: 8th December 2004. And:

Gergen, K.J. and Gergen, M.M. (1986) Narrative form and the construction of psychological science. In T.R. Sarbin (ed), *Narrative Psychology: the storied nature of human conduct.* New York: Praeger.

Gerhardt, S. (2010) *Why Love Matters: How affection shapes a baby's brain.* London: Routledge.

Gesch, C.B., Hammond, S.M., Hampson, S.E., Eves, A., and Crowder, M.J. (2002) Influence of supplementary vitamins, minerals and essential fatty acids on the antisocial behaviour of young adults. *British Journal of Psychiatry 81*: Pages 22–28. Available online: http://www.ncbi.nlm.nih.gov/pubmed/12091259

Gigerenzer, G. (2008) *Gut Feelings: The Intelligence of the Unconscious.* London: Penguin.

Gilliland, K. and Andress, D. (1981) Ad Lib caffeine consumption, symptoms of caffeinism and academic performance. *American Journal of Psychiatry, Vol 138 (4),* Pages 512-514.

Gladwell, M. (2006) *BLINK: The power of thinking without thinking.* London: Penguin Books.

Glasersfeld, E. von (1989) Learning as a constructive activity. In Murphy, P. and Moon, B. (eds) *Developments in Learning and Assessment.* London: Hodder and Stoughton.

Goldacre, B. (2007) Patrick Holford's untruthful and unsubstantiated claims about pills: http://www.badscience.net/2007/09/patrick-holdford-unsubstantiated-untruthful/ Accessed 14th April 2016.

Goldacre, B. (2012) *Bad Pharma: How drug companies mislead doctors and harm patients.* London: Fourth Estate.

Gomez, L. (1997) *An Introduction to Object Relations.* London: Free Association Books.

Gonçalves, O.F. (1995) Hermeneutics, constructivism and cognitive-behavioural therapies: from the object to the project. In: R.A. Neimeyer and M.J. Mahoney (eds) *Constructivism in psychotherapy.* Washington, DC: American Psychological Association.

Goleman, D. (1996) *Emotional Intelligence: why it can matter more than IQ.* London: Bloomsbury.

Gordon, A.M. (2013) Up all night: the effects of sleep loss on mood. Research shows just one bad night of sleep can put a damper on your mood. *Psychology Today Online.* August 15th 2013. Available here: https://www.psychology today.com/ blog/ between-you-and-me/201308/all-night-the-effects-sleep-loss-mood. Accessed: 20th January 2018.

Gottman, J. (1997). *Why Marriages Succeed or Fail: and how you can make yours last.* London: Bloomsbury.

Gray, J. (2003) *Straw Dogs: Thoughts on humans and other animals.* London: Granta Books.

Greger, M. (2016) *How Not To Die: Discover the foods scientifically proven to prevent and reverse disease.* London: Macmillan.

Griffin, J. and Tyrrell, I. (2004) *Human Givens: A new approach to emotional health and clear thinking.* Chalvington, East Sussex: HG Publishing.

Griffin, J. and Tyrrell, I. (2008) *Release from Anger: A practical handbook.* Chalvington, East Sussex: HG Publishing.

Gross, R. (2001) *Psychology: The science of mind and behaviour.* Fourth edition, London: Hodder and Stoughton.

Gullestad, S.E. (2001) Attachment theory and psychoanalysis: controversial issues. *Scandinavian Psychoanalytic Review, 24,* 3-16.

Haidt, J. (2006) *The Happiness Hypothesis: Putting ancient wisdom and philosophy to the test of modern science.* London: William Heinemann.

Hayes, N. (2003) *Applied Psychology (Teach Yourself Books).* London: Hodder and Stoughton.

Hellmich, N. (2013) The best preventative medicine? Exercise. Online: dailycomet.com. Accessed: 18th June 2016

Hill, D. (2015) *Affect Regulation Theory: A clinical model.* New York: W.W. Norton and Company, Inc.

Hobson, R.F. (1985) *Forms of Feeling: The heart of psychotherapy.* London: Routledge.

Hoffman, B.M., Babyak, M.A., Craighead, W.E., Sherwood, A., Doraiswamy, P.M., Coons, M.J., and Blumenthal, J.A. (2011) Exercise and pharmacotherapy in patients with major depression: one-year follow-up of the SMILE study. 2011 Feb-Mar; Vol.73(2): Pages 127-133. Cited in: Evans, J. (2016) Natural vs medical. *What Doctors Don't Tell You* (Alternative health magazine). London: WDDTY Publishing. April 2016 (Page 70).

Hofstadter, D. (2007) *I am a Strange Loop.* New York: Basic Books.

Holford, P. (2010) *Optimum Nutrition for the mind.* London: Piatkus.

Holmes, J. (1995) Something there is that doesn't love a wall. John Bowlby, attachment theory, and psychoanalysis. In: Goldberg, S. *et al* (eds) *Attachment Theory: Social, Developmental and Clinical Perspectives.* London: The Analytic Press.

Howatson, G., Bell, P.G., Tallent, J., Middleton, B., McHugh, M.P., Ellis J. (2012) Effect of tart cherry juice (Prunus cerasus) on melatonin levels and enhanced sleep quality. *European Journal of Nutrition. 2012 Dec; Volume 51(8):* Pages 909-916

Hubbard, B. (2018) Not sleeping? Write a to-do list before you go to bed. *What Doctors Don't Tell You.* January 2018. News.

Isold, K. (2010) Anger and exercise: Anger is a normal, adaptive human emotion. *Psychology Today blog.* Available online: https://www.psychologytoday.com/blog/hidden-motives/201008/ anger-and-exercise. Accessed: 16th June 2016.

Jacobs. E.E. (1993) *Impact Therapy.* Lutz, FL: Psychological Assessment Resources.

Jacobs, G. (1994) *Candida Albicans: A user's guide to treatment and recovery.* London: Optima.

Jahnke, R. Larkey, L. Rogers, C. Etnier, J. and Lin, F. (2012) A Comprehensive Review of Health Benefits of Qigong and Tai Chi. *American Journal of Health Promotion, Jul-Aug; Vol.24(6),* Pages e1-e25.

Jahnke, R. (2002) *The Healing Promise of Qi: Creating Extraordinary Wellness through Qigong and Tai Chi.* Chicago, Il: Contemporary Books.

James, O. (2002). *They F*** You Up: How to survive family life.* London: Bloomsbury.

Joines, V. and Stewart, I. (2002) *Personality Adaptations: A new guide to human understanding in psychotherapy and counselling.* Nottingham and Chapel Hill: Lifespace Publishing.

Kaplan, B.J., and S.G. Crawford, C.J. Field and J.S.A. Simpson (2007) 'Vitamins, minerals, and mood'. *Psychological Bulletin, Sept; 133(5):* Pages 747-760.

Kaplan, B.J., Julia J. Rucklidge, Amy Romijn, and Kevin Flood (2015) 'The emerging field of nutritional mental health: Inflammation, the microbiome, oxidative stress, and mitochondrial function'. *Clinical Psychological Science, Vol. 3(6):* 964-980.

Kashdan, T. and Biswas-Diener, R. (2015) *The Power of Negative Emotion: How anger, guilt and self-doubt are essential to success and fulfilment.* London: Oneworld Publications.

Keirsey, D. (1998) *Please Understand Me (II): Temperament, character, intelligence.* First edition. Del Mar, CA: Prometheus Nemesis Book Company.

Keirsey, D. and Bates, M. (1984) *Please Understand Me: Character and temperament types.* Fifth edition. Del Mar, CA: Prometheus Nemesis Book Company.

Kellogg, S. H. (2007). Transformational Chairwork: Five ways of using therapeutic dialogues. *NYSPA Notebook,* 19 (4), 8-9. Available online: http://transformationalchairwork.com/articles/transformational-chairwork/

Kiecolt-Glaser, J.K., Belury, M.A., Andridge, R., Malarkey, W.B., Glaser, R. (2011) Omega 3 supplementation lowers inflammation and anxiety in medical students: A randomised, controlled trial. *Brain, Behaviour, Immunity, Vol.25(8).* Pages 1725-1734

Kinchin, I.M. (1998) Constructivism in the classroom: mapping your way through. Paper presented at the British Educational Research Association (BERA), Annual Research Student Conference, The Queen's University of Belfast, August 26th. Available online: https://www.leeds.ac.uk/educol/documents/000000811.htm. Accessed: 28th May 2016.

Kitzinger, C. (1997) Born to be good? What motivates us to be good, bad or indifferent towards others? *New Internationalist, No.289, April 1997.*

Koffler, J. (2015) Donald Trump's 16 Biggest Business Failures and Successes. Time blog. Online: http://time.com/3988970/donald-trump-business/. Accessed: 25th January 2018.

Korn, L. (2016). *Nutrition Essentials for Mental Health: A complete guide to the food-mood connection*. New York: W. W. Norton & Company.

Krystal, P. (1994) *Cutting the Ties That Bind: Growing Up and Moving on*. Boston, MA: Red Wheel/Weiser Books.

Kurtz, A. and Coetzee, J.M. (2015) *The Good Story: Exchanges on truth, fiction and psychotherapy*. London: Harvill Secker.

Kyle, S. (2018) Sleepiness, fatigue and impaired concentration. Available online: https://www.sleepio.com/articles/insomnia/sleepiness-fatigue-and-impaired-concentration/. Accessed: 25th January 2018.

Larkey, L., Jahnke, R., Etnier, J., and Gonzalez, J. (2009) Meditative movement as a category of exercise: Implications for research. *Journal of Physical Activity & Health. 2009*; Vol.6: Pages 230–238.

Lawrence, F. (2004) *Not on the Label: What really goes into the food on your plate*. London: Penguin Books.

Lazarides, L. (2002) *Treat Yourself: With nutritional therapy*. London: Waterfall 2000.

LeDoux, J. (1996). *The Emotional Brain: the mysterious underpinnings of emotional life*, New York. Simon and Schuster.

LeDoux, J.E., and Gorman, J.M. (2001) A call to action: Overcoming anxiety through active coping. Volume 158, Issue 12, December 2001, Pages 1953-1955. Available online at: http://ajp.psychiatryonline.org/doi/10.1176/appi.ajp.158.12.1953

Lewis, T., Amini, F. and Lannon, R. (2001) *A General Theory of Love*. New York: Vintage Books.

Levine, A. and Heller, R. (2011) *Attached: Identify your attachment style and find your perfect match*. London: Rodale/Pan Macmillan.

Linder, K. and Svardsudd, K. (2006) Qigong has a relieving effect on stress. *Lakartidningen* (A Swedish Medical Journal). 2006; Vol.103 (24-25): Pages 1942-1945.

Little Black Classics (1973/2015) *The Dhammapada*. Taken from Juan Mascaró's translation and edition, first published in 1973. London: Penguin Books (Little Black Classics No.80)

Lopresti, A.L., and Sean D. Hood, and Peter D. Drummond (2013) A review of lifestyle factors that contribute to important pathways associated with major depression: Diet, sleep and exercise. *Journal of Affective Disorders, Vol.148(1)*, Pages 12-27.

Luborsky, L. and Crits-Christoph, P. (eds) (1990) *Understanding Transference: the CCRT method*. New York: Basic Books.

Lunzer, E. (1989) Cognitive development: Learning and the mechanisms of change. In: Murphy, P and Moon, B. (eds) *Developments in Learning and Assessment*. London: Hodder and Stoughton/Open University Press.

MacLachlan, G. and Reid, I. (1994) *Framing and Interpretations*. Carlton, Victoria: Melbourne University Press.

Mahler, M.S., Pine, F. and Bergman, A. (1975/1987) *The Psychological Birth of the Human Infant: Symbiosis and individuation*. London: Maresfield Library.

Mauss, I.B., Troy, A.S. and LeBourgeois, M.K. (2013) Poorer sleep quality is associated with lower emotion-regulation ability in a laboratory paradigm. *Cognition and Emotion, 2013; Vol.27(3):* Pages 567-76.

Mayo Clinic Staff (2014) Depression (major depressive disorder). Depression and anxiety: Exercise eases symptoms. Available online: http://www.mayoclinic.org/diseases-conditions/depression/in-depth/depression-and-exercise/art-20046495. Accessed: 19th June 2016.

Mayo Clinic Staff (2014) Anger management: 10 tips to tame your temper: Available online: http://www.mayoclinic.org/healthy-lifestyle/adult-health/in-depth/anger-management/art-20045434. Accessed 16th June 2016.

Mayo Clinic Staff (2016) Exercise and stress: Get moving to manage stress. Available online: http://www.mayoclinic.org/healthy-lifestyle/stress-management/in-depth/exercise-and-stress/art-20044469) Accessed: 23rd February 2016.

McCombs, J. (2014) *The Everything Candida Diet Book*. Avon, MA: Adams Media Corporation.

McGuiness, M. (2013) Poetry: "Sleep that knits up the ravell'd sleave of care". Poems and poetry blog. Available online: http://www.markmcguinness.com/ index.php/macbeth-sleep/. Accessed: 22nd January 2018.

McLeod, J. (1997/2006) *Narrative and Psychotherapy*. London: Sage.

McLeod, J. (2003) *An Introduction to Counselling*. Third edition. Buckingham: Open University Press.

McLeod, S. (2009/2015) Piaget's Theory of Moral Development. Simply Psychology blog. Available online: http://www.simplypsychology.org/piaget-moral.html

Medina, J. (2015) How Yoga is Similar to Existing Mental Health Therapies. Source: Psych Central website: http://psychcentral.com/lib/how-yoga-is-similar-to-existing-therapies/. Accessed: May 2016.

Mehrabian, A. (1981) *Silent messages: Implicit communication of emotions and attitudes*. Belmont, CA: Wadsworth (currently distributed by Albert Mehrabian, email: am@kaaj.com)

Mercola, J. (2010) Scientists Unlock How Trans Fats Harm Your Arteries. (Health Blog). Available online: http://articles.mercola.com/sites/articles/archive/2010/11/16/scientists-unlock-how-trans-fats-harm-your-arteries.aspx. Accessed: 20th May 2016.

Mercola, J. (2013) Vitamin D — One of the Simplest Solutions to Wide-Ranging Health Problems. Available online: http://articles.mercola.com/sites/articles/archive/2013/12/22/dr-holick-vitamin-d-benefits.aspx. Accessed 15 June 2016.

Mercola, J. (2016) The Fungal Etiology of Inflammatory Bowel Disease. Available online at this web address: http://articles.mercola.com/sites/articles/archive/2003/09/13/inflammatory-bowel-disease.aspx.

Messer, S. and Wampold, B. (2002) Let's face facts: Common factors are more potent than specific therapy ingredients. *Clinical Psychology: Science and Practice. 9:* 21-25.

Milgram, S. (1974) *Obedience to Authority*. New York: Harper and Row.

Miller, T. (1993) Self-Discipline and Emotional Control: How to stay calm and productive under pressure. Evansville, Indiana: A CareerTrack Seminar (audio program).

Minsky, M. (1975) A framework for representing knowledge. In: P. Winston (ed). *The Psychology of Computer Vision.* New York: McGraw-Hill.

Moyers, B. (1995) *Healing and the Mind.* New York: Doubleday.

Mozes, A. (2015) The Surprising Link Between Carbs and Depression. Online health blog. Available: http://www.health.com/depression/could-too-many-refined-carbs-make-you-depressed. Accessed: June 2016.

Myers, A. (2013) 9 Signs you have a leaky gut. On the Mindbodygreen Blog: Available online: http://www.mindbodygreen.com/0-10908/9-signs-you-have-a-leaky-gut.html. Accessed: 13th June 2016).

MySahana (2012) Common Causes for Anger Management Issues. MySahana blog post. Online: http://mysahana.org/2012/02/common-causes-for-anger-manage-ment-issues/. Accessed: 22nd January 2018.

Nauert, R. (2018) Sleep Loss Increases Anxiety — Especially Among Worriers. PsychCentral blog post. https://psychcentral.com/news/2013/06/27/sleep-loss-increases-anxiety-especially-among-worriers/56531.html

Nelson-Jones, R. (2001) *Theory and Practice of Counselling and Therapy.* Third edition. London: Continuum.

NHS (2007) NHS Quality Improvement Scotland. Understanding alcohol misuse in Scotland: Harmful drinking 3 – Alcohol and self-harm'. 2007. Available online at: http://bit.ly/TbBYAX. Accessed: 28th May 2016.

NHS (2016) Exercise for depression. Available online: http://www.nhs.uk/conditions/stress-anxiety-depression/pages/exercise-for-depression.aspx. Accessed: 23rd February 2016.

NHS choices (2015) Why lack of sleep is bad for your health. Online blog: https://www.nhs.uk/Livewell/tiredness-and-fatigue/Pages/lack-of-sleep-health-risks.aspx. Accessed: 25th January 2018.

NHS Choices (2016) Stress, anxiety and depression: How to control your anger. Available online: www.nhs.uk/conditions/anger-management. Accessed 16th June 2016.

Nierenberg, G.I. (1987) *The Complete Negotiator,* London, Souvenir Press Ltd.

NIH (2016) Folate: Dietary Supplement Fact Sheet; Published by the US Department of Health's National Institutes of Health, Office of Dietary Supplements. Available online: https://ods.od.nih.gov/factsheets/Folate-HealthProfessional/. Accessed: 14th June 2016.

Nisbet, M.C. (2016) Your Emotions Are What You Eat: How Your Diet Can Reduce Anxiety. Available online: http://bigthink.com/age-of-engagement/your-emotions-are-what-you-eat-how-your-diet-can-reduce-anxiety

Novak, J.D. and Gowin, B. (1984) *Learning How to Learn.* Cambridge: Cambridge University Press.

NSF (2018) Depression and sleep. Online blog: https://sleepfoundation.org/sleep-disorders-problems/depression-and-sleep. Accessed: 25th January 2018.

O'Beeve, D. (2015) *Obedience and Revolt: Volume 1: Learning to Conform.* (An autobiographical novel). Hebden Bridge: the Institute for E-CENT Publications.

Office for National Statistics (ONS) (1995) Surveys of Psychiatric Morbidity in Great Britain. Report 1 – The prevalence of psychiatric morbidity among adults living in private households. London: The Stationery Office. Cited on https://www.anxietyuk.org.uk/. Accessed 13th June 2016.

Omer, H. and Strenger, C. (1992) The pluralist revolution: From the one true meaning to an infinity of constructed ones. *Psychotherapy, 29:* Pages 253-261.

Panksepp, J. (1998) *Affective Neuroscience: The foundations of human and animal emotions*. Oxford University Press.

Panksepp, J. and Lucy Biven (2012) *The Archaeology of Mind: Neuroevolutionary Origins of Human Emotion*: W.W. Norton and Company.

Peck, M.S. (1998) *The Road Less Travelled: A New Psychology of Love, Traditional Values and Spiritual Growth*. New York: Touchstone.

Pennebaker, J.W. (2004) *Writing to Heal: A guided journal for recovering from trauma and emotional upheaval*. Oakland, Ca: New Harbinger Publications.

Perlmutter, D. (2015) *Brain Maker: The power of gut microbes to heal and protect your brain – for life*. London: Hodder and Stoughton.

Perls, F. S. (1969). *Gestalt therapy verbatim*. Lafayette, CA: Real People Press.

Perretta, L. (2001) *Brain Food: The essential guide to boosting brain power*. London: Hamlyn.

Perricone, N. (2002) *Dr Nicolas Perricone's Programme: Grow young, get slim, in days*. London: Thorsons.

Perry, P. (2012) *How to Stay Sane*. London: Macmillan.

Pilcher, J. J., Morris, D. M., Donnelly, J., and Feigl H. B. (2015) Interactions between sleep habits and self-control. *Frontiers in Human Neuroscience. Vol 9.* Pages 284. Available online: https://www.frontiersin.org/articles/ 10.3389/ fnhum.2015. 00284/ full. Accessed: 22nd January 2018.

Pinker, S. (2015) *How the Mind Works*. London: Penguin Random House.

Pinnock, D. (2015) *Anxiety and Depression: Eat your way to better health*. London: Quadrille Publishing.

Postman, N., and Weingartner, C. (1969), *Teaching as a Subversive Activity*. New York: Dell.

Poulter, S. (2016) Don't eat our pasta sauce more than once a week. *Daily Mail*. Pages 1 and 2, Friday April 15th. Available online: http://www.dailymail.co.uk/ health/article-3540217/When-sa-Dolmio-day-Just-week-Labels-advise-foods-high-sugar-salt-eaten-occasionally.html

Prochaska, J.O., Norcross, J.C. & DiClemente, C.C. (1998). *Changing for Good*. Reprint edition. New York: Morrow.

Radhakrishna, S. (2010) Application of integrated yoga therapy to increase imitation skills in children with autism spectrum disorder. *International Journal of Yoga, 3 (1); pp:26-30.*

Radhakrishna, S., Nagarathna, R., and Nagendra, H.R. (2010) Integrated approach to yoga therapy and autism spectrum disorders. *Journal of Ayurveda and Integrative Medicine, 1 (2); pp: 120-124.*

Rass, E. (ed) (2018) *The Allan Shore Reader: Setting the course of development*. Abingdon, Oxon: Routledge.

Ratey, J., and Hargerman, E. (2009) *Spark: The revolutionary new science of exercise and the brain.* London: Quercus.

Reder, A. (2007) Unmasking Anger. *Yoga Journal.* August 28th 2007. Available online: http://www.yogajournal.com/article/yoga-101/unmasking-anger/. Accessed: 17th June 2016.

Redfern, R. (2016) The importance of nutrition for mental health. *Naturally Healthy News.* Issue 30, 2016.

Reynolds, G. (2010) Phys Ed: Can Exercise Moderate Anger? August 11, 2010. Available online, on the New York Times blog: http://well.blogs.nytimes.com/2010/08/11/phys-ed-can-exercise-moderate-anger/?_r=0. Accessed: 16th June 2016.

Rickman, P. (2009) Is psychology science? *Philosophy Now, Issue 74,* July/August.

Rogers, C. (1983) *Freedom to Learn for the 80's.* Princeton, NC: Merrill.

Romm, A. (2014) 5 Steps to Heal a Leaky Gut Caused By Ibuprofen. *Huffpost Healthy Living*: Available online: http://www.huffingtonpost.com/aviva-romm/5-steps-to-heal-a-leaky-g_b_5617109.html. Accessed: 13th June 2016.

Ross, J. (2003) *The Mood Cure: Take charge of your emotions in 24 hours using food and supplements.* London: Thorsons.

Rumelhart, D.E. and Ortony, A. (1977) The representation of knowledge in memory. In: R.C. Anderson, R.J. Spiro and W.E. Montague (eds), *Schooling and the Acquisition of Knowledge.* Hillsdale, NJ: Erlbaum, pp. 99-135.

Russell, R.L. and van den Brock, P. (1992) Changing narrative schemas in psychotherapy. *Psychotherapy, 29:* 344-354.

Sadock, B.J. and Sadock, V.A. (2000) *Kaplan and Sadock's Synopsis of Psychiatry: Behavioural Sciences/Clinical Psychiatry, 7th Edition.* Lippincott Williams & Wilkins. USA

Sánchez-Villegas A, Verberne L, De Irala J, Ruíz-Canela M, Toledo E, Serra-Majem L. and Martínez-González, M.A. (2011) Dietary Fat Intake and the Risk of Depression: The SUN Project. PLoS ONE 6(1): Available online: http://journals.plos.org/plosone/article?id=10.1371/journal.pone.0016268. Accessed: 2nd May 2016.

Sánchez-Villegas, A., Almudena, M.A., et al. (2013) Mediterranean dietary pattern and depression: the PREDIMED randomized trial. *BMC Medicine* 2013, Vol.11: Article 208. Available online: http://bmcmedicine.biomedcentral.com/articles/10.1186/1741-7015-11-208. Accessed: 2nd May 2016.

Sandwell, H. and Wheatley, M. (2008) Healthy eating advice as part of drug treatment in prisons. *Prison Service Journal, Issue 182.*

Sansouci, J. (2011) Nutrition and anxiety. Healthy Crush Blog post. Available online: http://healthycrush.com/nutrition-and-anxiety. Accessed 20th May 2016.

Santer, M.J. (2015) Why Qigong Is So Effective Against Emotional Illnesses. Source: http://qigong15.com/blog/qigong-exercises/ why-qigong-is-so-effective-against-emotional-illnesses/. Accessed May 2015.

Sapolsky, R. (2010) *Why Zebras don't get Ulcers.* Third Ed. New York: St Martin's Griffin.

Sarbin, T. R. (1989) Emotions as narrative emplotments. In M. J. Packer & R. B. Addison (eds.) *Entering the circle: Hermeneutic investigations in psychology* (pp. 185-201). Albany, NY: State University of New York Press.

Sarbin, T. R. (2001) Embodiment and the narrative structure of emotional life. *Narrative Inquiry, 11*, 217-225.

Schank, R.C. and Abelson, R.P. (1977) *Scripts, Plans, Goals and Understanding.* Hillsdale, NJ: Lawrence Erlbaum Associates Inc.

Schmidt, K., Cowen, P.J., Harmer, C.J. ... et al (2014) Prebiotic intake reduces the waking cortisol response and alters emotional bias in healthy volunteers. *Psychopharmacology* (Berl.) (December 3rd 2014) [Epub ahead of print]. Online: http://www.ncbi.nlm.nih.gov/pubmed/25449699

Schoenthaler, S.C. (1983a) The Northern California diet-behaviour program: An empirical evaluation of 3,000 incarcerated juveniles in Stanislaus County Juvenile Hall. *International Journal of Biosocial Research, Vol 5(2),* Pages 99-106.

Schoenthaler, S.C. (1983b) The Los Angeles probation department diet behaviour program: An empirical analysis of six institutional settings'. *International Journal of Biosocial Research, Vol 5(2)*, Pages 107-17.

Schoenthaler, S., and Bier I. D. (2002) Food addiction and criminal behaviour – The California randomized trial. Food Allergy and Intolerance. 731–746. Saunders. Cited in Sandwell and Wheatley (2008).

Schoenthaler S. *et al.* (1997) The effect of randomized vitamin-mineral supplementation on violent and non-violent antisocial behaviour among incarcerated juveniles. *Journal of Nutritional & Environmental Medicine 7:* Pages 343–352.

Schore, A.N. (2003) *Affect regulation and the repair of the self.* New York: Norton.

Schore, A.N. (2015) *Affect Regulation and the Origin of the Self: The Neurobiology of Emotional Development.* London: Routledge.

Sicicurious (2010) If low serotonin levels aren't responsible for depression, what is? *The Guardian*: Blog post: Online: https://www.theguardian.com/science/blog/2010/sep/28/depression-serotonin-neuro-genesis. Accessed: 13th June 2016)

Scullin, M. K., Krueger, M. L., Ballard, H. K., Pruett, N., & Bliwise, D. L. (2018). The effects of bedtime writing on difficulty falling asleep: A polysomnographic study comparing to-do lists and completed activity lists. *Journal of Experimental Psychology: General, 147(1),* Pages 139-146.

Seligman, M.E.P. (2002). *Authentic Happiness: Using the New Positive Psychology to Realize Your Potential for Lasting Fulfillment.* New York, NY: Free Press.

Shapiro D., Cook I.A., Davydov, D.M., Ottaviani, C., Leuchter, A.F. and Abrams, M. (2007). Yoga as a Complementary Treatment of Depression: Effects of Traits and Moods on Treatment Outcome. *Evidence based complementary and alternative medicine, 4(4),* pp: 493-502.

Sharma, V.K., Das, S., Mondal, S., Goswampi, U. and Gandhi, A. (2005) Effect of Sahaj Yoga on depressive disorders. *Indian Journal of Physiological Pharmacology*, Oct-Dec, 49(4); pp:462-8.

Sharma V.K., Das, S., Monda,l S., Goswami, U. and Gandhi, A. (2006). Effect of Sahaj Yoga on neuro-cognitive functions in patients suffering from major depression. *Indian Journal of Physiological Pharmacology*, Oct-Dec, 50(4); pp:375-383.

Sher, B. (1995) *I Could Do Anything If I Only Knew What It Was: How to Discover What You Really Want and How to Get It*. New York: Dell.

Siegel, D.J. (2015) *The Developing Mind: How relationships and the brain interact to shape who we are*. London: The Guilford Press.

Small, G. (2010) Can Exercise Cure Depression? Exercise releases endorphins, the body's very own natural antidepressant. Posted Sep 25, 2010. *Psychology Today blog*: Available online: https://www.psychologytoday.com/blog/brain-bootcamp/201009/can-exercise-cure-depression. Accessed: 19th June 2016.

Smith, R. (2010) People who sleep for less than six hours 'die early'. *The Telegraph*. Online: http://www.telegraph.co.uk/news/health/news/7677812/People-who-sleep-for-less-than-six-hours-die-early.html. 5th May 2010. Accessed: 23rd January 2018.

Smith, P.K., Cowie, H., and Blades, M. (2011) *Understanding Children's Development*. Fifth edition. Chichester, West Sussex: Wiley.

Smith, M.L. and Glass, G.V. (1977) Meta-analysis of psychotherapy outcomes studies. *American Psychologist, 32*, 752-760.

Smith, M., Glass, G. and Miller, T. (1980) *The Benefits of Psychotherapy*. Baltimore, Maryland: The Johns Hopkins University Press.

Spector, T. (2013) *Identically Different: Why you can change your genes*. London: Phoenix.

Stanfield, M. (2008) *Trans Fat: The Time Bomb in your Food: The Killer in the Kitchen*. Souvenir Press: London.

Stevenson, S. (2016) *Sleep Smarter: 21 Essential Strategies to Sleep Your Way to a Better Body, Better Health, and Bigger Success*. London: Hay House UK.

Stewart, I. and Joines, V. (1987) *TA Today: A New Introduction to Transactional Analysis*. Nottingham: Lifespace Publishing.

Storr, A. (1989) *Freud: a very short introduction,* Oxford, Oxford University Press. (Pages 60-61). And:

Stress Management Society (2012/2016) Nutritional stress and health: The "Think 'nervous'" box. Available online: http://www.stress.org.uk/Diet-and-nutrition.aspx

Strine, T.W. and Chapman, D.P. (2005) Associations of frequent sleep insufficiency with health-related quality of life and health behaviours. *Sleep Medicine, Vol.6(1),* January 2005. Pages 23-27.

Strupp, H.H. and Binder, J.L. (1984) *Psychotherapy in a New Key: A guide to time-limited dynamic psychotherapy*. New York: Basic Books.

Taylor-Byrne, R., and Byrne, J. (2012) Exercise is good for your body, brain and general health. E-CENT Paper No.18: Hebden Bridge: The Institute for E-CENT. Available online: http://web.archive.org/web/20160322190430/http://www.abc-counselling.com/id373.html

Taylor-Byrne, R., and Byrne, J. (2012) Meditation: What is it, and how can you do it? ABC Coaching and Counselling Services. Available online: web.archive.org/web/20160323004156/ web.archive.org/web/*/http://abc-counselling.com/id260.html

Taylor-Byrne, R.E. and Byrne, J.W. (2017) *How to control your anger, anxiety and depression, using nutrition and physical activity*. Hebden Bridge: The Institute for E-CENT Publications.

Teychenne, M., Costigan, S., and Parker, K. (2015) The association between sedentary behaviour and risk of anxiety: A Systematic Review. *BMC Public Health, 2015*. Cited in *Medical Daily*, here: http://www.medicaldaily.com/constantly-sitting-down-being-sedentary-could-worsen-anxiety-and-mental-health-338952

The Brain Flux (2018) Can Sleep Increase Emotional Intelligence? Online blog: http://thebrainflux.com/can-sleep-increase-emotional-intelligence/. Accessed: 22nd January 2018.

Tkacz, J. Deborah Young-Hyman, Colleen A. Boyle, and Catherine L. Davis (2008) Aerobic Exercise Program Reduces Anger Expression Among Overweight Children. Cited in: *Paediatric Exercise Science*. 2008 Nov; Vol.20(4): Pages: 390–401. Available online: http://www.ncbi.nlm.nih.gov/pmc/articles/PMC2678873/#R28 Accessed 27th June 2016.

Trowbridge, J.P. and Walker, M. (1989) *The Yeast Syndrome*. London: Bantam Books.

Tse, M. (1995) *Qigong for Health and Vitality*. London: Piatkus.

Turner, J.H. (2000) *On the Origins of Human Emotions. A sociological inquiry into the evolution of human affect*. Stanford, CA: Stanford University Press.

Uebelacker, L.A., Tremont, G., Epstein-Lubow, G., Gaudiano, B.A., Gillette, T., Kalibatseva, Z. and Miller, I.W. (2010) Open trial of Vinyasa yoga for persistently depressed individuals: Evidence of feasibility and acceptability. *Behaviour Modification*, May, 34(3); pp: 247-264.

Vancampfort, D., De Hert, M., Knapen, J., Wampers, M., Demunter, H., Deckx, S., Maurissen, K. and Probst, M. (2011) State anxiety, psychological stress and positive well-being responses to yoga and aerobic exercise in people with schizophrenia: A pilot study. *Disability Rehabilitation, 33(8);* pp: 684-689.

Van der Helm, E., & Walker, M. P. (2009) Overnight Therapy? The Role of Sleep in Emotional Brain Processing. *Psychological Bulletin, 135*(5), Pages 731–748.

Van der Helm, E., Yao, J., Dutt, S. et al. (2011) REM Sleep Depotentiates Amygdala Activity to Previous Emotional Experiences. *Current Biology, Volume 21, Issue 23*, Pages 2029 – 2032.

Van der Veen, F.M., Evers, E.A.T., Deutz, N.E.P., Schmitt, J.A.J. (2006) Effects of Acute Tryptophan Depletion on Mood and Facial Emotion Perception Related Brain Activation and Performance in Healthy Women with and without a Family History of Depression. *Neuropsychopharmacology, Vol.32, Issue 1*. Pages 216-224.

Virkkunen, M. (1986) Reactive hypoglycaemic tendency among habitually violent offenders. *Nutrition Reviews, Vol.44 (Supplement)*. Pages 94-103

Visceglia, E. and Lewis, S. (2011) Yoga therapy as an adjunctive treatment for schizophrenia: A randomized, controlled pilot study. *Journal of Alternative and Complementary Medicine, 17(7)*: 601-607

Vitale, J. (2006) *Life's Missing Instruction Manual: the guidebook you should have been given at birth*. Hoboken, NJ: John Wiley and Sons Inc.

Wagner, E. (1996) *How to stay out of the doctor's surgery*. Carnell.

Waite, M. (2012) *Paperback Oxford English Dictionary*. Seventh edition. Oxford: Oxford University Press.

Walker, M. (2017) *Why We Sleep: The new science of sleep and dreams*. London: Allen Lane.

Wallin, D. (2007) *Attachment in Psychotherapy*. New York: The Guildford Press.

Wampold, B.E. (2001) *The Great Psychotherapy Debate: Model, methods, and findings.* Mahwah, NJ: Lawrence Erlbaum.

Wampold, B.E., Ahn, H., and Coleman, H.K.L. (2001) Medical model as metaphor: Old habits die hard. *Journal of Counselling Psychology, 48,* 268-273.

Warwick University (2016) '7 a day for happiness and mental health'. Press release: Available online at this address: http://www.2.warwick.ac.uk/newsandevents/presssreleases/7-a-day_for_happiness/ Accessed 2nd May 2016

Watts, A. (1962/1990) *The Way of Zen.* London: Arkana/Penguin.

West, W., and Byrne, J. (2009) Some ethical concerns about counselling research: *Counselling Psychology Quarterly,* 22(3) Pages 309-318.

White, M. and Epston, D. (1990) *Narrative Means to Therapeutic Ends.* New York: Norton.

Willson, R. and Branch, R. (2006) *Cognitive Behavioural Therapy for Dummies.* Chichester, West Sussex: John Wiley and Sons, Limited.

Wilson, T.D. (2011) *Redirect: The Surprising New Science of Psychological Change.* London: Allen Lane/Penguin.

Wood, D. (1988/1994) *How Children Think and Learn: the social contexts of cognitive development.* Oxford: Blackwell.

Woolfe, R., Dryden, W., and Strawbridge, S. (eds) (2003) *Handbook of Counselling Psychology.* Second Edition. London: Sage Publications.

Yu, W. (2012) High trans-fat diet predicts aggression: People who eat more hydrogenated oils are more aggressive. *Scientific American Mind,* July 2012. Available online: http://www.scientificamerican.com/article/high-trans-fat-diet-predicts-aggresion/

Zimbardo, P. (2007) *The Lucifer Effect: how good people turn evil.* London: Rider.

Zimbardo, P. G., Banks, W.C., Craig, H. and Jaffe, D. (1973) A Pirandellian prison: The mind is a formidable jailor. *New York Times Magazine, April 8th,* Pages 38-60.

~~~

Index

ABC model . xvii, 7, 19, 38, 133, 136, 137, 170, 171, 183, 185
   complex version - A12-B123-Y-yyy-C12 .... 134, 136, 137, 140
Acceptance of the inevitable or unavoidable ...... iii, 17, 49, 51, 109, 110, 113, 117, 121, 126, 137, 155, 158, 164, 189
Accurately rating your problems 116
Acting out childhood experiences 36
Active approaches to problem solving 119
Affect regulation
   mother regulates baby's affects 142
Affective neuroscience 4, 14, 41, 130, 131, 207
Ainsworth, Mary 215
Alcohol *See* Diet and nutrition: foods to avoid: alcohol
Amino acids 61
Anger .... 75, 78, *See* Managing anger and dietary considerations. 69, 70, 71, 72, 78
   and exercise benefits 73, 75
Anger and rage 132
Anger management
   Diet and nutritional links 151
   Using physical exercise 152
Anxiety...*See* Managing Anxiety: In and out of counselling and therapy
Anxiety management
   How physical exercise reduces anxiety 157
   The impact of diet and nutrition 155
APET model (Human Givens) 29, 185
Appreciation and gratitude
   forms of reframing 115
Attachment .... *See* Attachment Theory
Attachment in E-CENT 23
Attachment in psychotherapy 21
Attachment styles 51, 141, 171, 191, 210
Attachment theory .. xvii, 6, 18, 21, 23, 25, 37, 49, 165, 167, 207, 221
Aurelius, Marcus 9, 126, 215
Babies need external regulation (soothing) 147
Baby internalizes representations of social encounters and experiences 142
Bandler and Grinder 30
Basic description and origins of E-CENT 37
Basic theory of E-CENT counselling 38
Benefits of adequate sleep
   greater capacity to cope with stress 94
Blumenthal, James 76, 77
Body-brain-mind
   and alcohol 66
   and caffeine 66
   and gluten 66, 67
   and good and bad foods 78
   and nutrition 59
   and processed foods 66
   and sugar 66
   and the stress response 73
Body-mind, and emotions 37
Body-mind, integration, and social environment 4
Body-mind, needs sleep, good diet, physical exercise .... xviii, 40, 209
Bowlby, John ...4, 6, 15, 18, 19, 20, 21, 22, 23, 25, 124, 125, 147, 165, 167, 216, 221, 241
Brief introduction to the E-CENT models of mind 40
Brogan
   Dr Kelly 71, 72, 217
Buddha, and Buddhism
   on human emotions 130
Buddhism and Stoicism on emotion 123
Caffeine 78, 80
Carbohydrate
   refined carbs
     and depression 62
Case studies, the case against them 8, 10, 11, 17, 207
Childhood, The impact of 49
China Study, The 218
Coates, Gordon 130
Co-enzyme-Q-10
   and brain health 64
Cognitive psychology 50, 108
Cognitive science 7, 38, 108
Colonization of baby, by mother 140
Controllable and uncontrollable situations and problems 3, 5, 8, 11, 16, 20, 31, 40, 41, 54, 105, 116, 117, 118, 126, 129, 134, 138, 139, 143, 146, 149, 153, 155, 218, 225
Cortisol
   and the stress response 70, 72
Counseling clients towards
   healthy exercise 73, 195
Counselling and therapy revolution xix

Counselling clients towards
  healthy diet 59, 195
  healthy emotions 121, 195
  healthy self-talk.......................... 101, 195
  healthy sleep 83, 195
Counselling individuals in E-CENT 163
  A quick tutorial on 'how to do it' 163
  Imaginary 'typical' session structure .. 166
Counsellor
  'good enough'
    E-CENT counsellor........................... 21
Cutting the ties from destructive parents .. 56
Dairy 80, 81
  butter 65
Damasio, Antonio..5, 7, 8, 122, 133, 136, 138, 219, 241
Darwin, Charles 129, 130, 153, 219
Defining Attachment Theory 18
Delusional beings
  humans... 103
Depression ... xviii, xix, 3, 17, 40, 47, 108, 132, 146, 158, 159, 175, 183, 216, 217, 218, 221, 224, 225, 226, 227, 228, 229, 230
  and alcohol 66
  and carbohydrates 62
  and gluten 67
  and healthy gut bacteria 72
  and inflammation................................ 72
  and medication 71
  and nutrient deficiencies 81
  and physical exercise 76
  and processed food....................... 67, 72
  diet, nutrition, and lifestyle factors 72, 78
  How depression can be reduced by
    exercise 161
  How diet and nutrition can reduce and
    eliminate depression..................... 160
  multiple causes 71
Diet and nutrition
  and anxiety.. 69
  and depression.................................... 71
  and gut health 69, 72
  and mental health 68, 78
  and personalized dietary guidelines 64
  and stress 70
  as prebiotics and probiotics 70
  balanced diet.2, 6, 63, 68, 69, 78, 80, 154, 199
    and supplements............................ 69
    difficulty of defining 63
  foods to avoid
    alcohol.xviii, 36, 66, 70, 72, 78, 80, 84, 87, 88, 155, 157, 204
    caffeine... 66

    gluten 67
    junk food 37, 47, 63, 66, 199, 200, 209
    sugar 16, 17, 64, 66, 70, 71, 72, 74, 78, 79, 80, 87, 97, 151, 154, 157, 159, 200, 202, 218
    trans-fats....65, 66, 151, 154, 160, 224
  no universally agreed approach 63
  personalized to the individual 63
  raw salads very nutritious.................... 80
  supplements and healthy foods 62
Diet types
  Mediterranean and Nordic diets 63
  Personalized diet 64
inflammation....67, 72, 81, 157, 159, 160, 222
Inflammation 62, 63, 66
Drinks and drinking
  alcohol.. 66, 78
  caffeine 66, 70, 78, 80
  water... 66, 80
E-CENT counselling ... 3, 4, 5, 6, 11, 12, 21, 25, 26, 31, 37, 40, 49, 121, 123, 129, 140, 153, 163, 165, 166, 171, 174, 178, 186, 193, 207
E-CENT models
  A brief summary 25
  Hindu/Buddhist binary model 43
  The complex ABC model.............. 136, 140
  The dialectical interaction of the mother and baby....................................... 43
  The dialectical nature of the individual/social ego. 44
  The emergent ego of the child, an illustration 144
  The Event-Framing-Response model (EFR) 27, 107, 183, 210
  The Good and Bad Wolf model............. 25
  The holistic SOR model 26, 173, 193
  The Jigsaw-story model 29
  The Mind Hut model........................... 108
  The mother-baby dyad model 140
  The neo-behaviourist's Stimulus-Organism-Response model............... 42
  The neo-behaviourist's Stimulus-Organism-Response model............... 38
  The OK-Corral model from TA 140
  The Parent-Adult-Child (or PAC) model (from TA).. 29
  The Six Windows Model 26, 101, 107, 181, 193
  The social individual, A relational model 140
  Tripartite (or three-part) models........... 41
E-CENT models and processes
  A brief Anxiety inventory 175

A more holistic version of the Stimulus>Organism>Response model. 171
A puberty rite - Cutting the Ties that Bind 191
And the importance of pursuing a virtuous life.................................. 170
APET model from the Human Givens school 185
Attachment system work 191
Dangers of questioning! 176
Depression inventory 175
Education of the client 180
Gerard Nierenberg's question grid 178
Gradual desensitization....................... 190
Holistic SOR model
    Diet, exercise, self-talk, relaxation, meditation, good relationships. 171
Jigsaw-story model............................. 186
Meditation... 191
Narrative inquiry 184
Parent-Adult-Child (PAC) model of Transactional Analysis 187
Personality-styles - The Keirsey Temperament Sorter..................... 192
Questioning strategies 168
The E-CENT holistic SOR model 173
The Egan model................................. 169
The emotional needs assessment questionnaire 175
The Event-Framing-Response (EFR) model 183
The Gestalt Chair-work model 190
The OK Corral model (from TA)........... 188
The original SOR model of neo-Behaviourism................................ 170
The WDEP model................................ 168
Various questioning strategies............ 175
E-CENT theory xix, 4, 8, 12, 14, 15, 18, 19, 23, 25, 35, 41, 47, 49, 51, 52, 57, 103, 123, 146, 148, 153, 158, 173, 185, 207, 208, 210
    Key Learning Points and Applications . 208
    The core theory of E-CENT 207
Ekman, Paul................................ 129, 130, 219
Ellis, Albert.... 9, 19, 35, 38, 52, 122, 124, 133, 134, 136, 170, 189, 217, 218, 219
Embodied-narratives about something 14
Emotion, The importance of 40
Emotional availability and sensitive mothering.. 20
Emotional brain-mind, The 50
Emotional distress or disturbance

and junk food 64, 81
and lifestyle factors 72
Emotional vulnerability 55
Emotional, motivational and automatic control systems 133
Enders, Dr Giulia....................................... 219
Epictetus........................... 9, 105, 126, 219
Eric Berne's Parent-Adult-Child model 41
Essential fatty acids (EFA's) 66, 81
    omega 3
        and fish oil supplements 64
        omega 3/6 ratio.............................. 81
    omega 6
        and animal products 81
        and inflammation 81
Evolutionary psychology and human emotion 127, 131
Exaggerating the degree of 'badness' of your problems 115
Exercise systems
    aerobic exercise 70
    Indian yoga 78
    running 77
    walking 78
Failure to process earlier experiences 56
Fear Response, The 132
Fibre... 61, 67, 80
Fight or flight response 73
    parasympathetic nervous system 74
    sympathetic nervous system 73
Fish
    oily fish
        and omega-3 64
Food......*See* Diet and nutrition: balanced diet
    and anger 70
    and nutrition .... 69, *See* Diet types
Frame theory 106
Frames
    and perception 26, 30, 103, 105, 106, 107, 108, 109, 111, 114, 115, 116, 120, 125, 181, 183, 184, 185
    of reference.................................. 12, 104
Framing
    an illustrative example 108
Freud, Sigmund xvii, xix, 4, 7, 8, 18, 19, 20, 23, 37, 38, 41, 43, 122, 124, 130, 144, 170, 171, 172, 187, 217, 220, 229
Freud's 'It', 'Ego' and 'super-ego' model 41
Gergen, Kenneth 6, 13, 165, 220
Gladwell, Malcolm.......................... 10, 220
Gluten..... 67, *See* Diet and nutrition: foods to avoid: gluten
    case study (Martina) 70
    intolerance and gluten sensitivity 67

is a body-mind toxin 78
linked to anxiety and depression 67, 68
Grains 62, 68, 80, 81
Gray, John 10, 221
Greger
    Dr Michael
        and the omega-3-to-6 ratio 81
        high veg diet cuts depression 81
        How Not to Die 221
Grief and depression 132, 158
Gut bacteria
    and curative diet changes 64
    and human health and illness 69
    and probiotic supplements 69
Haidt, Jonathon 105, 133, 221
Healing the Inner Child 57
Hill, Daniel
    A four-part model of mind 138
    Affect regulation theory. xviii, 4, 5, 10, 21,
        31, 103, 133, 138, 148, 176, 182, 221,
        225, 241
Hoffman, Benson, PhD
    exercise and major depression 76
Holistic SOR model .... xiii, 26, 102, 173
Human beings as emotional beings 50, 145,
146
Human emotions
    origins .... xix, 121, 123, 124, 130, 131, 146
Human stories, The nature of 50
Human story tellers 35, 54, 209, 212
Humans are body-minds .... xviii, 37, 51, 209
Humans are primarily social animals 52
Humans as primary non-conscious beings . 53
Humans need love and acceptance 52
Humans operate from one of three so-called
    'ego states' 53
Individual and the effects of his/her family
    history, The 146
Inflammation
    physical disease and anxiety and
        depression 81
    physical disease and depression 72
    physical disease and emotional disorders
        ....62, 63, 66, 81, 159
    linked to omega-6 grain fed meat .. 81
Insufficient sleep 87–92
interpersonal neurobiology xviii, 4, 14, 24, 42,
    133, 207
Interpersonal neurobiology and the tripartite
    model of mind 42, 138
Interpretations and frames 104
Interpretations and frames and perception
    .... 103, 106, 109
Jigsaw-story model 29

Kaplan, Dr Bonnie 222
    on nutritional mental health 222
    on vitamins, minerals and mood 222
Keirsey, David 171, 181, 192, 210, 222
Korn, Dr Leslie
    and our level of nutritional need 80
    Nutritional Essentials for Mental Health
        223
    the case for personalized diet 64
Language and mentation
    Verbal and non--verbal communication in
        counselling and therapy 138
Leaky gut syndrome
    and the link to gluten 67
LeDoux, Joseph 137, 223
Limbic system 22, 103, 106, 122, 133, 134,
    136, 137, 138, 142, 144
Lust and desire 132
Managing Anger
    Healthy anger 149
    In and out of counselling and therapy .148
Managing anger, anxiety and depression ..148
Managing Anxiety
    In and out of counselling and therapy .153
    Practical strategies 154
Managing Depression 158
    And transient grief 158
    Diet and depression 159
    Distinguishing grief and depression 158
Managing human emotions 146
Margaret Mahler 20
McLeod, John ....xviii, 3, 12, 13, 27, 30, 31, 36,
    224, 241
Meat
    grain fed meats, omega-6 imbalance, and
        depression 81
    meat tolerance may be linked to genetic
        heritage 64
Meditation ..... iii, 4, 38, 40, 51, 139, 150, 153,
    175, 180, 181, 191
Mindfulness 21, 51, 125
Minerals and vitamins ....*See* Vitamin and
    mineral supplements
Mother and child, The relationship between
    them 20
Mothering
    the normal 'good enough' mother .. 21, 44
Mother's influence over baby, The 51
Narrative therapy
    The cognitive/constructivist approach .. 13
    The E-CENT approach 12
    The psychodynamic approach 13
    The social constructionist approach 13
Narratives and stories 12, 54, 217

National Health Service (NHS - UK) guidelines regarding depression.............................. 77
Non-conscious framing
and interpretation...... 107, 108, 114, 139, 141, 163, 164, 171, 181, 188, 208, 212, 213, 217
Non-conscious framing, and interpretation, and perception 2, 8, 11, 21, 31, 35, 36, 53, 105, 120, 139, 141, 147, 183, 184, 185, 186, 208
Nutritional deficiency or insufficiency
and emotional problems.................. 69, 81
nutritional treatment of........................ 70
Object Relations 7, 18, 19, 20, 37, 38, 52, 220, 241
Origin of human emotions 129
Our adult relationships mimic earlier relationships..................... 21, 36, 208, 210
Panksepp, Jaak . 5, 8, 11, 14, 23, 41, 122, 129, 130, 131, 133, 134, 135, 136, 137, 146, 153, 226
Pattern matching
and frames.. 105
and perception, and interpretation; ... 105
Pennebaker, James............................... 26, 226
Perfinking
Perceiving-feeling-thinking in one grasp of the mind 139
Perlmutter, Dr David 226
and probiotic and prebiotic supplements 68, 69
on probiotics, prebiotics and the stress response 70
on the link between inflammation XE "Inflammation: physical disease and depression" and depression............ 72
the gut as source of most illness..... 69, 72
Perls, Fritz ....xvii, 38, 226
Personality of mother
and care of baby................................... 140
Piaget, Jean.............................. 5, 15, 30, 224
Plato's model of the psyche 41
Probiotics
and stress reduction............................... 70
for a healthy gut and brain..................... 69
Processed foods
and aggression, irritability and impatience... 71
as legally available toxins 78
avoidance of, reduces risk of depression 67, 72
what to eat and what to avoid. 61, 62, 66, 80
Protein

and complex carbohydrates.................. 62
and personalized diet............................ 64
and the anti-Candida diet 80
and the Paleo diet 62
grains and inflammation, the argument 67
recommended proportion of diet......... 80
Proximal cause of emotional disturbance 130
Rational Emotive Behaviour Therapy xvii, 5, 7, 19, 21, 38, 42, 125, 133, 153, 166, 170, 179, 185, 207, 217
REBT ...... 179, 218, 241, *See* Rational Emotive Behaviour Therapy
Reframing *See* Framing, frame theory, frames
Life is difficult for everybody............... 109
Relationship connection and support 14
Relationship of mother and baby 7
Relationship with mother, and attachment theory... 18
Relationship, and the Internal Working Model 14
Relaxation........ iii, 2, 4, 14, 38, 40, 48, 51, 150, 153, 164, 180, 181, 190, 191
Ross, Dr Julia... 227
on gluten and mood problems.............. 68
on serotonin and anger........................ 70
Salt
reduce and restrict................................ 67
Sapolsky, Robert.. 227
on exercise for stress 77
Sarbin, Theodore............. 6, 13, 165, 220, 228
Schemas
and frames; and interpretations;105, 108, 185
Schoenthaler, Prof Stephen
on healthier diet and reduction in violence and anti-social behaviour . 71
Schoenthaler, Stephen 228
Schore, Allan.............. 8, 14, 22, 146, 147, 228
Secure attachment style 141, 150
Secure base
attachment, mothering......................... 2
Self-talk, or inner dialogue, how to change it 181
Seligman, Martin 114, 228
Serotonin
and the link to anger and aggression.... 71
Sher, Barbara.. 229
Siegel, Daniel .. xviii, 5, 7, 8, 11, 14, 21, 24, 26, 42, 122, 128, 133, 138, 142, 146, 147, 229
Sleep hygiene
and sleep disrupters....................... 86–87
Benefits of adequate sleep
better mood control........................ 95
better physical health 96

greater capacity to cope with stress 94
greater enjoyment of life 96
improved emotional intelligence 95
improved willpower and self-control
.... 95
less anxiety and depression 95
fundamental need for sleep 84
hours of sleep
impact of less than 6-7 hours ... 83, 92
importance of 8-9 hours, Walker 88
need for 8 hours, James Maas 83
insomnia, and how to cure it 96–98
a winding-down process 98
avoid stimulants, like caffeine 97
by using sleep-promoting
supplements 98–99
by writing out worries before bedtime
.... 98
develop a flexible philosophy of life 99
eat a healthy diet 97
have suitable bedroom conditions . 98
need for physical exercise 97
with sleep-promoting supplements 99
insufficient sleep is linked to
anger 91
anxiety 91
depression 90
early death 92
physical illnesses 92
poor concentration 90
reduced emotional intelligence 89
particularly bad
and relaxation, warm bath,
meditation 98
the common sense perspective 85–86
the scientific perspective 94–96
Sleep hygiene famously ignored by
Silvia Plath 92
Rhianna 92
David Ortiz 93
Jay Leno 93
Margaret Thatcher and Ronald
Reagan 93
Donald Trump 93
Snacks
as blood-sugar management 80
Social environment, The role of the 19
Social individual, The 7
Socialized humans, The nature of 144
SOR Model .... See Holistic SOR model
Stoicism 7
Stories in E-CENT counselling and therapy ... 2
Stories, and human habit patterns xviii

Stories, scripts, frames, beliefs, attitudes, and
values 4
Stress and strain 54
Stress management
and Sopolsky on exercise 77
and vitamin and mineral supplements .. 80
Sugar .. See Diet and nutrition: foods to avoid:
sugar
and anger and aggression 71
and anxiety 70
and blood-sugar management 80
and depression 72
as a body and mind toxin 78
as an enemy of the body-brain-mind 66
in low-sugar vegetables 80
Supplementation of vitamins and minerals
.... 155
Supplements
vitamins B, C and E for stress 64, 80
Tasks of counselling
And typical client problems 46
Taylor-Byrne, Renata .... i, xviii, 40, 229
The core beliefs of E-CENT philosophy 49
The E-CENT approach 14
The EFR model 183
The Jigsaw-story model 29, 30, 186, 193
The Mind Hut 109
The relationship between mother and child
.... 20
The status of E-CENT theory 6
The use of metaphor 13
Thinking straight and crooked 55
Transactional Analysis (TA) theory 7
Turner, Jonathan 122, 130
Two fundamental human potentials
Pro-social and anti-social tendencies 52
Understanding emotive-cognitive
interactionism 133
Understanding human emotions 121
Validity of the E-CENT models and processes
The 'common factors' research 165
Views of science 7
Vitamins B, C and E
for stress 64, 80
Wallin, David ... 6, 20, 21, 22, 23, 50, 147, 165,
167, 230
Wampold, Bruce 6, 38, 165, 224, 231, 241
Wanter-fall chart
and human emotions 131
Wanting, and desiring
and emotional disturbance 130, 131
We are bodies as well as minds 51
What is E-CENT counselling? 3
White and Epston 6, 12, 13, 165

Working Models of relationship 36, 39, 46, 145, 146
Zen Buddhism 7

Zimbardo, Philip 179, 231
Zinc
    depleted by caffeine 66

Endnotes

[1] Woolfe, R., Dryden, W., and Strawbridge, S. (eds) (2003) *Handbook of Counselling Psychology*. Second Edition. London: Sage Publications.

[2] McLeod, J. (2003) *An Introduction to Counselling*. Third Edition. Buckingham: Open University Press. Chapter 21 of 21; section 6 of 9 within that final chapter! No references to diet. This is the totality of his commentary on physical exercise: "The therapeutic value of physical exercise is well established. But, for the most part, counselling remains centred on talking rather than doing". (Page 523 of 527!)

[3] In attachment theory, a child is seen to use his/her mother (or main carer) as a **secure base** from which to explore its environment, and to play. If the child's stress level rises, or s/he becomes anxious, s/he can scurry back to mother for a feeling of being in a sensitive and responsive relationship of care and reassurance. This reassurance can also be sought and given nonverbally from a distance. And in counselling and therapy, that role of being sensitive and caring, and reassuring the client, is also seen as providing a new form of secure base from which the client can explore difficult and challenging memories and feelings.

[4] The British 'Object relations' tradition was a breakaway from the Freudian psychoanalytic theory - pioneered by of Melanie Klein, Ronald Fairbairn, Donald Winnicott, Michael Balint, Harry Guntrip and John Bowlby - which emphasized *interpersonal relations*, primarily in the family and especially between mother (the 'object') and child (the 'subject'). In Object Relations theory, 'object' actually means a person, or part of a person, which is internalized by the subject (normally a baby or child). The concept of 'relations' refers to interpersonal relations, and suggests *the residue of past relationships* that affect a person in the present. The internalization of 'objects' results in the formation of *an Inner Working Model* of relationship.

[5] Hill, D. (2015) *Affect Regulation Theory: A clinical model*. New York: W.W. Norton and Company, Inc.

[6] Damasio, A. R. (1994). *Descartes' Error: emotion, reason and the human brain*. London, Picador.

[7] Glasersfeld, E. von (1989) Learning as a constructive activity. In Murphy, P. and Moon, B. (eds) *Developments in Learning and Assessment*. London: Hodder and Stoughton.

[8] See my page on 'REBT and Research', Available here: web.archive.org/web/*/http://abc-counselling.com/id113.html

[9] West, W., and Byrne, J., (2009) 'Some ethical concerns about counselling research': *Counselling Psychology Quarterly*, 22(3) 309-318.

[10] Smith, M.L. and Glass, G.V. (1977) Meta-analysis of psychotherapy outcomes studies. *American Psychologists*, 32, 752-760.

Smith, M., Glass, G. and Miller, T. (1980) *The Benefits of Psychotherapy*. Baltimore, Maryland: The Johns Hopkins University Press.

[11] Wampold, B.E. (2001) *The Great Psychotherapy Debate: Model, methods, and findings*. Mahwah, NJ: Lawrence Erlbaum.

Wampold, B.E., Ahn, H., and Coleman, H.K.L. (2001) Medical model as metaphor: Old habits die hard. *Journal of Counselling Psychology*, 48, 268-273.

[12] Bowlby, J. (1988/2005) *A Secure Base*. London: Routledge Classics.

[13] Beauchamp, T.L. and Childress, J.F. (1994) *Principles of Biomedical Ethics*. Fourth edition. New York. Oxford University Press. And:

Bond, T. (2000) *Standards and Ethics for Counselling in Action*. Second edition. London: Sage.

[14] Watts, A. (1962/1990) *The Way of Zen*. London: Arkana/Penguin. And:

The Dhammapada (1973/2015) Taken from Juan Mascaró's translation and edition, first published in 1973. London: Penguin Books (Little Black Classics No.80)

[15] Wilson (2011); and:

Sarbin, T. R. (1989). Emotions as narrative emplotments. In M. J. Packer & R. B. Addison (eds.) *Entering the circle: Hermeneutic investigations in psychology* (pp. 185-201). Albany, NY: State University of New York Press. And:

Sarbin, T. R. (2001). Embodiment and the narrative structure of emotional life. *Narrative Inquiry, 11,* 217-225.

Gergen, K. (1985) The social constructionist movement in modern psychology. *American Psychologist, 40:* 266-275. And:

Gergen, K. J. (1994). *Toward Transformation in Social Knowledge*. London: Sage Publications. And:

Gergen, K. (2004) When relationships generate realities: therapeutic communication reconsidered. Unpublished manuscripts. Available online: http://www.swarthmore.edu/Soc.Sci/kgergen1/printer-friendly.phtml?id-manu6. Downloaded: 8th December 2004. And:

Gergen, K.J. and Gergen, M.M. (1986) Narrative form and the construction of psychological science. In T.R. Sarbin (ed), *Narrative Psychology: the storied nature of human conduct.* New York: Praeger. And:

Chapter 4 – 'What's the story' – in Philippa Perry (2012) *How to Stay Sane*. London: Macmillan.

~~~

[16] The ABC model of REBT states that the adversities (or 'A's) which happen to us are responded to by our beliefs (or 'B's) which gives rise to our Consequent emotions (or 'C's). This model ignores two major factors: (1) That we are creatures of habit, and thus we respond to adversities on the basis of how we responded to those same adversities in the past; which also tends to be how we were trained by our social environment to respond to such adversities. And (2) that in addition to our beliefs, we are also influenced by our blood sugar level; our gut flora health or lack of heath; our general level of stress; and how fit our bodies are. It is not all about beliefs.

[17] Hofstadter, D. (2007) *I am a Strange Loop*. New York: Basic Books.

[18] Ellis, A. (1962) *Reason and Emotion in Psychotherapy*. New York: Lyle Stuart.

[19] Byrne, J. (2013) *A Wounded Psychotherapist: Albert Ellis's Childhood, and the strengths and limitations of REBT/CBT*. Hebden Bridge: The Institute for CENT Publications/CreateSpace.

[20] Goleman, D. (1996) *Emotional Intelligence: why it can matter more than IQ*. London: Bloomsbury.

[21] Beck, A.T. (1976/1989). *Cognitive Therapy and the Emotional Disorders*. London: Penguin Books.

[22] Rugby League and Rugby Union are "two distinctly different forms of rugby football".

[23] White, M. and Epston, D. (1990) *Narrative Means to Therapeutic Ends*. New York: Norton.

[24] Sarbin, T. R. (1989). Emotions as narrative emplotments. In M. J. Packer & R. B. Addison (eds.) *Entering the circle: Hermeneutic investigations in psychology* (pp. 185-201). Albany, NY: State University of New York Press. Sarbin, T. R. (2001). Embodiment and the narrative structure of emotional life. *Narrative Inquiry, 11,* 217-225.

[25] Gergen, K. (1985) The social constructionist movement in modern psychology. *American Psychologist, 40:* 266-275.

Gergen, K. J. (1994). *Toward Transformation in Social Knowledge*. London: Sage Publications.

Gergen, K. (2004) When relationships generate realities: therapeutic communication reconsidered. Unpublished manuscripts. Available online: http://www.swarthmore.edu/ Soc.Sci/kgergen1/printer-friendly.phtml?id-manu6. Downloaded: 8th December 2004.

Gergen, K.J. and Gergen, M.M. (1986) Narrative form and the construction of psychological science. In T.R. Sarbin (ed), *Narrative Psychology: the storied nature of human conduct*. New York: Praeger.

[26] McLeod, J. (2003) *An Introduction to Counselling*. Third edition. Buckingham: Open University Press.

[27] Strupp, H.H. and Binder, J.L. (1984) *Psychotherapy in a New Key: A guide to time-limited dynamic psychotherapy*. New York: Basic Books.

[28] Luborsky, L. and Crits-Christoph, P. (eds) (1990) *Understanding Transference: the CCRT method*. New York: Basic Books.

[29] Russell, R.L. and van den Brock, P. (1992) Changing narrative schemas in psychotherapy. *Psychotherapy, 29:* 344-354.

[30] Byrne, J. (2009d) A journey through models of mind - The story of my personal origins. E-CENT Paper No.4. Hebden Bridge: The Institute for E-CENT. https://ecent-institute.org/e-cent-articles-and-papers/

[31] Gonçalves, O.F. (1995) Hermeneutics, constructivism and cognitive-behavioural therapies: from the object to the project. In: R.A. Neimeyer and M.J. Mahoney (eds) *Constructivism in psychotherapy*. Washington, DC: American Psychological Association.

[32] Quoted on page 27 of McLeod (1997/2006).

[33] White, M. and Epston, D. (1990) *Narrative Means to Therapeutic Ends*. New York: Norton.

[34] The baby's attachment relationship to their mother (or primary caregiver) – and layers of cumulative, interpretive experience of encountering them - leads to the development of an **'internal working model'** (Bowlby, 1969). This internal working model is an emotive-cognitive framework comprising mental representations for understanding the world, self and others. ("How they related to me; and how I felt I had to relate to them"). (Bowlby, J. [1969] *Attachment. Attachment and loss: Vol. 1. Loss*. New York: Basic Books.)

[35] See Dr Mercola's web site here: http://www.mercola.com/

[36] You can subscribe to the alternative health magazine, *What Doctors Don't Tell You*, here: https://www.wddty.com/

[37] See the link between mood and food in Part 1 of Taylor-Byrne and Byrne (2017).

[38] Gomez, L. (1997) *An Introduction to Object Relations*. London: Free Association Books. Chapter 7.

[39] Gullestad, S.E. (2001) Attachment theory and psychoanalysis: controversial issues. *Scandinavian Psychoanalytic Review, 24,* 3-16.

[40] Bowlby, J. (1988/2005) *A Secure Base*. London: Routledge Classics.

[41] Ainsworth M.D. (1969) Object relations, dependency, and attachment: a theoretical review of the infant-mother relationship". *Child Development, 40 (4):* 969–1025.

[42] Bowlby J (1958). The nature of the child's tie to his mother. *International Journal of Psychoanalysis* 39 (5): 350–73.

[43] Ainsworth M (1967). *Infancy in Uganda: Infant Care and the Growth of Love*. Baltimore: Johns Hopkins University Press.

[44] Mahler, M.S., Pine, F. and Bergman, A. (1975/1987) *The Psychological Birth of the Human Infant: Symbiosis and individuation.* London: Maresfield Library.

[45] Bowlby, J. (1988/2005) *A Secure Base: clinical applications of attachment theory.* London: Routledge Classics.

[46] This use of the word 'thinking' is a mistake. **Perfinking** should become the central concept used in E-CENT, to the exclusion of feeling, thinking, etc. We perfink all in one grasp of the mind. Our feelings and our linguistic stories (taken over from our family, community and society, become braided together as the foundation of our 'mentalizing' capabilities – which expresses our 'social/ emotional intelligence'. Our **mentalized stories** about our social experiences are braided into the core of our being as social-individuals.

[47] Wallin, D. (2007) *Attachment in Psychotherapy.* New York: The Guildford Press.

[48] Fonagy, P., Gergeley, G., Jurist, E.J., and Target, M.I. (2002) *Affect regulation, mentalization, and the development of the self.* New York: Other Press.

[49] Schore, A. N. (2003) *Affect regulation and the repair of the self.* New York: Norton.

[50] Hofstadter, D. (2007) *I am a Strange Loop.* New York: Basic Books.

[51] Holmes, J. (1995) Something there is that doesn't love a wall. John Bowlby, attachment theory, and psychoanalysis. In: Goldberg, S. et al (eds) *Attachment Theory: Social, Developmental and Clinical Perspectives.* London: The Analytic Press. (Pages 19-43).

[52] Byrne, J.W. (2010a) *Therapy after Ellis, Berne, Freud and the Buddha: the birth of Emotive-Cognitive Embodied-Narrative Therapy (E-CENT).*

[53] Bloom, P. (2013) *Just Babies: the origins of good and evil.* London: The Bodley Head. Pages 18 to 31, describing a range of very clever experiments with very young babies. "These experiments suggest that babies have a general appreciation of good and bad behaviour, one that spans a range of interactions, including those that the babies most likely have never seen before..." (Page 30).

[54] Bowlby, J. (1988/2005) *A Secure Base.* London: Routledge Classics.

[55] Pennebaker, J.W. (2004) *Writing to Heal: A Guided journal for recovering from trauma and emotional upheaval.* Oakland, Ca.: New Harbinger Publications.

[56] Bucci, W. (1993) The development of emotional meaning in free association: a multiple code theory; in A. Wilson and J.E. Gedo (eds) *Hierarchical Concepts in Psychoanalysis: Theory, research and clinical practice.* New York: Guilford Press. Pages 3-47.

[57] Bandler, R. and Grinder, J. (1975) *The Structure of Magic, Vol.1: A book about language and therapy.* Palo Alto, Calif.: Science and Behaviour Books Inc.

[58] Lunzer, E. (1989) Cognitive development: learning and the mechanisms of change. In: Murphy, P and Moon, B. (eds) *Developments in Learning and Assessment.* London: Hodder and Stoughton/Open University Press.

[59] Omer, H. and Strenger, C. (1992) The pluralist revolution: from the one true meaning to an infinity of constructed ones. Psychotherapy, 29: 253-261.

[60] Docherty, R.W. (1989) Post-disaster stress in the emergency rescue services. *Fire Engineers Journal, August.* Pages 8-9.

[61] Hofstadter, D. (2007) *I am a Strange Loop.* New York: Basic Books.

[62] Wampold, B.E. (2001) *The Great Psychotherapy Debate: Model, methods, and findings.* Mahwah, NJ: Lawrence Erlbaum.

[63] Messer, S. and Wampold, B. (2002) Let's face facts: Common factors are more potent than specific therapy ingredients. *Clinical Psychology: Science and Practice.* 9: 21-25.

[64] Byrne, J. (2009e) How to analyse autobiographical narratives in Cognitive Emotive Narrative Therapy. Hebden Bridge: The Institute for E-CENT Studies. https://ecent-institute.org/e-cent-articles-and-papers/

[65] Byrne, J. (2009b) The 'Individual' and his/her Social Relationships - The E-CENT Perspective. E-CENT Paper No.9. Hebden Bridge: The Institute for E-CENT. Available online: https://ecent-institute.org/e-cent-articles-and-papers/

[66] An 'affective state' is a state of the body-brain-mind of an individual, in which there is physiological arousal and a felt sense of emotional attraction ('positive affect') or aversion ('negative affect'). For most practical purposes, among counsellors, the word affect may be used interchangeably with 'feelings' and 'emotions'.

[67] Bruner, J. (1986) Actual Minds, Possible Worlds. Cambridge, MA: Harvard University Press.

[68] (For example: John Money's failure to 'reassign' the sexual identity of David Reimer. Source: https://samanthakatepsychology.wordpress.com/ 2012/ 04/ 28/david-reimer-possibly-the-most-unethical-study-in-psychological-history/. Accessed: 30th December 2015.)

[69] Spector, T. (2013) *Identically Different: Why you can change your genes*. London: Phoenix.

[70] Bargh, J.A. and Chartrand, T.L. (1999) The unbearable automaticity of being. *American Psychologist,* 54(7): 462-479.

[71] Gray, J. (2003) *Straw Dogs: thoughts on humans and other animals.* London: Granta Books.

[72] Gladwell, M. (2006) *BLINK: The power of thinking without thinking.* London: Penguin Books.

[73] Stewart, I. and Joines, V. (1987) *TA Today: A New Introduction to Transactional Analysis*. Nottingham: Lifespace Publishing.

[74] Boseley, S. (2018) Half of all food bought in UK is ultra-processed. *The Guardian.* Saturday 3rd February 2018. Issue No. 53,323.

[75] Watch the movie: 'All Jacked Up': The explosive junk food documentary the food companies hope you never see; by Mike Adams, 2008: https://www.naturalnews.com/022510.html

[76] And see also Morgan Spurlock's documentary - ('Super Size Me', 2004) - about trying to live on McDonald's burgers for 30 days, and the medically confirmed negative impact on his physical and mental health! Source: http://watchdocumentaries.com/super-size-me/. Accessed: 21st November 2017.

[77] Coenzyme Q10 may be important for general health. According to the Mayo Clinic: "Coenzyme Q10 (CoQ10) is an antioxidant that your body produces naturally. Your cells use CoQ10 for growth and maintenance.

"Levels of CoQ10 in your body decrease as you age. CoQ10 levels have also been found to be lower in people with certain conditions, such as heart disease.

"CoQ10 is found in meat, fish and whole grains. The amount of CoQ10 found in these dietary sources, however, isn't enough to significantly increase CoQ10 levels in your body.

"As a supplement, CoQ10 supplement is available as capsules, tablets and by IV. CoQ10 might help treat certain heart conditions, as well as migraines and Parkinson's disease." Source: https://www.mayoclinic.org/ drugs-supplements- coenzyme-q10/ art-20362602. Accessed: 30th October 2017.

[78] According to NHS choices: "Probiotics (like Acidophilus) are live bacteria and yeasts promoted as having various health benefits. They're usually added to yoghurts or taken as food supplements, and are often described as 'good' or 'friendly' bacteria.

"Probiotics are thought to help restore the natural balance of bacteria in your gut (including your stomach and intestines) when it has been disrupted by an illness or treatment." (Source: https://www.nhs.uk/Conditions/probiotics/Pages/Introduction.aspx. Accessed: 30th October 2017.

According to Enders (2015) changing the variety of live bacteria in the guts of lab mice can change their behaviour so radically that it is thought they could change character and temperament (in human terms)." And gut bacteria have been shown to be involved in communication between the gut and the brain in humans. (Enders, 2015).

[79] "Essential fatty acids are, as they sound, fats that are necessary within the human body. Though you've probably often heard the word "fats" and associated it with bad health, there are some essential fatty acids that are necessary for your survival. Without them, you could cause serious damage to different systems within the body. However, essential fatty acids are also not usually produced naturally within the body. This means that you have to obtain essential fatty acids by adding them to your diet. There are two basic types of essential fatty acids": Omega-3 and Omega-6. And it is argued that we need more of the 3's than the 6's; or, at least, we have to get the balance right (which could be as low as 1:1). Too much omega-6 seems to be bad for our health (and western diets currently include too much omega-6). Sources: Friday Editor (2017) 'What are essential fatty acids?' The Fit Day Blog. Available online at: http://www.fitday.com/fitness-articles/nutrition/fats/what-are-essential-fatty-acids.html. And, Dr Michael Greger (2016).

[80] Dr Michael Greger (2016) gives the following source for his conclusion that eating more vegetables may help to reduce depression:

Agarwal, U, Suruchi Mishra, Jia Xu, Susan Levin, Joseph Gonzales, and Neal D. Barnard (2015) 'A Multicentre Randomized Controlled Trial of a Nutrition Intervention Program in a Multi-ethnic Adult Population in the Corporate Setting Reduces Depression and Anxiety and Improves Quality of Life: The GEICO Study. *American Journal of Health Promotion, Vol 29, Issue 4*, pp. 245 - 254.

~~~

[81] Professor Colin Espie: Online: https://www.sleepio.com/articles/sleep-basics/sleep-basics-intro/. Accessed: 25th January 2018).

[82] Walker (2017) conducted an experiment in his sleep lab, to show how the lack of sleep affects people's emotional intelligence. He took two groups of people and placed them under two different experimental conditions. One group had a full night's sleep, and then were shown a range of pictures of individual human faces, which displayed a wide range of emotions, varying from friendliness through to intense dislike and anger. The participants had to individually assess this range of facial expressions, to decide if they were displaying threatening or friendly messages. While they were engaged in this activity, their brains were being scanned in a Magnetic Resonance Imaging (MRI) machine. (The following night, this group was deprived of sleep, particularly rapid eye movement (REM) sleep).

The second groups in Walker's research had the sleep deprivation condition first, and then examined the pictures, and had to assess the emotions on display. (They had a full night's sleep the following night, and did a similar visual assessment the following day).

The results of Walker's experiments were as follows: If participants had had a good night's sleep beforehand, then they had no difficulty in distinguishing facial expressions ranging from hostility through to benevolence. Their assessments (spoken, and neurological, confirmed by the MRI scans) – unlike those of the sleep deprived condition - were accurate, showing that the quality of their sleep had helped them in their reading of facial expressions.

But in the sleep deprived condition, participants found it much harder to differentiate between the facial expressions displayed on in the range of pictures shown to them. Their ability to quickly spot and decipher facial expressions accurately had deserted them. And their errors were far from minor. For example, they perceived facial expressions of kindliness and welcome as hostile and menacing. According to Walker (2017):

"Reality and perceived reality were no longer the same in the 'eyes' of the sleepless brain. By removing REM sleep we had, quitter literally, removed participants' level-headed ability to read the social world around them". (Page 217).

For an illustration of why this kind of loss of emotional intelligence might be very serious indeed, it is the kind of ability to read social signals which has to be used by police officers in situations of social conflict, to decide whether or not to use gunfire, or to use a lesser form of response. And it is crucial in making judgements in sales and negotiation situations; and in managing personal and professional relationships. Thus lack of adequate sleep is clearly a very costly form of poor self-management!

~~~

[83] According to the NHS Choices (UK) website, lack of sleep affects physical health as much as emotional wellbeing: "Many effects of a lack of sleep, such as feeling grumpy and not working at your best, are well known. But did you know that sleep deprivation can also have profound consequences on your physical health?"

The bottom line of this statement was this: "Regular poor sleep puts you at risk of serious medical conditions, including obesity, heart disease and diabetes – and it shortens your life expectancy." (See NHS Choices, 2015).

"One in three of us suffers from poor sleep, with stress, computers and taking work home often blamed.

"However, the cost of all those sleepless nights is more than just bad moods and a lack of focus.

"Regular poor sleep puts you at risk of serious medical conditions, including obesity, heart disease and diabetes – and it shortens your life expectancy."

"It's now clear that a solid night's sleep is essential for a long and healthy life." Available online: https://www.nhs.uk/Livewell/tiredness-and-fatigue/Pages/lack-of-sleep-health-risks.aspx. Accessed: 25th January 2018.

~~~

[84] Calm-Clinic (2018) How Sleep Debt Causes Serious Anxiety. Online blog: https://www.calmclinic.com/anxiety/causes/sleep-debt. Accessed: 25th January 2018.

[85] NSF (2018) Depression and sleep. Online blog: https://sleepfoundation.org/sleep-disorders-problems/depression-and-sleep. Accessed: 25th January 2018.

[86] Kogan, N. (2018) The magic of a good night's sleep: Because an exhausted person is never a happy person. Happier. Online: https://www.happier.com/blog/the-magic-of-sleep. Accessed: 25th January 2018.

~~~

[87] Byrne, J. (2011) Completing your experience of difficult events, perceptions and painful emotions. E-CENT Paper No.13. Hebden Bridge: The Institute for E-CENT. Available online: http://web.archive.org/web/20160519163415/

[88] Griffin, J. and Tyrrell, I. (2004) *Human Givens: A new approach to emotional health and clear thinking.* Chalvington, East Sussex: HG Publishing.

[89] To *frame a problem* means to look at it through a particular frame of reference, or interpretative lens. If you look at an event through the frame which asserts that 'This should not be happening', then you are likely to be much more distressed or angry than if you looked at it through a frame that asserts, 'This seems to be unavoidable'.

[90] Mono-focal means 'single viewpoint'; or 'one way of looking at things'. Is it ever true that there is only one way of looking at anything? (I don't think so!)

[91] Seligman, M.E.P. (2002). *Authentic Happiness: Using the New Positive Psychology to Realize Your Potential for Lasting Fulfillment.* New York, NY: Free Press.

[92] Ervine, W. (2009) *A Guide to the Good Life: The ancient art of Stoic joy.* Oxford: Oxford University Press.

[93] This frame was created by Renata Taylor-Byrne. What she did not realize at the time was that this perspective had already been attributed to the Native American Cherokee people: "Everything in life comes to you as a teacher. Pay attention. Learn Quickly". Old Cherokee woman to her grandson; cited in Baran (2003).

[94] Pinker, S. (2015) *How the Mind Works.* London: Penguin Random House.

[95] Hobson, R.F. (1985) *Forms of Feeling: The heart of psychotherapy.* London: Routledge. Page 88.

[96] Paul Ekman (1993) identified the most universal, basic emotions - from a detailed international study - as: anger, fear, disgust, sadness, and enjoyment. See: Ekman, P. (1993) Facial expression and emotion. *American Psychologist 48 (4):* Pages 384-392.

[97] Turner, J.H. (2000) *On the Origins of Human Emotions. A sociological inquiry into the evolution of human affect.* Stanford University Press. See the book outline at this website: http://www.sup.org/books/title/?id=436

[98] *The Dhammapada* (1973/2015) Taken from Juan Mascaró's translation and edition, first published in 1973. London: Penguin Books (Little Black Classics No.80)

[99] *The Dhammapada* (1973/2015)

[100] See page 245 of Cardwell, M. (2000) *The Complete A-Z Psychology Handbook.* Second edition. London: Hodder and Stoughton.

[101] Bretherton, I. (1992) The Origins of Attachment Theory: John Bowlby and Mary Ainsworth. *Developmental Psychology 28:* 759.

[102] Ayya Khema quotation taken from: Josh Baran (ed) (2003) *365 Nirvana: Here and now.* London: HarperCollins/Element.

[103] Epictetus (1991) *The Enchiridion.* New York: Prometheus Books.

[104] Aurelius, M. (1946/1992) *Meditations.* Trans. A.S.L. Farquharson. London: Everyman's Library.

[105] **First example**: 'Painkillers (are) behind most mass killings, say researchers' from a news item in the magazine, *What Doctors Don't Tell You*, dated August 2015, page 14. (This report is based on a published research study from the University of East Finland, published in *World Psychiatry, 2015; 14*:245-247). **Second example**: DrugWatch, an advocacy organization which supports people damaged by drugs, reports that people who take antidepressants: "...may experience side effects such as violent behavior, mania or aggression, which can all lead to suicide." Source: https://www.drugwatch.com/ssri/suicide/. And **Third example**: Patrick Holford has found evidence that brain allergies to particular foods and chemicals can cause emotional dysfunctions: "The knowledge that allergy to foods and chemicals can adversely affect moods and behaviour in susceptible individuals has been known for a very long time. Early reports, as well as current research, have found that allergies can affect any system of the body, including the central nervous system. They can cause a diversity of symptoms including fatigue, slowed thought processes, irritability, agitation, aggressive behaviour, nervousness, anxiety, depression, schizophrenia, hyperactivity and varied learning disabilities." Source: http://www.alternativementalhealth.com/brain-allergieshow-sensitivities-to-food-and-other-substances-can-effect-the-mind/

[106] Darwin, C. (1872/1965) *The Expression of the Emotions in Man and Animals*. Chicago: University of Chicago Press.

[107] Evans, D. (2003) *Emotion: a very short introduction*. Oxford. Oxford University Press.

[108] Turner, J.H. (2000) *On the Origins of Human Emotions. A Sociological Inquiry into the Evolution of Human Affect*. Stanford University Press. See the book outline at: http://www.sup.org/books/title/?id=436

[109] **Sociality** is a measure of the extent to which individuals in an animal population tend to associate in social groups, and to form cooperative communities or societies.

[110] Panksepp, J. and Lucy Biven (2012) *The Archaeology of Mind: Neuroevolutionary Origins of Human Emotion*: W.W. Norton and Company. See the book description here: http://www.amazon.co.uk/The-Archaeology-Mind-Neuroevolutionary-Interpersonal/dp/0393705315

[111] Coates, G. (2008) *Wanterfall*: A practical approach to the understanding and healing of the emotions of everyday life. An online e-book. Available at this website: http://www.wanterfall.com/Downloads/Wanterfall.pdf. Section 1: The origins of emotions.

[112] Damasio, A. R. (1994). *Descartes' Error: emotion, reason and the human brain*. London, Picador.

[113] Siegel, D.J. (2015) *The Developing Mind: How relationships and the brain interact to shape who we are*. London: The Guilford Press.

[114] Byrne, J. (2009a) Rethinking the psychological models underpinning Rational Emotive Behaviour Therapy (REBT). E-CENT Paper No.1(a). Hebden Bridge: The Institute for E-CENT. Available online: https://ecent-institute.org/e-cent-articles-and-papers/

[115] Ellis, A. (1958). Rational Psychotherapy, *Journal of General Psychology, 59*, 35-49. And: Ellis A. (1962). *Reason and Emotion in Psychotherapy*, New York, Carol Publishing.

[116] From a PowerPoint presentation by Jaak Panksepp, regarding his book: Panksepp, J. (1998) *Affective Neuroscience: The foundations of human and animal emotions*. Oxford University Press. Slide 12.

[117] LeDoux, J. (1996). *The Emotional Brain: the mysterious underpinnings of emotional life*, New York. Simon and Schuster.

[118] Mehrabian, A. (1981) *Silent messages: Implicit communication of emotions and attitudes*. Belmont, CA: Wadsworth (currently distributed by Albert Mehrabian, email: am@kaaj.com)

[119] Byrne, J. (2009b) The 'Individual' and his/her Social Relationships - The E-CENT Perspective. E-CENT Paper No.9. Hebden Bridge: The Institute for E-CENT. Available online: https://ecent-institute.org/e-cent-articles-and-papers/.

[120] Bowlby, J. (1988/2005) *A Secure Base*. London: Routledge Classics.

[121] Lewis, T., Amini, F. and Lannon, R. (2001) *A General Theory of Love*. New York: Vintage Books.

[122] Gerhardt, S. (2010) *Why Love Matters: How affection shapes a baby's brain*. London: Routledge.

[123] Siegel, D.J. (2015) *The Developing Mind: How relationships and the brain interact to shape who we are*. London: The Guilford Press.

[124] Hobson, R.F. (2000) *Forms of Feeling: the heart of psychotherapy*. London: Routledge.

[125] Panksepp, J. (1998) *Affective Neuroscience: The foundations of human and animal emotions*. Oxford University Press.

[126] Schore, A.N. (2015) *Affect Regulation and the Origin of the Self: The Neurobiology of Emotional Development*. London: Routledge.

[127] Smith, P.K., Cowie, H., and Blades, M. (2011) *Understanding Children's Development*. Fifth edition. Chichester, West Sussex: Wiley.

[128] Siegel, D.J. (2015) *The Developing Mind: How relationships and the brain interact to shape who we are*. London: The Guilford Press. Pages 152-153.

[129] Wallin, D.A. (2007) *Attachment in Psychotherapy*. New York: Guildford Press.

[130] Erwin, E. (1997) *Philosophy and Psychotherapy: Razing the troubles of the brain*, London, Sage.

[131] Kashdan, T. and Biswas-Diener, R. (2015) *The Power of Negative Emotion: How anger, guilt and self-doubt are essential to success and fulfilment*. London: Oneworld Publications.

[132] Teychenne M, Costigan S, Parker K. (2015) The association between sedentary behaviour and risk of anxiety: A Systematic Review. *BMC Public Health, 2015*. Cited in *Medical Daily*, here: http://www.medicaldaily.com/constantly-sitting-down-being-sedentary-could-worsen-anxiety-and-mental-health-338952

[133] Borchard, T. (2015) 10 Ways to Cultivate Good Gut Bacteria and Reduce Depression. Everyday Health Blog. Available online: http://www.everydayhealth.com/columns/therese-borchard-sanity-break/ways-cultivate-good-gut-bacteria-reduce-depression/

[134] See Chapter 3 – 'Shaping our narratives' – in Wilson, T.D. (2011) *Redirect: The Surprising New Science of Psychological Change*. London: Allen Lane/Penguin.

[135] See Appendix G of Byrne (2016).

[136] See this blog post: Your Emotions Are What You Eat: How Your Diet Can Reduce Anxiety, by Matthew C. Nisbet, Available here: http://bigthink.com/age-of-engagement/your-emotions-are-what-you-eat-how-your-diet-can-reduce-anxiety

[137] Siegel, D.J. (2015) *The Developing Mind: How relationships and the brain interact to shape who we are*. London: The Guilford Press.

[138] Peck, M.S. (1998) *The Road Less Travelled: A New Psychology of Love, Traditional Values and Spiritual Growth*. New York: Touchstone.

[139] See our web page – 'What is Transactional Analysis (TA)?' - here: https://abc-counselling.org/transactional-analysis/

[140] See my page on 'REBT and Research', Available here: web.archive.org/web/*/http://abc-counselling.com/id113.html

[141] West, W., and Byrne, J., (2009) 'Some ethical concerns about counselling research': *Counselling Psychology Quarterly*, 22(3) 309-318.

[142] Smith, M.L. and Glass, G.V. (1977) Meta-analysis of psychotherapy outcomes studies. *American Psychologists*, 32, 752-760.

Smith, M., Glass, G. and Miller, T. (1980) *The Benefits of Psychotherapy*. Baltimore, Maryland: The Johns Hopkins University Press.

[143] Wampold, B.E. (2001) *The Great Psychotherapy Debate: Model, methods, and findings*. Mahwah, NJ: Lawrence Erlbaum.

Wampold, B.E., Ahn, H., and Coleman, H.K.L. (2001) Medical model as metaphor: Old habits die hard. *Journal of Counselling Psychology*, 48, 268-273.

[144] Bowlby, J. (1988/2005) *A Secure Base*. London: Routledge Classics.

[145] Beauchamp, T.L. and Childress, J.F. (1994) *Principles of Biomedical Ethics*. Fourth edition. New York. Oxford University Press. And:

Bond, T. (2000) *Standards and Ethics for Counselling in Action*. Second edition. London: Sage.

[146] Watts, A. (1962/1990) *The Way of Zen*. London: Arkana/Penguin. And:

The Dhammapada (1973/2015) Taken from Juan Mascaró's translation and edition, first published in 1973. London: Penguin Books (Little Black Classics No.80)

[147] Epictetus (1991) *The Enchiridion*. New York: Prometheus Books. And:

Aurelius, M. (1946/1992) *Meditations*. Trans. A.S.L. Farquharson. London: Everyman's Library.

~~~

[148] Wilson (2011); and:

Sarbin, T. R. (1989). Emotions as narrative emplotments. In M. J. Packer & R. B. Addison (eds.) *Entering the circle: Hermeneutic investigations in psychology* (pp. 185-201). Albany, NY: State University of New York Press. And:

Sarbin, T. R. (2001). Embodiment and the narrative structure of emotional life. *Narrative Inquiry*, 11, 217-225.

Gergen, K. (1985) The social constructionist movement in modern psychology. *American Psychologist*, 40: 266-275. And:

Gergen, K. J. (1994). *Toward Transformation in Social Knowledge*. London: Sage Publications. And:

Gergen, K. (2004) When relationships generate realities: therapeutic communication reconsidered. Unpublished manuscripts. Available online: http://www.swarthmore.edu/Soc.Sci/kgergen1/printer-friendly.phtml?id-manu6. Downloaded: 8th December 2004. And:

Gergen, K.J. and Gergen, M.M. (1986) Narrative form and the construction of psychological science. In T.R. Sarbin (ed), *Narrative Psychology: the storied nature of human conduct*. New York: Praeger. And:

Chapter 4 – 'What's the story' – in Philippa Perry (2012) *How to Stay Sane*. London: Macmillan.

[149] In the **Master Therapist Series** of video tapes produced by the Albert Ellis Institute, each of the 'master therapists' used the A-B-C-D-E model as the ***invariable structure*** of their sessions.

[150] Definition of **rapport** = "A close and harmonious relationship, in which the counsellor and client understand each other's words, attitudes, feelings or ideas, and communicate well with each other".

[151] Nelson-Jones, R. (2001) *Theory and Practice of Counselling and Therapy*. Third edition. London: Continuum.

[152] Jacobs. E.E. (1993) *Impact Therapy*. Lutz, FL: Psychological Assessment Resources.

[153] We use a *secular* definition of 'karma' as meaning the **results** of all of our actions in the real world of *this (the only) life* we have lived so far (or the only life we can know about!) This combines both earned merit/demerit, plus accidents of being in the right or wrong place at a particular point in time. "Your karma is what happens to you. You don't have to be very *wise* about that!" Werner Erhard.

[154] The Golden Rule, which goes back to ancient China, and is preserved in both Catholic dogma and in the thinking of Immanuel Kant, goes like this: Do not do unto others what you would not want them to do to you in similar circumstances. Or: Treat other people in ways that you would like to be treated.

[155] *The Dhammapada* (1973/2015) Taken from Juan Mascaró's translation and edition, first published in 1973. London: Penguin Books (Little Black Classics No.80)

[156] The British National Health Service (NHS) supports the view that exercise is good for mood disorders, like anxiety and depression. Here's their comment specifically on depression:

"Exercise for depression

"Being depressed can leave you feeling low in energy, which might put you off being more active.

"Regular exercise can boost your mood if you have depression, and it's especially useful for people with mild to moderate depression.

'Any type of exercise is useful, as long as it suits you and you do enough of it,' says Dr Alan Cohen, a GP with a special interest in mental health. 'Exercise should be something you enjoy; otherwise, it will be hard to find the motivation to do it regularly.'

"How often do you need to exercise?

"To stay healthy, adults should do 150 minutes of moderate-intensity activity every week." In E-CENT we recommend 30 minutes of brisk walking every day, minimum. Source: http://www.nhs.uk/conditions/stress-anxiety-depression/pages/ exercise- for- depression.aspx) Accessed: 23rd February 2016.

~~~

[157] Keirsey, D. and Bates, M. (1984) *Please Understand Me: Character and temperament types*. Fifth edition. Del Mar, CA: Prometheus Nemesis Book Company.

[158] 'The healing environment': An interview with Dr Ron Anderson, in Bill Moyers' (1995) book: *Healing and The Mind*. New York: Doubleday. Page 25.

[159] Burns, D. (1999) *The Feeling Good Handbook*. London: Plume/Penguin Books.

[160] Gottman, J. (1997). *Why Marriages Succeed or Fail: and how you can make yours last*. London: Bloomsbury.

[161] Byrne, J. (2012) *Chill Out: How to control your stress level and have a happier life*. Hebden Bridge: CreateSpace.

[162] Nierenberg, G.I. (1987) *The Complete Negotiator,* London, Souvenir Press Ltd.

[163] Asch, S.E. (1956) A minority of one against a unanimous majority. *Psychological Monographs, 70 (416).* And:

Zimbardo, P. G., Banks, W.C., Craig, H. and Jaffe, D. (1973) A Pirandellian prison: The mind is a formidable jailor. *New York Times Magazine, April 8th*, 38-60. And:

Milgram, S. (1974) *Obedience to Authority*. New York: Harper and Row.

[164] Please see Appendices E(1) and E(2) above.

[165] E-CENT Paper No.18: Exercise is good for your body, brain and general health. By Renata Taylor-Byrne and Jim Byrne. Available online, here: https://ecent-institute.org/e-cent-articles-and-papers/

[138] Please see our web page on 'How to meditate - A brief introduction', by Renata Taylor-Byrne and Jim Byrne, at ABC Coaching and Counselling Services. Available online: web.archive.org/web/20160323004156/web.archive.org/web/*/http://abc-counselling.com/id260.html

[167] Keirsey and Bates (1984); An online questionnaire on character and temperament: Available here: http://www.keirsey.com/sorter/register.aspx

[168] What is your attachment style? Online Questionnaire: http://www.web-research-design.net/cgi-bin/crq/crq.pl

[169] Our approach to stress management is outlined in Byrne, J. (2012) *Chill Out: How to control your stress level and have a happier life*. Hebden Bridge: CreateSpace.

[170] See our web page – 'What is Transactional Analysis (TA)?' - here: https://abc-counselling.org/transactional-analysis/

[171] Byrne, J. (2010b) Self-acceptance and other-acceptance in relation to competence and morality. E-CENT Paper No.2(c). Hebden Bridge: The Institute for E-CENT. Available online: https://ecent-institute.org/e-cent-articles-and-papers/

[172] 'Transformational Chairwork: Five Ways of Using Therapeutic Dialogues'. A blog by Scott Kellogg, PhD; New York University. Available online: http://transformationalchairwork.com/articles/transformational-chairwork/ . And:

Perls, F. S. (1969). *Gestalt therapy verbatim*. Lafayette, CA: Real People Press.

[173] We often use relaxation processes which were developed by Paul McKenna. For an example, please watch this video clip at YouTube: https://www.youtube.com/watch?v=6prbVluob5E

[174] For a description of Rational Emotive Imagery, by Dr Albert Ellis, please go to: http://www.billhanshaw.com/My_Office_Web_Page/Blog/Entries/2009/3/19_REBT_Rational_Emotive_Behavior_Therapy_%22Rational_Emotive_Imagery%22.html

[175] Paul McKenna has been involved in the recent development of Havening, a psycho-sensory technique for processing trauma, anxiety and stress. You can find a video introduction to this new technique at YouTube, here: https://www.youtube.com/watch?v=0C1liEFCZm4

[176] Krystal, P. (1994) *Cutting the Ties That Bind: Growing Up and Moving on*. Weiser Books.

[177] Taylor-Byrne and Byrne: 'How to meditate - A brief introduction'. Available online: web.archive.org/web/20160323004156/web.archive.org/web/*/http://abc-counselling.com/id260.html

[178] Wallin, D. (2007) *Attachment in Psychotherapy*. New York: The Guildford Press. And:

Levine, A. and Heller, R. (2011) *Attached: Identify your attachment style and find your perfect match*. London: Rodale/Pan Macmillan.

[179] Keirsey, D. and Bates, M. (1984) *Please Understand Me: Character and temperament types*. Fifth edition. Del Mar, CA: Prometheus Nemesis Book Company.

[180] Postman, Neil, and Weingartner, Charles (1969), *Teaching as a Subversive Activity*. New York: Dell.

[181] Rogers, C. (1983) *Freedom to Learn for the 80's*. Princeton, NC: Merrill.

[182] Bastable, S.B. (2008) *Nurse as Educator*. Burlington, Mas: Jones & Bartlett Learning

[183] Novak, J.D. and Gowin, B. (1984) *Learning How to Learn*. Cambridge: Cambridge University Press.

[184] Prochaska, J.O., Norcross, J.C. & DiClemente, C.C. (1998). *Changing for Good*. Reprint edition. New York: Morrow.

Made in the USA
Lexington, KY
09 April 2018